FOUNDATIONS OF HEALTH AND SOCIAL CARE

Also by Robert Adams:

A Measure of Diversion? Case Studies in IT (co-author)
Prison Riots in Britain and the USA (2nd edition) *
Problem-solving with Self-help Groups (co-author)
Protests by Pupils: Empowerment, Schooling and the State
Quality Social Work *
Self-help, Social Work and Empowerment *
Skilled Work with People
Working With and Within Groups (co-author)
Social Work and Empowerment (4th edition) *
The Abuses of Punishment *
The Personal Social Services: Clients, Consumers or Citizens?
Social Policy for Social Work *
Social Work: Themes, Issues and Critical Debates (co-editor) *
Critical Practice in Social Work (co-editor) *
Social Work Futures: Crossing Boundaries, Transforming Practice (co-editor) *

* Published by Palgrave Macmillan

Foundations of Health and Social Care

Edited by
ROBERT ADAMS

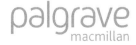

First published 2007 by
PALGRAVE MACMILLAN
Houndmills, Basingstoke, Hampshire RG21 6XS and
175 Fifth Avenue, New York, N.Y. 10010
Companies and representatives throughout the world

PALGRAVE MACMILLAN is the global academic imprint of the Palgrave
Macmillan division of St. Martin's Press, LLC and of Palgrave Macmillan Ltd.
Macmillan® is a registered trademark in the United States, United Kingdom
and other countries. Palgrave is a registered trademark in the European
Union and other countries.

ISBN-13: 978–1–4039–9886–6
ISBN-10: 1–4039–9886–8

This book is printed on paper suitable for recycling and made from fully
managed and sustained forest sources. Logging, pulping and manufacturing
processes are expected to conform to the environmental regulations of the
country of origin.

A catalogue record for this book is available from the British Library.

10 9   8   7   6   5   4   3   2   1
16 15 14 13 12 11 10 09 08 07

Printed in China

Brief Contents

Full Contents

List of Resource Files

List of Figures and Tables

Figures

Tables

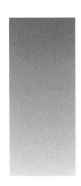

Notes on Contributors

JON ADAMS has worked as an occupational therapist in the NHS for over six years, specialising in adult mental health. His specialist areas include vocational rehabilitation and assertive outreach. Jon has published work on the role of occupational therapy in crisis resolution and home treatment and co-authored a study exploring the role of occupational therapists in community mental health services.

ROBERT ADAMS is professor in the School of Health and Social Care, University of Teesside. He was editor of the first half-dozen titles of the Health and Nursing Active Learning series published by Churchill Livingstone, about 80 open learning titles in social work, the Working with People series published by CollinsEducational and three well-known co-edited texts on social work. He was co-writer of the first block of six books in the NHSTD/Open University Advanced MESOL programme for senior managers in the health and social services. He has researched and written on social work and social care, including *Skilled Work with People*, *The Personal Social Services* and *Social Work and Empowerment*, written 20 years ago and in its fourth edition, and several books on social policy and criminal justice. He is currently involved in research in service user and carer participation and is preparing a book on working with children.

SUE BALDWIN is the programme manager of the advanced Diploma in Nursing Learning Disability Branch at the University of Leeds. Her input to the curriculum for the past few years has been on health and social care aspects of learning disability to a multiprofessional audience. Sue has a particular interest in the mental health and welfare of people with a learning disability, and has published on risk assessment and the role of the learning disability nurse. Her research interests include the management of change, with particular reference to institutional care, and, more recently, eugenic attitudes of care staff towards people with a learning disability.

JAN DARGUE is a senior lecturer at the University of Teesside, teaching across both pre- and post-registration nursing programmes within the School of Health and Social Care. Her clinical background was in community nursing. Having a special interest in tissue viability, she worked as the tissue viability lead for the PCT, taking forward new initiatives, providing wound care education and developing wound care strategies, prior to moving into education.

LIZ DAVIES has many years of practice experience as a child protection manager and now teaches social work at undergraduate, postgraduate and post-qualifying levels. She has a particular interest in training police and social workers in joint investigation and interview skills and has developed an online multiagency child protection training resource with Akamas Publishing. Liz writes widely on the subject and contributed to a *Real Story* BBC television documentary *Saving Becky* on the subject of the sexual exploitation of children.

DAVE FOUNTAIN is a former instructor in the army who spent time as a patient in intensive hospital care and as a resident in Victoria House, Hull, which caters for people with physical disabilities. He lives independently and works part time at Mires Beck Nurseries, North Cave where he is taking his NVQ in horticulture.

RUTH GILI has over 12 years' experience working as an occupational therapist in both adult and elderly mental health multidisciplinary teams. She is currently working as an independent occupational therapy practitioner and life coach. Ruth's specialist areas include training occupational therapists on occupational therapy theory and its application to practice and life coaching. Ruth has worked extensively in the public and private sector.

MARION GRIEVES is a principal lecturer within the University of Teesside, School of Health and Social Care and teaches across the nursing programme. Her research interests include the use of IT in nursing, interprofessional learning and developing communication skills. Her publications include *Patient and Person: Empowering Interprofessional Relationships in Nursing* (with Stevenson and Stein-Parbury).

CAROL HAIGH is senior lecturer in research at the School of Nursing, University of Salford. She has published widely in the field of pain management and has recently contributed to the book *Research Ethics in the Real World: Issues and Solutions for Health and Social Care* and is a member of the working party reviewing the Royal College of Nursing's ethical guidelines.

RUTH HAMILTON is lecturer in social care at Northumberland College, Ashington. She has a background in practice and research and teaches social work and foundation degree students in health and social care.

JACQUIE HORNER is a senior lecturer in the School of Health and Social Care at Teesside University. Prior to this, she was employed as a district nursing sister in a local PCT.

DIANE HOWARD has taught on social care, counselling and education programmes. She is currently teaching on the Social Work Degree at Northumbria University and the Foundation Degree in Applied Social Care and Health Studies at Northumberland College, and is also currently working on a Dementia Diagnosis project with the Alzheimer's Society. Her research interests include user participation in the evaluation of residential services, the impact of training on practice and widening higher education participation for social care workers. She has previously worked as a NISW consultant to residential care homes and published findings on staff development and the inspection process.

LYN JACKSON is a senior lecturer in nursing at the University of Teesside. Her teaching interests include a variety of pre-registration nursing skills, along with post-registration education modules for healthcare professionals learning to be mentors. Her research interests include the use of reflection in learning and first year student nurses' experiences of higher education.

MAGGIE JACKSON has been a senior lecturer at the University of Teesside since 1999. Previously she worked as a senior practitioner for the County Psychological Service in Cleveland. Her research interests are loss and death and death education.

TONY LONG is professor of child and family health in the University of Salford School of Nursing and Centre for Nursing, Midwifery and Collaborative Research. He leads on research with children and families, publishing widely in this field as well as on health professional education and regulation. His book *Excessive Crying in Infancy* has received international acclaim, while *Research Ethics in the Real World: Issues for Health and Social Care*, co-edited with Martin Johnson, has become a core text for many programmes.

RUTH MCDONALD is currently employed at the University of Teesside as a senior lecturer in service improvement. Prior to joining the university, she was employed as a clinical lead for continence, developing and providing integrated continence services for people with bladder and bowel problems. She has conducted research examining the experiences of living with urinary incontinence and the challenge of implementing an integrated continence service. She continues to work as a practitioner in a local PCT and her interests include continence care, leadership and service improvement and research.

RACHEL MORRIS is senior lecturer in nursing in the School of Health and Social Care, University of Teesside.

BERNARD MOSS is professor of social work education and spirituality at Staffordshire University, where he has been leading the Social Work Degree for the past four years. His particular interests are communication skills, the links between religion, spirituality and social work/social care practice, and death, dying and bereavement. He teaches on the Foundation Degree in Social Care, and also serves as a link tutor.

ALLISON MULVIHILL is senior lecturer in the School of Health and Social Care, University of Teesside.

JENNIFER NEWTON coordinates postgraduate teaching in the Department of Applied Social Sciences at London Metropolitan University, and lectures on mental health and community care. Her books include *Preventing Mental Illness* while working for MIND, *Care Management: Is It Working?* for the Sainsbury Centre for Mental Health, and chapters and papers on community care services.

JULIETTE OKO is senior lecturer in social work at the University of Teesside where she teaches on the professional social work degree.

TERENCE O'SULLIVAN is principal lecturer in social work at the University of Lincoln. He has written a number of articles with particular regard to practice. He is the author of *Decision Making in Social Work*.

MARTIN PAGE is a psychotherapist and a senior lecturer in health studies at the University of Lincoln. He is programme leader of the MSc Trauma and Disaster Management Studies in the School of Health and Social Care. His research and writing focus on the psychological needs of professionals who work in dangerous, hostile and threatening environments.

MALCOLM PAYNE is director of psychosocial and spiritual care, St Christopher's Hospice, Sydenham, emeritus professor, Manchester Metropolitan University and honorary professor, Kingston University/St George's Medical School. He is the author of many books including *Social Work and Community Care*, *Teamwork in Multiprofessional Care*, *The Origins of Social Work: Continuity and Change* and the best-selling *Modern Social Work Theory*.

JAMES REID is a senior lecturer in social work at the University of Teesside where he teaches on qualifying and post-qualifying programmes. He studied social work in Durham before working as a children and families social worker in Essex. He has made contributions to the development of social work education regionally as an adviser to a number of post-qualifying consortia, and nationally, through papers at conferences.

MARGARET REITH has worked in health-related social care settings for many years. In addition to several articles, she has written a mental health resource book *Community Care Tragedies: A Practice Guide to Mental Health Inquiries*. She is currently working as a palliative care social worker in a hospice in Surrey.

JO SMITH is a senior lecturer in nursing skills development at the University of Teesside. Her research interests are education, facilitating learning and clinical skills development.

ELIZABETH STUART-COLE is a medical practitioner with specialist qualifications in diabetes. She has lectured in health studies at Northumberland College and worked as a clinical assistant in diabetes at Newcastle General Hospital. She is undertaking sociomedical studies at Northumbria University.

TERRY THOMAS is reader in criminal justice studies in the School of Social Sciences, Leeds Metropolitan University. He has researched and published widely on policing, sex offending and criminal justice.

NEIL THOMPSON is professor of social work and well-being at Liverpool Hope University and a director of Avenue Consulting Ltd. He has over 100 publications to his name, including bestselling texts such as *Anti-Discriminatory Practice* (4th edn) and *People Skills* (2nd edn). His latest book is *Understanding Social Care* (2nd edn, co-authored with Sue Thompson).

SUE THOMPSON is an independent social worker, practice teacher and mentor. She is a director of Avenue Consulting Ltd, a company offering training and consultancy around social and workplace wellbeing issues. She has experience in both nursing and social work and is the author of *Age Discrimination* and *From Where I'm Sitting*, a training manual for staff working with older people.

WADE TOVEY is programmes director of social work in the School of Health and Social Care at the University of Teesside. He has leadership and consultancy interests in participation by people who use services and carers, youth inclusion, adult protection, partnership working and flexible learning, as chair of the Learning Resource Network and the executive of Skills for Care and board member of the Open Learning Foundation. He is the editor of the *Handbook of Postqualifying Practice*.

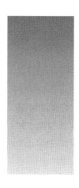

Introduction

ROBERT ADAMS

I have brought together a large team of authors, expert in their own fields, to write this book to provide you, the reader, with the kind of learning support and help with study that I would have appreciated when I started on my first degree course. I hope the way it is laid out encourages you to learn and gives you scope to study beyond the covers of this book.

'Health and social care' has one of the largest workforces in the UK. The health services in the UK are reputedly one of the largest employers in Europe; more than a million people out of a total workforce of about 25 million are employed in health and social care and although estimates vary, it seems likely that more than five million people are informal, that is, unpaid, carers. Health and social care includes the range of medical and other healthcare services, alongside all the different kinds of personal support that people need in order to live as safely, fully and independently as possible throughout their lives, from residential through daycare to community services aiming to maintain people in their own homes. Government-funded health trusts and local authorities work with voluntary, not-for-profit and private organisations to provide this vast array of services.

There are tensions between hospital and community services, between health and social care, and between the relatively huge NHS annual budget of over £70 billion and the relatively small cost of social care. Just as people receiving services need social care and health, so the managers and practitioners in health service and social services need each other. This is what makes the challenge of developing these services so exciting and this book so rewarding to prepare.

What This Book Will Do for You

This book will help your journey through health and social care, whether you are a practitioner or a student and whether you are a beginner at learning or are already fairly experienced. It aims:

- to provide study skills for learners who have limited time and want to develop their learning skills
- to indicate where and how you can find support, as you learn and study
- to provide the underpinning knowledge for the Foundation Degree in Health and Social Care and other courses requiring equivalent levels of knowledge.

What This Book Contains

You will find three main kinds of material in this book:

- Collections of useful information, such as *abbreviations* and *key terms* at the start, and *website addresses* in the appendices at the end, which may be helpful at any point in your studies.
- *Chapters* discussing the topics of relevance to your studies in health and social care and *resource files*. The purpose of the resource files is to give you stimulus material to start you thinking about a topic. They include information, further reading and on occasions activities. Resource files sometimes relate to and complement the chapters nearest them. Other files, such as those concerned with studying, learning and preparing assignments, are grouped in two parts. The first group, on basic learning and study topics, follow Chapter 2. The second group follow Chapters 37, 41, 43, 44 and 46 and tackle topics linked with the more challenging material in the later parts of the book.
- *Activities, practice studies* and *review questions* in the chapters for you to think about, respond to and check out against your experience, knowledge and understanding.

How to Use This Book

You can:

- Dip into a particular resource file to kick start study of a topic
- Read the related chapter for broader coverage of the topic
- Check facts by referring to the start of the book for abbreviations and the key terms, and the appendices for contact details, important government publications, inquiries, reports and legislation.

The structure of the book makes it possible for you to find your way quickly to particular topics. The content of the book is divided into nine major parts.

Part I, Preparing to Learn, underpins your entire learning and studying, equips you to learn and offers you some core study skills. Parts II to VIII cover essential aspects of values, knowledge and skills, which are vital to your competence as a health and social care practitioner. Part IX invites you to move on and engage in further personal and professional development, on an open-ended basis.

Two final points:

1. Most of the examples used in this book are fictitious. Any references to real people are indicated at the time and unless otherwise indicated with their permission, their names and other details have been changed to preserve anonymity.

2. It is significant that there are no universally agreed terms for the two main stake-holders in health and social care work – the 'worker' and the 'client'. In this book, we usually refer to the person doing the work as the worker or the practitioner, although sometimes we group them together with other 'professionals'. We usually refer to the 'client' as the service user, the person using services or the patient. It is quite common to fall into the phrase 'service users and carers' as though carers are tacked on to service users, but we try to avoid doing this automatically because it becomes meaningless. Sometimes, we place carers first – 'carers and service users' – to emphasise their distinctive importance. It isn't an answer but it shows we are aware of the problem.

Abbreviations

ACMD	Advisory Council on the Misuse of Drugs		DAS	Director of Adults Services
			DCS	Director of Children's Services
ADAS	Association of Directors of Adult Services		DfES	Department for Education and Skills
ADCS	Association of Directors of Children's Services		DNA	deoxyribonucleaic acid
			DoH	Department of Health
ADSS	Association of Directors of Social Services		DRC	Disability Rights Commission
			DTI	Department of Trade and Industry
ARC	Association for Residential Care		DWP	Department for Work and Pensions
BCODP	British Council of Disabled People			
BMA	British Medical Association		ECCA	English Community Care Association
BRC	Better Regulations Commission			
BRE	Better Regulations Executive		FACS	Fair Access to Care Services
BRTF	Better Regulation Task Force		GP	general practitioner (doctor)
CAMHS	Children and Adolescent Mental Health Service		HAZ	Health Action Zone
			HCAI	healthcare-associated infection
CAT	complementary and alternative therapies		HCC	Health Care Commission (full name: Commission for Healthcare Audit and Inspection)
CBT	cognitive-behaviour therapy			
CDNA	Community and District Nursing Association		HFEA	Human Fertilisation and Embryology Authority
CHAI	Commission for Healthcare Audit and Inspection (now known as Health Care Commission)		HMCI	Her Majesty's Chief Inspector of Schools
			HMCS	Her Majesty's Courts Service
CHI	Commission for Health Improvement (functions now transferred to Health Care Commission)		HMICA	Her Majesty's Inspectorate of Court Administration
			HPA	Health Protection Agency
			ICO	Independent Care Organisations
CMHT	community mental health team		ICS	Integrated Children System
CPA	care programme approach		IMCA	independent mental capacity advocate
CPAG	Child Poverty Action Group			
CPR	child protection register		ISA	information sharing and assessment
CRB	Criminal Records Bureau			
CRE	Commission for Racial Equality		LAC	local authority circular
CSCI	Commission for Social Care Inspection		MDT	multidisciplinary team

MRSA	methicillin-resistant Staphylococcus Aureus	POVA	Protection of Vulnerable Adults
MS	multiple sclerosis	RCA	Residential Care Association (now SCA)
NAHRS	National Alcohol Harm Reduction Strategy	RNHA	Registered Nursing Home Association
NCHA	National Care Homes Association	RNID	Royal National Institute for Deaf and Hard of Hearing People
NCSC	National Care Standards Commission	SAP	single assessment process
NFER	National Foundation for Educational Research	SCA	Social Care Association
		SCIE	Social Care Institute for Excellence
NHSCCA	National Health Service and Community Care Act 1990	SfC	Skills for Care
		SfH	Skills for Health
NICE	National Institute for Clinical Excellence	SIPs	Social Inclusion Partnerships
		SSD	social services department
NRT	nicotine replacement therapy	SSI	Social Services Inspectorate
NSF	National Service Framework	STD	sexually transmitted disease
Ofsted	Office for Standards in Education	STI	sexually transmitted infection
OFT	Office of Fair Trading	TFI	Tobacco Free Initiative
OHS	Occupational Health Service	TSO	The Stationery Office
PCP	person-centred planning	UKHCA	UK Home Care Association
PCT	Primary Care Trust	UTI	urinary tract infection
PHCT	Primary Health Care Team	VCS	voluntary and community sector
PNS	peripheral nervous system	WHO	World Health Organization
PACE	Police and Criminal Evidence (Act 1984)	YJB	Youth Justice Board
		YOT	youth offending team

Key Terms

Alzheimer's disease	A progressive condition in which the person's brain degenerates, leading to a general decline in mental capacity and a weakening of the body, which may itself lead to fatal illness
Anti-discriminatory practice	Practice that aims to achieve equality by countering discrimination and oppression and promoting diversity and inclusion of people
Aphasia	Loss of speech, as after a stroke
ADSS	The Association of Directors of Social Services, which represents all the Directors of Adults Services (DAS) and Directors of Children's Services (DCS) in England, Wales and Northern Ireland
Carer	A person not paid apart from any 'direct payments', who, as a partner, other family member, friend or neighbour, is informally looking after or providing a substantial amount of help on a regular basis for a sick, disabled or elderly person living on their own or in another household
Cerebral palsy	Not an illness or disease but a physical impairment that affects movement and not mental abilities
Clinical audit	Process of quality improvement through reviewing against stated criteria and the extent of change
Cognitive-behavioural therapy	Encouraging desired behaviour by replacing undesirable thinking
Crisis	An unplanned, unanticipated event or moment that disrupts a person's life and functioning
Crisis intervention	A range of actions and treatments aiming to tackle the crisis
Dilemma	A choice between two options, neither of which 'remedies' the situation or solves the problem
Direct payments	Payment by social services direct to the service user for her or him to buy services
Disability living allowance	An allowance for people who need additional resources in order to look after themselves
Ecological public health	Public health that links achieving health with economic and environmental factors and sustainable development
Ethical practice	Standards of practice considered acceptable and desirable

Governance	A system for ensuring the accountability of the organisation as it manages itself
Health promotion	The provision of information about healthy living, which enables individuals and communities to make rational and informed choices about improving lifestyles and health
Incapacity benefit	A weekly benefit for people under state pension age who are unable to work because of illness or disability
Integration	Bringing together, for example 'bringing together' theory and practice
Model	A representation, image or description of the main features of a problem, scheme or initiative, which often simplifies it, to show how key features of it work, or could work
Multidisciplinary practice	Practice involving several different professional groups working together, drawing on different bases of knowledge and skills
Pension credit	A means-tested benefit to top up income to a minimum level, for single people and those with a partner, where at least one is over 60
Primary care	'The science and art of promoting health, preventing disease, and prolonging life through the organised efforts of society' (Nutbeam, 1998, p. 14, adapted from the Acheson Report, 1988)
Psychosomatic illness	An illness brought about by psychological factors
Risk management	The process of identifying, assessing and managing risks and monitoring and reviewing progress in this
Quality assurance	A systematic process of verifying that the product or service is being delivered according to a specified standard
Senility	A condition whose symptoms included progressive memory loss, disorientation and loss of control over basic bodily functions
Service user	A person receiving adult care services or direct payments
Stigmatisation	The process by which somebody attracts a negative label
Stroke	Damage to the brain caused most often by a blood clot in an artery supplying it (ischaemic stroke) and less often by a burst blood vessel leaking blood into brain tissue causing damage or death (haemorrhagic stroke)
Theory	A theory is a statement of principles and ideas with the aim of explaining something and possibly predicting how it will work or change in the future, for example theory about how the body works may be used to explain the effectiveness of a particular drug

Preparing to Learn

Part I
Preparing to Learn

Introduction

We are all learners, throughout our lives. Some of us only experience formal study during our school years. If you are reading this book, you are likely to have returned to study as an adult. You may be working and studying at the same time. Students on foundation degrees are normally working and studying in the same field, which enables them to make links between their studies and their work experiences.

Becoming a student is difficult at the best of times. It is even more stressful when you have been working full time, away from formal study, for a considerable time. Returning to study, becoming a student, are challenges.

If you are finding it daunting to consider yourself as returning to learning as a student, Part I of this book is written with you in mind. The two chapters in this first part offer you the means to build up your knowledge, confidence and skills. Chapter 1 equips you to manage your own learning. Chapter 2 provides study skills, at the end of which you will find Resource Files that summarise key areas of study skills.

This book is for health and social care practitioners. It contains material designed for use across the entire field of health and social care. In order to make this material work for you, you need to cross and recross the boundary between health and social care. It will not work if you go through the book as a care worker ignoring anything with the words 'health' and 'nursing' attached. Similarly, it will not work if you are a healthcare worker and you ignore anything referring to 'social care', 'social work' or 'social services'.

Resource file

Experiences of two students

Denise

Denise works with looked after children and wanted to continue to work to support her family while moving towards a qualification in social work. Her local college runs a Foundation Degree in Applied Health and Social Care which suited those needs.

She had been away from academic life for some time and so was anxious about the particular demands of academic work – understanding academic language and then putting it into her own language, making sure she had met the learning outcomes, writing objectively rather than subjectively and using counter-arguments effectively.

Denise experienced 'feelings of dread at not being able to do it', but talking to other students who understood made her feel less isolated and gave her the space to adjust to these new demands. Other strategies that enabled her to approach the work feeling less overwhelmed were reflecting back on lectures to check understanding, reading different texts, discussing assignment plans with tutors, planning each piece of work systematically and remaining focused.

Denise also felt that it was made more manageable by keeping a healthy balance between college, family, work and a smattering of social life. Getting stressed may have motivated her to do the work in the short term, but it could easily get out of hand if she didn't manage her commitments carefully and then it proved far from helpful.

Denise didn't realise how in-depth her job was until she started to understand the theory behind her actions and has now started to use her practice to help her understand her college work. While the course continues to be demanding, it is also rewarding, both personally and professionally.

Kris

Kris is working in a hospital as a healthcare assistant. He has taken courses to improve written English, his second language, and studied A levels part time. He began his Foundation Degree in Health and Social Care last year and cannot believe how much more enthusiastic he feels now.

For the first few weeks at college he floundered and nearly gave up. He learned to wait behind after lectures and tutorials and continually ask about things he didn't understand. He failed his first assignment, but in a meeting with his tutor learned to use this to identify his weak points – presentation, references and bibliographies – and tackle them.

The turning point came when he started to choose topics which really interested him and found out how to use the internet, and links to the college and university library, to study at home after work. He is starting his second year in an altogether more positive and confident frame of mind than when he began the course. It has been hard work, but worth it.

1 Managing Yourself and Your Learning

JAMES REID with RUTH HAMILTON and DIANE HOWARD

Is This the Right Course for Me?

Before you enrol on a course or programme of study you need to be sure that it is the right course for you in order to be able to learn effectively. In order to make this decision, you need to know what your motivation is for undertaking the course – what do you want from the course? This might be many different things for different people, in that the course might offer:

- an opportunity for personal and/or professional development
- a qualification that will further your career
- a qualification that will enable you to progress onto another course that offers further opportunities, personal or work-oriented
- a range of subjects that interest you
- an opportunity to prove something to yourself (or your family/housemates/friends)
- an opportunity to develop knowledge and/or intellectual skills that are relevant to your current role or a future role
- new or different social opportunities

■ a challenge!

Whatever your motivation, make sure the course you have chosen will fulfil your personal and/or professional expectations. You can do this by:

■ studying the prospectus/website carefully
■ talking to tutors
■ talking to former students.

My Previous Educational Experiences

It is normal for students beginning a new course to experience a range of feelings including excitement and anxiety. One reason for the presence of these feelings is your previous experiences of education, and although you may have had very positive experiences in the past, almost everyone can identify something from their previous education that they would like to change or do differently. It is therefore important for you to think about your previous educational experiences and what you are feeling in order that you can take account of any issues that may arise.

Activity 1.1

1. Think about your previous educational experiences. Write your own lists of what you did and didn't enjoy.

   The example below will help.

   What I enjoyed
   ■ Learning new things
   ■ Being a student
   ■ Some lecturers
   ■ Other students
   ■ Feeling valued
   ■ Potential to develop

   What I didn't enjoy
   ■ Too much homework
   ■ Pressures from elsewhere
     – home
     – work
   ■ Not feeling valued
   ■ Lack of support

2. Next consider the lists you made and note the factors (that is, things affecting you) that are internal to you, for example feelings, and the factors that are external, for example pressures at work.

This activity is about identifying the things that have helped with or impeded your learning in the past. You are also being explicit about the experiences and the associated feelings that can affect your motivation and attainment. It is important that you consider the potential blocks to your learning. If, for example, you have identified 'too much homework' as an issue, ask yourself what you can do to deal with this. The answer perhaps lies in good time management. You should do this for all the potential blocks, and don't worry if the answers are not immediately apparent as the work you have done on the activity will be a good foundation for a discussion about these issues with your course tutor.

The next activity will also help you to think about things further.

My Strengths and Weaknesses, Opportunities for, and Threats to, Learning

First of all recognise the positives, for example you were motivated enough to consider your development needs and apply for and get a place on the course.

Some students begin their studies feeling highly motivated and enjoy their course until pressures from elsewhere, including home and work, begin to impact on the time given over to study, and consequently lectures and other learning activities may be missed. This can lead to feelings of not being in control and of lost confidence in the ability to succeed. This in turn will affect motivation and studies may end prematurely. It is therefore extremely important to plan effectively for your course and a good way of beginning to do this is to apply an analysis based on your strengths and weaknesses, and the opportunities and threats (SWOT) to your studies. The lists you did in Activity 1.1 will help you to complete the analysis; a sample of a SWOT analysis is provided below.

Example of a SWOT analysis

Strengths	*Weaknesses*
Good reader	Not studied for a number of years
Can use the library	Writing essays
Support from work and family	Managing time
Motivation to succeed and progress	Anxiety about failing
Get on with others	Study skills
	Space at home to study
Opportunities	*Threats*
Progression and promotion	Work demands
Up-to-date knowledge	Home demands
Financial support from work	Attitude of co-workers
Agency needs qualified staff	Losing contact with service users
Meeting new people	Loss of social life
Recognition by other people	

You may notice that strengths and weaknesses concentrate on a range of issues internal to you, including your personal motivation, skills, feelings and values. Opportunities and threats concentrate on the range of external issues that can affect your studies, including finance, career demands and problems that may arise in work or at home.

Activity 1.2

1. Complete a SWOT analysis for yourself.
2. What does the analysis tell you? What are the positives and what issues do you need to tackle?

You may find the following prompts useful to help you complete the activity:

- *Strengths:* What qualities and skills do you possess to be a good student?
  What do you do well now, having studied previously?
  What do others tell you that you do well?

- *Weaknesses:* What skills do you need to develop?
  What doesn't work well or what should you avoid doing?
  What things do you need to improve?

- *Opportunities:* What financial and policy developments will support your learning?
  Will opportunities include the support of others?
  Will they include your aims and objectives or future plans?

- *Threats:* What are the factors in your home and working life?
  What other obstacles are you aware of?

Having identified your strengths and weaknesses, and the opportunities and threats to your learning, it is necessary to think how to minimise the impact of both weaknesses and threats. Look at the weaknesses and consider how these could be developed into strengths. Similarly, threats should be developed into opportunities. You can also ensure that your strengths and opportunities are used to their maximum potential.

It may be helpful to understand that the points you have identified extend to many other students undertaking new study. Common themes will include your ability to meet the demands of the course through study skills and managing time effectively, recognising your learning behaviour, and balancing the demands of study with home and work. The remainder of this chapter will concentrate on your learning.

My Study Skills

The example of the SWOT analysis above shows that the student has some confidence in her or his abilities but is concerned about study skills including using time well and about having appropriate space to study. Study skills include reading, writing, note-taking and the use of computers (see Chapter 2).

Universities and colleges put a lot of effort into providing assistance in these areas and many provide study skills programmes or packages for students who feel they need help. If this applies to you, ask your tutor about available support. Whether you are a confident learner or feel that you need further support, it is important that you are aware of the essential study skills for university or college (Burns and Sinfield, 2003).

How Best will you Learn?

For many people, undertaking a health and social care course will mean returning to education after a significant period has elapsed and any new activity will naturally be accompanied by some anxiety. Starting a new course can evoke both positive and negative memories of that last encounter with education, which may affect how you approach this new endeavour. You need to reflect on these experiences and learn how to use them positively to inform this period of study – both the positive and negative experiences. What did they tell you about how you learned then? What may be the same and what has changed? It is a type of skills audit.

Activity 1.3 aims to enable you to recognise how to reflect on previous educational experiences and learn from them, acknowledging and building on the positives and recognising the changes you need to make to ensure that the negative aspects can be turned into positive ones.

Activity 1.3

Part 1

Think back to your last *negative* experience of study and reflect on the following questions:

- List what was negative about this experience.
- What else was happening in your life at that time? (Did this support or distract you from your studies?)
- What did you not enjoy about the lectures/taught sessions – the content and the delivery – and what contributed to that? (This may include the teacher/lecturer, the presentation of material, the way you examined the material, that is, activities in class, what other students contributed to the sessions.)
- How did you prepare for your studies? (How did you allocate time? How much time did you spend on your studies? Where did you study? Did did you do additional reading? Did you plan in advance for assignments, submitting plans to tutors or working in groups. Did you have someone to proofread drafts?)
- Whose support was available to you during your studies? (This could be from partner, family, friends, colleagues, organisation, or a combination of these). Be clear about what they did that you found supportive (or unsupportive).

Looking at each of your responses, can you identify what has changed, or what could you change and who could help you to achieve this change, to make this experience a more positive one now? Write the answers down next to the original responses so they stand out (for example use a different coloured pen).

Part 2

Now reflect on a *positive* experience of study and answer the same set of questions including things that you enjoyed about being a student and what your strengths were.

Again, looking at each of your responses:

■ Identify what, if anything, has changed?

■ What could you change?

■ What could help you to achieve this change, to build upon this positive experience and use it to good effect this time?

Write the answers down next to the original responses so they stand out (for example use a different coloured pen).

From the two lists, compile an *action list* of what you need to make sure is in place, or you can work towards, to support your completion of this course and then what you need to do to make sure each one happens. If you think of strategies that you have used in the past to help you overcome difficulties, this may give you the confidence to tackle these. Remember, many students experience the same hurdles to studying and colleges/universities recognise this. There are often many forms of support and guidance available to students to overcome obstacles to studying so don't be afraid to ask for advice either from your tutor or the college advice services. These can range from support with literacy (spelling, punctuation, structuring assignments) and numeracy skills to financial support for childcare.

The example below may help you structure this effectively.

Action list

What helped/ hindered in previous studies?	What do I need to do to maintain/ change this?	Who could help me to achieve this?	When do I need to do this by?

My Learning Style

Just as you each have individual experiences that can impact on your learning, you also possess influential learning attributes. One common framework for thinking about these is to discover your own learning style. Honey and Mumford (1992) have identified four learning styles – activist, reflector, theorist and pragmatist – and their research shows that a majority of students tend to have one or two favoured ways of learning from among the four learning styles:

■ *Activists* are open-minded and enthusiastically pursue new experiences. They enjoy the immediacy and excitement of these new experiences but will become bored over time.

- *Reflectors* like to think about their experiences and listen to others before making their own views known. They will tend to postpone reaching definitive conclusions for as long as possible.
- *Theorists* will think issues through in a methodical logical way. They are rational and prefer objectivity to subjectivity or ambiguity. They are analytical and seek out principles, theories and models.
- *Pragmatists* like to find out whether things work in practice. They have a practical, problem-solving approach and they will want to get on with things quickly and will become distracted if things carry on for too long.

You may favour one or two of these learning styles over the others and discovering this will enable you to consider which style you would benefit from developing. As an activist or a pragmatist you may be keen on getting on and writing essays or doing practical work but will be less happy with reading and reflective tasks. Theorists will enjoy reading, researching and attending lectures but can take time to complete an assignment. Reflectors will enjoy discussion activities and mulling over ideas but will also require time to complete a task.

Activity 1.4

1. Think of a lesson, meeting or group that you were recently involved in and consider your behaviour.
2. Ask yourself some questions about your involvement in this activity:
   - Did you participate fully or did you let other people lead the way?
   - Did you become bored? If so, when and why?
   - Were you anxious to get things done rather than talk or think about them?
   - Did things appear rational or were they tenuous and ambiguous?
   - What do you think is your preferred learning style?

Having identified the learning style or styles that you favour, it is important to understand that this is simply an aid and your preferred style may change with time or in particular situations. Nonetheless there will be aspects of your study style that you need to develop and it will be worthwhile setting aside some time to do this; for example as an activist, you may want to read more. Remember to incorporate any activity that you intend to undertake into your study plan.

Activity 1.5

In order to discover more about your learning style visit this website:

www.campaign-for-learning.org.uk/aboutyourlearning/whatlearning.htm.

Fitting Studying into your Life

Using Supervision to Support your Learning

Foundation degrees have been developed to allow students to develop and learn while they continue to work. It is therefore essential that anyone undertaking a foundation degree recognises the competing demands of study and work and takes steps to ensure effective communication with their manager about needs, progress and attainment on the course. The most obvious place for these discussions will be within supervision.

Supervision has a long history in the helping professions and is essential in ensuring effective and competent practice. As such, supervision should not only cover issues of performance but should also consider the development of the worker. Indeed, most supervision policies and procedures identify four major functions for discussion: management, education, support, and mediation (Richards et al., 1990). Management concerns effective, accountable practice, whereas education focuses on the professional development of the worker in becoming an effective practitioner. This is helped by support to consider the impact of that on practice, either internal or external to work. Mediation allows issues to flow between frontline workers and higher management.

Activity 1.6

1. Think about your last supervision and the topics discussed. Which supervision functions were in evidence?

It is not essential that all the functions are evident within a particular supervision session; however, you should be able to identify instances where discussion took place under the umbrella of each function over a period of time.

There are a number of things that you can do to ensure that supervision is effective for you. For example, *read your employer's supervision policy* in order that you understand your rights and responsibilities and discuss with your supervisor your wish to have your progress on your course as a regular item for discussion. Furthermore, it is good practice to arrive at supervision with your own agenda of items to be discussed.

To do this, develop a *list of the key activities* that you are involved with at work. Do not list more than 10 and remember to include your personal development as an issue. These may also change over time so it is important to ensure the continuing relevance of the list. Another good idea is to ask your supervisor to do the same about you. This will give you the opportunity to develop a fuller understanding of your role and to consider similarities and differences in expectations. The example below is a list of key activities for a residential social worker.

KEY ACTIVITIES	Managerial	Educational
	1. Keyworker	5. Supervision
	2. Administration	6. Foundation degree
	3. Assessments	
	4. Team member	
	Supportive	**Mediation**
	7. Shift work	9. Introduction of new policies
	8. Team leader	

Complete a list of your key activities at work. Remember, list no more than 10 and
include your studies as a topic.

Maintaining a balance between work and study is important in ensuring a positive
outcome for you from your course. Supervisors need to understand the demands
being placed upon you by college or university and it is your responsibility, in part,
to create the opportunity for discussion and effective communication.

For most people, starting a course means taking on a new commitment in addition
to the others they currently manage. These may include commitments at work and
to colleagues, family commitments, care commitments, trade union activities and/or
social networks, often a combination of these and many more besides. Being clear
about what the course will require of you will help you to decide how well you can
manage this new commitment. Check this out with the course leader and current
students in terms of attendance, assignments, homework and independent
reading/research, with the approximate number of hours you will be expected to
spend on each and what support is available in order to manage this.

You will then need to be clear with your employer, your family/housemates and
friends about the time you will need to devote to your studies.

Negotiating Study Time at Work

If you are being 'supported' on the course by your employer, you will need to
confirm in what ways and to what extent they are supporting you:

- Are they paying for the course fees?
- Are they giving you time off work to attend (and making sure this is seen as a
  priority by your team)?
- Are they giving you study time in addition to attendance?
- Are they reducing your workload to reflect time away for your studies?
- Are they providing formal support during supervision to enable you to reflect on
  your studies in relation to your work?

Negotiating Study Time with Family/Housemates and Friends

This may mean changing not only the amount of time you spend with them, but
when you spend time with them too. You need to examine your weekly routine and
work out the amount of hours you need for your studies and when this will best fit
in. Remember, the time you allocate to your studies will need to be concentrated
time, with minimal interruptions. It will also mean spending time on your studies
when you're feeling alert and able to think clearly about the task in hand, setting
targets so the time doesn't drift without achieving anything. That may mean going

to the library to avoid distractions, which may take more planning. Decide what will be the most effective strategies for you and then take note of what works best.

Negotiating Space to Study

Family members or housemates moving your carefully arranged piles of books and notes off the dining table in order to eat at it may cause you frustration and cost you additional time reorganising the piles. Spending time on the computer may cause resentment in housemates or other family members who are used to monopolising it. Sorting out the right space, and enough of it (that will allow you to spread out, organise and store notes, books and papers), will indicate to your cohabitants (whether housemates, family or fellow students) how important studying is to you.

Being clear from the outset about how the course will impact on your life will mean other people can make the necessary changes to their lives and readjust their expectations of you, reducing the potential for conflict and stress, so that you can then focus on the course. By being clear about both the challenges and opportunities that the programme will bring, you will be more likely to be able to sustain your studies rather than allowing stress to build and overwhelm you.

The planning of this is something you need to take responsibility for and marks the start of taking responsibility for your own learning. This is part of what is described as the 'adult learning model' – being more responsible for managing your own learning rather than expecting to be 'spoon-fed' as was traditionally the case in most schools.

Conclusion

This chapter has introduced you to the issues that support and inhibit learning. You have considered yourself as a learner and the impact of previous experiences on your behaviour. You should be aware of the tools and activities required to study well, including the need to develop an effective study plan that balances the range of demands you face within the limited number of hours in a week. In the next chapter we shall consider the study skills you need to develop in order to maximise the effectiveness of your learning.

REVIEW QUESTIONS

1 How can a SWOT analysis help you to learn more effectively?

2 What are the main characteristics of Honey and Mumford's different learning styles?

3 What is work-based supervision and how may it help you to learn?

2 Skills for Studying

RUTH HAMILTON and DIANE HOWARD with JAMES REID

By the end of this chapter, you should be able to understand how to:

- MAKE time to study
- USE learning resources effectively
- MAKE the most of lectures and seminar groups
- DO a written assignment
- MAKE sense of feedback
- TACKLE the challenges of work-based learning.

Making Time to Study

In the previous chapter we examined what is involved in coming to grips with learning. In this chapter, we enable you to identify the issues involved in studying. It will be important for you to discuss your learning and study needs and seek support from your tutor and employer. As a work-based student, you should try to negotiate a high profile for your studies in supervision at work and clarify what you and your supervisor expect from them. Undertaking a foundation degree makes demands on your study skills, for example reading and writing, and your time. You will be expected to fit study into an already busy week and commit yourself to the university's or college's expectations for the study time required to pass your course. Most universities or colleges will calculate this on the basis of, for example, 10 hours of study per credit. A 20-credit module will therefore require 200 hours of notional effort from you over the year. This includes not only time spent poring over books but also time spent in lectures, tutorials, at work and in individual study activity. A good way of beginning to manage your time effectively is to list everything you spend time on in a typical week.

Activity 2.1

1. List the activities you do and the time spent on these in a typical week. Remember that you only have 168 hours.
2. Make a weekly plan, making sure you provide sufficient time for work, friends, family and study. Have a goal for your study time.

The template below might be useful but arrange the timings to suit you.

	Mon.	Tues.	Wed.	Thurs.	Fri.	Sat.	Sun.
0700							
0800							
0900							
1000							
1100							
1200							
1300							
1400							
1500							
1600							
1700							
1800							
1900							
2000							
2100							
2200							
2300							

There will be obvious opportunities to study using the resources of the university or college including the library, but it is unlikely that you will do all your studying there and there will be times when you study at home or work. Most students will not have the use of a dedicated study area at either home or work, having to use the dining table, for example. This is fine as long as it is not a meal time and your children/housemates aren't using it to do their homework. You will need to find a place to study where you are not likely to be interrupted.

Using Learning Resources Effectively

The Library/Books and Journals

The library, or learning resource centre, is an important source of books, journals, collections of archived material, tapes and information and communication technology (ICT). A library induction session will help you gain most from this resource. Despite the increasing use of websites, books and journals remain a vital source of information, although journals can often be accessed via the internet, through internet accounts such as Athens. Ask a library assistant for help to access journals.

In order to make the best use of books and journals, you need to:

- *Understand your purpose:* Clarify the task first and keep checking that what you are reading is relevant to the task in hand.
- *Select the appropriate texts:* If you can't find the book on the reading list, look around the same shelf for similar books. Read the back cover and scan the list of contents to assess their relevance. If you're in any doubt about which books to use, ask your tutor, other students (or the subject librarian at the library) what they would recommend.
- *Be realistic about how much you can read:* Academic books often take longer to read than other books, partly because of their formal language and the way they present complex ideas and practices. In academic assignments you don't usually need to read a book from cover to cover. With practice, you can develop the skill of selective reading. To begin, try picking the most relevant chapters by reading the introductions and conclusions. Find relevant sections using the subheadings for guidance and set yourself a time limit for each piece.
- *Choose up-to-date texts if possible, unless you know a particular text is a classic:* Journals and periodicals give the most up-to-date account of recent research and thinking on subjects and are more condensed due to the length of articles. A journal article usually has an abstract at the beginning, which is a summary of what it will cover. This will give you an idea if the article is pitched in a way that will be useful to you. (See Resource File: Finding Information, at the end of this chapter.)
- *Take notes when reading:* Always take notes when reading as this will help to trace ideas and enable you to review your understanding. Make notes, spider diagrams or concept maps (visual ways of making connections between ideas starting with the subject matter at the centre) or highlight sections in chapters in the text, whichever way you find most useful. Don't squeeze your notes too closely together. You may want to add bits from subsequent books at the relevant place. (See Resource File: Organising Information, at the end of this chapter.)
- *It will also help your 'academic' style if you read critically:* Always ask questions about what you're reading. Do you agree with the author or not, and if so, why? What point is the author trying to make? Have you read something that disagrees with this point of view? What are the key points to the argument overall? (See Resource File: Reading Critically, at the end of this chapter.)
- *You may want to quote from a piece of writing:* Be very careful that you copy the quote accurately and reference it appropriately, otherwise you can be accused of 'plagiarism' – presenting someone else's ideas as yours – which in academic life is tantamount to theft and viewed just as seriously. Your selected quote should be no more than a few lines and, if longer, you should really paraphrase it (rewrite it in your own words and then reference the idea to the original author). You may initially lack confidence in doing this, worrying that you'd never be able

to say it as well as the author has and it can be tempting to copy down chunks, word for word. However, you may forget later on and use it in the same form without acknowledging the author, and you could then be accused of plagiarism, which, depending on the extent and perceived intent to deceive, could result in work being disqualified or, at worse, expulsion from the programme. Read your college/university regulations regarding this.

Activity 2.2

Paraphrasing is the art of summarising and is an important skill in academic writing.

1. Practise paraphrasing by choosing a book you are familiar with (it could be a novel or even a newspaper article) and selecting a section you are confident that you understand.
2. Read it several times, then turn the book/paper over and in your own words summarise what that section was attempting to tell you.
3. Return to the passage and see how accurate your summary was. Remember you are only summarising so you aren't trying to record every detail.

Repeating this exercise several times will help you to develop not only your skills at paraphrasing and summarising but also those of recall. (See Resource File: Organising Information, at the end of this chapter.)

Computers and the Internet

Computers give access to the internet, which offers an increasingly wide range of information, some sources more credible than others. This can all happen at the touch of a button, but it can feel daunting unless you know how to use it effectively. To do this it will help if you become familiar with the language of computers and the functions they offer.

You can use 'browsers', 'search engines' and 'subject gateways' to produce a vast range of 'hits' (potential sources of relevant information) but you need to choose from these selectively. Some subject gateways offer a more focused search covering particular subject areas. Finding reliable sources on the internet can be difficult. (See Resource File: Finding Information, at the end of this chapter.) Not all information has been vetted and you therefore need to develop your ability to scrutinise and select from the options judiciously. Some academic institutions have their own search engines which only select credible databases. These search engines will often organise the databases into subject categories, both saving time used searching the web and aiding your selection of reliable material.

For more general searches, using a search engine such as 'Google' and 'Yahoo!' will require you to first enter a general topic area or keywords (if you don't know the exact web address you are after) and it will then offer often hundreds, or sometimes thousands, of web addresses that contain potentially relevant information. Being as precise as possible will limit the number of sites that are thrown up.

Making the Most of Lectures and Seminar Groups

Lectures and seminar groups:

- form the hub of most college courses
- offer you the opportunity to benefit from the lecturer's expertise
- can take many forms depending on the size of the group, the content of the module and the style of the lecturer
- provide an introduction or framework for understanding the subject
- signpost further reading to broaden your understanding.

To gain the most from lectures, you should:

- find out before each lecture what it is about and do some preparatory reading
- attend punctually, sit near the front and note the main points rather than trying to write down everything
- after each lecture, reread your notes and rewrite them more fully and coherently.

You and your Student Group(s)

Other members of your student group will offer a wealth of knowledge and experience that you can share and draw upon from both personal and professional experience of a subject. Lecturers recognise this and often plan sessions that encourage this pooling of understanding and may involve discussions or presentations – these can be in sessions such as seminars, support groups, tutorials, group projects and skills groups. (See Resource File: Doing a Presentation, at the end of Chapter 41.)

The benefits of this type of groupwork are many. They may include:

- presenting ideas in a more practical, recognisable way
- offering a broader range of perspectives, realising there is no 'right' or 'wrong' answer, but many ways to approach a subject
- clarifying your own thinking by taking time to discuss the detail until it falls into place
- encouraging more critical thinking around a topic when faced with opposing ideas
- encouraging a greater understanding of your fellow students – the building block for effective study together
- developing your interpersonal skills, particularly active listening, negotiating and discussing a subject with objectivity (whenever possible)
- reducing isolation and offering support to you when trying to grapple with a subject – you will discover that you're not the only one confused
- sometimes reducing the workload (although often getting everyone together can itself be quite time-consuming)
- an opportunity to develop groupwork or teamwork, which is excellent preparation for future employment.

If your groupwork is being assessed, you need to monitor progress as carefully as you do all assessed work, keeping to agreed deadlines and ensuring all elements are present, each person being clear what their responsibilities are.

Working in groups and being part of group discussions can be an intimidating environment where you think everyone knows more than you or can articulate it better than you, using more appropriate language. Some people will feel a lot more confident about contributing to a group discussion than others, whether the contribution is relevant or not. Join in. Take the plunge and make a simple contribution to begin with – ask a question or offer a straightforward example. You have as much right to exercise your ideas as the next person and it is as important a part of academic learning as any other. Remember, once you have made your first contribution, your confidence will grow. Another tip is to do some preparatory reading beforehand so that you are familiar with the subject matter – you should feel a lot more confident making a contribution to a discussion that you're keeping pace with.

Doing a Written Assignment

Assessment can take many forms – essays, presentations, posters, groupwork, exams and many others. Written work is the most common form of assessment. Undertaking your first piece of written work can be daunting, but is potentially satisfying and rewarding.

Writing requires many different skills – spelling, punctuation, grammar, sentence structure, paragraph structure, developing an argument, appropriateness of content, reflection, applying theory to practice and referencing. Try following the five stages below to help you through the task.

1. Understanding the Task

Some tasks and titles for essays may seem a lot more straightforward than others. In any case, read and reread the task several times before you take the next step and if necessary seek clarification from the tutor. As the level of study increases from year one to year two (level 4 to level 5), so will the complexity of the activity required of you; for example evaluating is considered a more complex task than describing.

2. Making a Time Plan

Make a rough time plan of what you need to do to complete the task. Working back from the submission date will focus you on the appropriate time frame and when you need to start. Your plan should include time allocated to the following stages:

- information-gathering, including visits to the library and time researching the internet
- confirming your outline of the assignment and checking it out with the tutor (if possible submitting a written plan for comment)

- reading around the subject
- writing the first draft of the assignment
- writing second and subsequent drafts
- compiling the reference list/bibliography
- getting someone to proofread it who, if possible, can understand what you're trying to say and has reliable written skills themselves
- making the appropriate alterations after proofreading
- allowing plenty of time to leave your final draft for a few days and return to read it afresh.

3. Planning the Structure

Once you sit down to sketch out the structure of your assignment (the plan) you need to organise your thoughts. Include in your written plan an introduction and conclusion and then begin to group related points together in sections. Allow an estimated amount of words for each section, giving more words to the sections that should make up the main thrust of the discussion.

4. Reading and Research

We covered reading and research earlier under Using Learning Resources Effectively. Be patient, selecting and reading appropriately is a skill you will develop with time. Don't spend too much time on the research and leave too little time for actually writing your assignment.

5. Writing your Assignment

Gather your notes; organise them into sections and prepare to write:

- Review your notes and decide what arguments you want to present from them. Decide how you can compose them in a logical and coherent argument.
- Get started by writing anything to begin with – you can always change it later.
- Begin with whatever seems easiest and write in short, simple sentences.
- Include your most creative ideas. You can always delete or modify them later. This is your draft, to get you thinking and structuring your ideas.

The content: Each section should have its own purpose. It should include:

- establishing the link with the task
- evidence and references to support your assertions and opinions, stating what type of evidence it is, for example research, recent statistical evidence and so on, and how reliable it is
- alternative points of view on the subject and some evaluation of these – you should be prepared, where possible, to state what you think is the most persuasive point of view, and why

- acknowledgement of the strengths and weaknesses of an argument and questions that remain unanswered
- reflections on your experiences, which you may have been asked to give. If so, this may mean reflecting on relevant personal or professional experiences. Before mentioning other people in these accounts, check the requirement for using practice examples and ensure confidentiality is upheld. Make the links between theory and practice clear – explain how each supports and develops the understanding of the other and what general conclusion can be drawn from this.

The introduction: This doesn't necessarily have to be written first. Once you have drafted the sections and feel happy at this stage with the content – your arguments and the evidence (quantity and quality) – try writing the introduction. This should say how you interpret the task and inform the reader from the beginning what your assignment is attempting to address, that is, its content and its main argument(s). There should be a logical sequence to your reasoning that is easily followed by the reader.

The conclusion: Once you have read the whole thing and made the links, try drafting your conclusion. This should refer back to the task set and sum up the main arguments, identifying the most significant ones and why you think they are significant. It should also contain a critical element and provide a platform for posing new questions about where the debate should go from here. (See Resource File: Writing an Essay, at the end of Chapter 43.)

Bibliography: At the end of your assignment, present an alphabetical list of all the work you have quoted, or paraphrased. This is called a bibliography. We recommend that you use the Harvard convention for referring to, and quoting from, authors of books and journal articles in your work. (See Resource File: References and Bibliography, at the end of Chapter 44.)

Types of Feedback

Assessment of work comes usually in two stages – formative and summative. *Formative* assessment measures your progress within a certain unit/module with the emphasis on marking being developmental. *Summative* assessment is the final assessment for a unit/module and the mark is designed to assess your overall achievement.

Passing an assignment is one thing, but to know how you can improve your mark, you need to make sense of the feedback given by the marker. If you don't know how to improve your work, also ask for clarification and advice – that is part of a tutor's role.

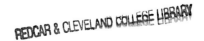

Work-based Learning

Some health and social care courses will include a work-based learning component. This is where you as the student can learn about practice settings, exercise appropriate skills and understand the relevance of, and relationship between, theory and practice.

Work-based learning components can either take place as part of an organised placement (found by the student or the university/college) or, if you are on a work-based route, by using your current place of work as a learning resource for practice. In either case, it is important to establish the boundaries of the work-based learning and clarify what knowledge, skills and values you are expected to demonstrate. It is also important to recognise and understand the partnership that will be established between the student, practice placement and tutor and what the roles of the respective participants will be. This should be established within a practice agreement prior to the commencement of the practice period. The role of the placement and the partners may include elements of the following:

- identifying your needs as a student in relation to practice and reviewing and adapting these as the practice period progresses
- identifying the sequence of learning opportunities to be provided
- identifying and establishing links between the academic and practice elements of the programme
- enabling you as a student to recognise and transfer existing knowledge, skills and values to the current practice and academic setting
- assessing knowledge, skills and values which the placement aims to meet, how these will be assessed and at what level
- giving feedback to you as a student – when and in what format
- supervising you, the student: who will do this and what this will focus on.

If you are a seconded student, that is, supported on the programme as part of your work role, you also need to be aware of what this means contractually. For example, what will happen if you change jobs – will you be required to repay fees – and how will absences from college be viewed by employers?

Conclusion

The purpose of this chapter was to round off the two-chapter sequence of Part I, giving you a measure of learning support and providing some study skills. You should now be in a position to tackle the chapters in the main part of the book. The way Part I and the other parts are laid out will enable you to dip into different chapters and come back to these beginning chapters as required.

REVIEW QUESTIONS

1   What preparation will help you to gain the most from lectures and seminars?

2   What are the main points you need to consider when preparing to write an assignment?

3   What key tasks will you face when carrying out a work-based learning placement?

FURTHER READING

Burns, T. and Sinfield, S. (2003) *Essential Study Skills: The Complete Guide to Success at University*, London, Sage

Collins, S.C. and Kneale, P.E. (2003) *Study Skills for Psychology Students: A Practical Guide*, London, Arnold
One of a great many useful, practical guides to studying.

Resource file

Finding information

Sources of information

You will find information about health and social care in many places, because health and social care services are prominent in so many people's lives. Here are some of the main sources. You can probably add one or two more of your own:

- Government departments' websites and publications, such as official reports
- Professional bodies
- Research and conference reports
- Reports by research bodies, voluntary agencies and, for example, service user or carer groups, many with their own websites
- Academic books and textbooks
- Journals
- Newspaper articles
- Fiction, such as novels, poems and short stories about health and social care issues.

Gathering information

Searching books, journals, reports and other publications

- Choose a subject for your search
- Limit the scope (too wide and it will be unmanageable)
- Clarify the broad category of information, for example academic, fiction, biographies
- Narrow down the types of information, for example statistics, official reports, books, journal articles based on research
- Arrive at keywords to use, for example young carers, empowering disabled people, teenage pregnancy
- Identify where to find the information, for example on databases in the library
- Leave enough time, for example spend a regular amount of time each day for a week, allowing extra time because searching generally takes longer than you anticipate
- Do the search
- Write down a summary of each item and take a full note of the reference to it – see details on creating references in Resource File: References and Bibliography, at the end of Chapter 44
- Evaluate your search, that is, look back at the search and ask four questions:
  - How adequate were my sources?
  - How well did I carry out the search?
  - Am I very pleased, pleased, displeased or very displeased with the result?
  - Why is this?

Searching on the internet

- Identify keywords before you start
- Remember to try to focus your search and not become side-tracked
- List the main words you think are useful, for example for abuse in residential care, your keywords might be adult, social, care, sexual abuse, physical abuse, financial abuse, protection, inquiries, care standards
- Type your topic in the search box in lower case
- If you think a particular word is especially important, type a plus (+) before it
- Enclose a whole phrase in double inverted commas, for example "multidisciplinary groupwork"
- Use 'not' to exclude a word from the search, for example abuse, not sexual
- Use 'or' to broaden the search, for example abuse or protection
- Use 'and' to link two ideas, for example sensory and physical disability.

Clarifying the topic

Don't be afraid to narrow the topic down. Most people start with too broad and ambitious a topic. For instance, rather than older people, focus on older people in residential care. Or rather than disability, focus on people with a learning disability. Linking two subjects narrows down the topic. Linking three narrows it down still more, for instance black lone mothers with a learning disability.

Your aim now is to gather as full a list as you can of articles, publications – books and reports – relevant to the topic.

Go to your nearest library – usually the college or university library is best – and ask for help at the IT or learning resources desk if you are unsure. The best way of searching the internet is to go straight to one of the websites listed below, or another website you already know about. Alternatively, use a 'search engine'. A search engine does a lot of the work of searching for you. You can type in keywords to one of

these. The disadvantage is it often produces a huge number of results and you will need to learn to narrow down the choice by using very specific terms. Try the search engine Google first and www.scie-socialcareonline.org.uk and the Royal College of Nursing (RCN) library (www.rcn.org.uk/library/catalogue) and the National Library for Health (www.library.nhs.uk). For more detailed searches, try Cinahl (accessed through university and college libraries), Medline (www.infor.medline@bma.org.uk) and Proquest and the Cochrane Library (www.cochrane.org).

Here are some of the most commonly used search engines:

- Google   http://www.google.co.uk
- Excite   http://www.excite.com
- Yahoo!   http://www.yahoo.com
- Altavista   http://www.altavista.digital.com

Subject gateways

You can narrow down your search by using a subject gateway. Subject gateways are internet-based sources of information in specific subject areas:

- Galaxy Medicine: http://www.einet.net/galaxy/Medicine.html
- NMAP – Internet Resources on Nursing, Midwifery and Allied Health Professions: http://www.nmap.ac.uk
- Health On the Net Foundation: http://www.hon.ch/
- Healthfinder: http://www.healthfinder.org
- Social Care Institute for Excellence: http://www.scie.org.uk
- Research mindedness in social work and social care: http://resmind.swap.ac.uk.

Use keywords from your topic. If your topic is 'causes of alcoholism among men with a physical impairment', try using the main nouns from your topic as keywords, on their own at first and then together. I used Google and typed in 'alcoholism' and received 729,000 hits. This is far too many for your search. I then added 'men' to the first word and this reduced the hits to 232,000. Adding 'physical impairment' massively reduced the hits to 19,700.

Many of the hits on Google will not be articles you can include in your review. You should ignore them. When you have identified an item you want to include, follow up the reference and open it. Print it out if possible.

Read the article through and use the notes in the Resource File: Evaluating Research, at the end of Part 5 Introduction, to guide you through the process of doing the review. Remember, you should read and review each item and then add a general conclusion, summarising what you have found at the end.

Resource file

Reading critically

Do not be intimidated by the book or journal article sitting on the desk in front of you. Take charge of the material. Critical reading is about having a clear goal and managing the time you have available to reach that goal.

Reading a book

There are three main ways of reading a book. You can:

1. Go through slowly, reading every word, rereading sentences, paragraphs and pages as you go. That is how many people read novels. Few people read academic books, textbooks and reference books that way. This may take you a week or two, at a chapter a day.
2. Go straight to the list of *contents* at the start and read a section or chapter on the topic you want. This may take you two or three hours to complete.
3. Go to the *index* at the back and follow page references to the topic or name you want. This may take you half an hour to complete.

Whichever approach you choose, take notes on any aspects that interest you, taking care to keep on your notepad details of the title, date, author and page number of each entry you note. You can always refer to them later in what you write without having to return to the book.

Decide on your reason for wanting to read the book and focus on your goal. If it is a narrow goal – finding out about a particular concept or item – use point 3

above. You may be able to finish with the book in a few minutes.

Forming habits to help you read critically

1. *Develop a questioning attitude:* Take the idea you have read about and sit for a few minutes thinking about it. Do you agree with it? Does it agree with your own experience? Has it particular strengths or weaknesses? Jot down notes on this, under your notes on the ideas from the book.
2. *Put the idea in the wider context:* Spend time thinking about the wider context. Does the idea link with other ideas of other people you have read or heard about? Jot their names down.
3. *Doodle on a sheet of paper:* Put the original idea in the centre and put a circle round it. Jot down related ideas on the sheet, putting closely related ideas nearer and more important ones in larger letters. You may find it helpful to use a concept map (where you jot down related ideas on a page and link them up) or a spider diagram (where you start with a core idea at the centre and draw lines radiating out from it to related ideas). Make links between the ideas using lines. You can use different colours for ideas that correspond and differ.
4. *Go networking for ideas:* Have a look in the library for the names of people who have written about these other ideas. Or go to the internet and type the ideas in. For instance, if you are studying user participation, you can access the SCIE library (socialcareonline.org.uk) (see Resource File: Finding Information, above).

5. *Make links with other ideas:* Use the above procedures so that you follow the original idea along threads of reference until you decide you have enough.

6. *Review your work:* Spend a few minutes looking back over the notes you've made and jot down any thoughts that occur to you. Try to relax and let thoughts bubble to the surface. Jot down 'off the wall' ideas as well as the more 'rational' thoughts. This will help you when you come to discuss, present or write about the topic later.

7. *Sign off your work:* Put the date either at the top or the bottom of your notes.

Resource file

Organising information

Don't rely on your memory alone when you come across interesting or relevant information. You should try to take notes on the information you gather, whether *from a book or article* or *in class*. Bear in mind the following when taking notes:

- Don't leave writing something until later. You may have forgotten it then. Write it down now.
- Carry a memo pad or notebook with you all the time, night and day, in your bag or pocket.
- Transfer information at home onto A4 sheets in folders or ring binders.
- Label these separate folders with subjects such as 'Law' or 'Essays' and divide each into sections, labelled with the different topics in a subject, such as 'Material for case study on ... '.
- Summarise the information in note form.
- Use bullet points or numbered lists to help you to summarise points.
- Try to summarise arguments in a word or phrase which strikes you as easy to remember. Have confidence in your ability to recall a point from that single word or phrase.

Contexts for Practice

Part II
Contexts for Practice

Introduction

Health and social care services are delivered in rapidly changing social, legal and policy contexts. This part of the book examines the relationship between these changing contexts and the conditions in which services are delivered. The consequences of rapid change are important to managers, practitioners, carers and people who use services. Each of them is a stakeholder in the vast industry of health and welfare that we call the health and social services. Some are involved in the public provision of services, others are involved in private provision, whether as providers, patients or service users. More than one million people are service users of adult care. Local authorities spend more than £8 billion annually on personal social care services; in 2004/05 £1.66 billion of this was recouped in means-testing, a further £3.7 billion was paid in non-means-tested benefits and more than £3.86 billion per annum was paid by people in fees to the private sector providers of care services (Wanless, 2006, p. xxi). Another huge group of people – perhaps as many as six million in the UK – are involved as informal, that is, unpaid, carers. They spend a significant amount of each working day, throughout the year, often with little or no respite, looking after another person. The majority – almost 60 per cent – are women, although a significant minority are children and young people, caring for other children and young people and, sometimes, for adults in their own household.

The range of health and caring services has to be as broad as the huge variety of human experiences leading to people becoming ill, vulnerable or otherwise unable, through physical, emotional or mental difficulties, to manage their lives without help. This enormous variety is affected by the broader and deeper divisions and splits in society, which follow from some people being more healthy, better housed, better educated, better off than others. Part II of the book examines the effects of these differences on health and social care. It:

■ sets the scene for health and social care work

■ looks at the physical, physiological and social contexts for health and wellbeing

■ examines equal opportunities, equality perspectives and human rights

■ deals with relevant policies and legislation

■ covers major questions arising about values and ethics

■ discusses ideas about human growth and development through the life course.

Resource file

Linking the past and present of health and social care

One of my students returned from collecting memories from an older person who was resolutely opposed to entering a residential home, because, it emerged, she remembered it as a former workhouse for the town, before 1930, and said 'I'm not one of those paupers'. Old values and memories die hard, long after the policies that created them. The past of the health and social care system lives on in people's memories and is reflected in current practices.

Activity II.1

Go to the public library and ask where to find records of the location of your nearest local workhouse.

When the workhouse system ended in 1930, many of these grim institutions from the Victorian era became old people's homes, 'Part III accommodation' under the Public Assistance Act 1948. It is still possible to encounter old people who remember the workhouse master and the board of guardians who ran the local workhouse until 1930.

In mental health, girls who became pregnant could be sent to an institution. I met a woman in a locked ward in Stanley Royd hospital in 1966 who was in her sixties and had lived there since she had become pregnant as an unmarried minor and sent away by her parents, labelled as a 'moral imbecile' (the definition of moral imbecility was incorporated into the Mental Deficiency Act 1913). She said she didn't want to leave the hospital because she'd lost contact with everybody outside and there was nobody to return to.

Activity II.2

Spend some time talking to older people, disabled people, children and young people about their experiences of being users of services and carers.

Activity II.3

Read what you can about the history of health and social care services, including Chapter 3 of this book. The task is to try to link your own experiences and those of other people with what you know of past and present policies and practice.

FURTHER READING

Adams, J., Bornat, J. and Prickett, M. (1998) 'Discovering the Present in Stories About the Past', in A. Brechin, J. Walmsley, J. Katz and S. Peace (eds) *Care Matters: Concepts, Practice and Research in Health and Social Care*, London, Sage, pp. 27–41

RESOURCE FILE: Life Experiences and Biographical Research, at the end of Chapter 35

WEBSITE: www.workhouses.org.uk

3 The Development of Health and Social Care

MALCOLM PAYNE

Health and Social Care: Early Development

All societies have arrangements for healthcare and social welfare, because good health and social relations are crucial to a satisfying human life and a successful economy. Health and social care in the UK have developed in tandem, often separately but linked. Change in the links and divisions between them is a historical influence on present services, which practitioners need to understand in order to make sense of the pattern of services in which they work.

Modern health and social care provision in the UK starts from the creation of the National Health Service (NHS) in 1948, bringing into force the National Health Service Act 1946. At the same time, the National Assistance Act and Children Act 1948 created local government social welfare services (Note: to avoid a common grammatical error, Children Act is correct because the Act is about children, Children's Act is not correct because the children do not own the Act). In this first section, I trace some of the forerunners to this major social change.

Since the 1600s, England had extensive provision, compared with other European countries, for the poor through its Poor Law (Kidd, 1999). Although this provided help for people afflicted by poverty, it also aimed to control poor people in order to prevent social disorder. The UK was mainly an agricultural country and people who could not find farm work in their home village travelled around finding casual jobs, for example at harvest time. Mechanisation of agriculture and industrialisation of the manufacture of goods brought people together in cities to find work, and this led to a disruption in traditional moral and social control, which was replaced by public services provided through local government. The close proximity of people in poor housing led to increasing problems of communicable diseases.

The economic policy of laissez faire associated with this Industrial Revolution meant that the Poor Law was reformed in 1834 so that people applying for help were to be supported in workhouses, which formed a substantial group of important institutions. People in them were separated from spouses and families and generally treated oppressively as 'less eligible' for care than people who worked, to ensure that they had an incentive to work. Workhouses began to develop as long-term care institutions and hospitals, since most poor people were elderly, sick and disabled. Workhouses developed alongside the charity hospitals already in existence, and all these institutions were merged into the NHS when it was formed, or provided the first old people's homes in the local authority welfare services.

The first successful health interventions were in public health, improving water quality, drainage and sewage, starting from the Public Health Act 1848, and associated with the reforming zeal of the civil servant Edwin Chadwick and pioneering doctors. Efforts were made to organise effective care for mentally ill people, and there was considerable investment in asylums to keep ordinary people safe from them, while also protecting them from exploitation. Jones (1993) argues that we can understand the development of these services as a continually changing balance between medical and legal responses to mental illness; incorporating a social treatment model as part of the ongoing debate. Prisons and industrial schools (for young offenders) also grew up to deal with increasing social problems. All these provisions, often starting from charitable action, increasingly came within the ambit of the state, as 'idealist' philosophy gained influence. This view proposes that the state should intervene in private lives to protect and help citizens, while laissez-faire policy argues that people should look after themselves and their families, helped by local communities rather than the state.

During the late 1800s, the Christian churches withdrew from providing welfare. Instead, welfare organisations with a Christian philosophy grew up, such as Dr Barnardo's, the children's charity, often reflecting an evangelical Christianity, which was more radical than the Established Church of England because it sought to convert working-class people from amoral lives towards a moral Christian life. This meant that welfare became secularised. As the influence of Christianity declined during the 1900s, most social charities became completely secular (Payne, 2005a) and formed an important voluntary sector of provision, offering alternatives, critiques and additions to public provision.

In Germany, a system of social insurance developed after it became a unified nation in 1870: this influenced other countries. It was taken up in important legislation in Britain and began to replace the Poor Law. The Liberal government from 1906 until the First World War in 1914 organised the first general system of retirement pensions and unemployment benefits (Thane, 1996, Ch. 4). Alongside German insurance, a women's movement developed social assistance to provide practical personal help for people in poverty and radical philosophers created 'social pedagogy', which emphasised self-improvement in community groups as a form of social work. Social assistance and social pedagogy have become linked to social work, but are distinct groupings of social work employees in many European countries (Lorenz, 1994).

The medical and nursing professions emerged during the 1800s, and social work grew up in the early 1900s. Medicine and surgery developed as scientific understanding of human biology developed throughout the 1800s. Nursing was strongly influenced by the experience of pioneers such as Florence Nightingale (Dossey, 2000) and Mary Seacole (Robinson, 2005) in the Crimean War in the mid-1850s.

Social work method developed through two important influences: 'charity organisation' and reform, so it always contains elements of social help and social change, which are sometimes in tension. The 'charity organisation movement' of the late 1800s tried to organise rich people's donations to the poor, to encourage the poor to provide for themselves rather than relying on charity. One aspect of charity organisation was to give alms only after an assessment of character. This encouraged friendly visiting to help families in their own homes and efficient recording of information about people applying for assistance and is one origin of social work. A welfare role in hospitals grew up, where 'almoners' were employed to check people's eligibility for the free healthcare provided from charity hospitals. This led eventually to medical social work.

Social conditions for poor people in urban areas led to reform movements to publicise scandals and rescue those affected. Children, truants from school and 'fallen women' were rescued from the streets; crime, drunkenness, immorality and poor family management were combated by the involvement of friendly visitors to people's homes or the supervision of offenders and drunks (Young and Ashton, 1956). This strengthened children's homes, schools promoting work and reform for delinquent youngsters and probation work. Both sources of method contained elements of social control: through assessment and classification of people's efforts at trying to solve their own problems, and through moral judgements about ways in which their own behaviour contributed to their social problems.

These ideas transferred to the Poor Law, as it became a health and welfare service for the poor, and in local education and probation services. They were placed under strain by the worldwide economic Depression of the early 1930s, so that, after the Second World War, there was political and social pressure for major improvements.

Health and Social Care in the Postwar Welfare State

After the Second World War, the Labour government elected in 1945 created a welfare state, whereby for the first time people had a reasonable degree of security in social provision. The state accepted the responsibility for universal social provision in health, housing, social security and education, with the implication that this was a right accorded to citizens, rather than a residual service for those who were unable for moral or practical reasons to manage their own lives.

The NHS was a centrepiece of the new welfare state, initially created in three elements (Jones, 2000, Ch. 10). Public health provision remained the responsibility of local authorities. Doctors, called general practitioners (GPs), became private contractors to the NHS, providing family healthcare and primary care, the first place people called on to receive health services. If GPs were unable to deal with the problem, patients were referred on to hospitals, which were separately administered. The asylums were incorporated, but remained largely separate until the Mental Health Act 1959 brought them fully into the system.

The Poor Law was broken up and welfare elements of it incorporated into local government social services, which employed social workers in:

- children's departments to 'board out' or foster children from the large children's homes left over from the Poor Law
- welfare departments for homeless, elderly and disabled people.

Increasingly, social workers used the social casework method developed in the USA (Payne, 2005a).

At first, it was assumed that health problems would decline with the welfare state and the NHS. However, improvements in medical care and rising standards of living always led to increasing demands on the service. Old institutions taken over from the Poor Law and charity hospitals were unsatisfactory for both medical and welfare care, and there was rising concern about the quality of long-term residential care provision (Jones and Fowles, 1984). Compared with acute care in the NHS, these were often called 'cinderella' services, because they were neglected by policy developments. During the 1960s, coordinated planning of NHS services began (Ministry of Health, 1962).

The 1950s saw the culmination of a movement away from residential and institutional care towards helping elderly people and people with mental illnesses and learning and physical disabilities in ordinary life in the community (community care). This was most influenced by an explicit community care policy in the mental health services, introduced by the Mental Health Acts of 1959 and 1983, and attempts to discharge long-stay patients from mental hospitals, which continued into the 1990s.

Organisational Change in the 1970s

During the Labour government of the 1960s, these movements came to a head. It was thought that local government and the NHS would become more efficient by being provided in larger units and combining local authority community health and hospital services. Demands for unification of the separate local government social work services came from the influence of the 'generic' social work technique of casework, and through a wish in the 1960s to coordinate provision for young

offenders through a comprehensive, preventive family service focused on deprivation rather than delinquency. There were a few experiments with combined public
health and social services departments in local government in the 1960s.

These movements led to the formation of social services departments (SSDs)
(social work departments in Scotland) in 1971, as a result of the implementation of
the recommendations of the Kilbrandon (1964) and Seebohm Reports (1968). These
large local government agencies brought together social workers from different
specialisms and had a general responsibility (in Scotland, by law) for improving
social wellbeing.

In 1974, a major reorganisation of local government and health services created a
more coordinated system, but still separated, administratively, legally and financially,
social services from healthcare. Hospital and local community health and public
health services were merged into one system, although GPs remained independent
contractors. For the first time, consumer representation in the health service was
possible via community health councils, elected from local voluntary organisations
and local government.

Policy Change in the 1980s

When a Conservative government was elected in 1979, further reorganisation
became constant in the NHS, with the aim of limiting public expenditure by introducing business management techniques into the health service to achieve greater
service and financial efficiency. Management of GPs was brought within the NHS
administration, maintaining their independent contractual status. Then, in the late
1980s, the Conservative view that the state should be an enabler of social provision
rather than a provider of unified services led to the introduction of a quasi-market
in the NHS by the NHS and Community Care Act 1990. This divided provision
between state 'commissioners', who planned and managed the service system, and
service providers in the private, voluntary or state sectors.

Provision of long-term care for adults developed in the unified SSDs. By the 1990s,
the closure of NHS long-stay hospitals for older people and people with learning
disabilities and mental illnesses had extended community care with local support
services and provision for former patients to live a more normal life outside hospitals. Changes in funding allowed a significant growth in private residential care
mainly for elderly people during the 1980s and 90s. Thus, the 1990 Act also introduced the 'purchaser–provider split' in a quasi-market similar to that of the NHS.
Local government commissioned or purchased services from a wide range of
providers. Care management, borrowed from the social work 'case management'
techniques with American origins, implemented this for individuals. Services for
disabled, elderly and other people in the community are designed as a 'package'
tailored to specific needs. There are criticisms that care management reduces the
professional role of social work, by emphasising efficient administration and financial control over social change and the personal wellbeing of service users.

Health and social care developed an important role in public and social protection, particularly as child abuse became a public issue in the 1970s and led to concerns about professional decisions by and coordination between doctors, healthcare workers and social workers. However, a radical or critical view of social work criticised UK social work's alignment with the protective and social policing functions of the state (Bailey and Brake, 1975), and this led to a decreasing confidence in their official role by social workers. Failures in public protection in childcare during the 1980s (DoH, 1991a) and mental health during the 1990s (Reith, 1998) led to public disquiet and a series of inquiries into professional and organisational failures.

This led to a swing towards, first, in the Children Act 1989, engaging parents and, second, earlier and more positive intervention during the 1990s. During the late 1990s, the idea of preventive work developed through family support, particularly in children's centres, where parents were supported to strengthen their childcare skills. Also during the 1990s, there was a significant development in service user and carer involvement in planning services, particularly where people were receiving services long term. This was associated with the development of advocacy and self-help services allied to a philosophy of empowerment (Adams, 2007). Another development of care management in this context was making direct payments to service users to buy their own care services, with the support of care managers, rather than having it all organised for them.

The Current Network of Services

These general trends continued with the election in 1997 of a Labour government committed to investment in modernised education and healthcare services. Its 'New Labour' policies sought to balance continued promotion of service effectiveness through encouraging service user choice between various providers, with a greater emphasis on social justice in resource allocation. Effectiveness was promoted by encouraging greater partnership between public, private and voluntary sector agencies and different professions and between service management, professionals and service users (DoH, 1998a, 1998b, 1998c). There has been a strong emphasis on coordination and joint working for people with long-term needs, especially older people (Glasby and Littlechild, 2004). Single assessment processes have been developed for adults. The NHS Plan (DoH, 2000e) and the White Paper on community healthcare (DoH, 2006a) both emphasise co-location of health and social care in ways that are more accessible to service users, in local clinics and GP surgeries.

The Children Act 2004 lays a 'duty to cooperate' on many public bodies, requires local authorities to take the lead in creating an agreed 'children and young persons plan', to establish representative 'safeguarding children' panels and to take part in establishing a common assessment framework (DfES, 2004b). However, private sector innovations continued, with the introduction in the NHS from 2006 of 'payment by results', where finance followed success in providing good quality services to patients.

The priority given to education and healthcare led to the division of social services departments into family and children's services within education departments of local authorities and encouragement of structures for joint cooperation between adult social services provision and healthcare agencies. However, the social work profession was finally recognised in the Care Standards Act 2000 with the establishment of regulatory councils. Regulation of social care workers started with the registration of social workers, in England from 2004, and 'protection' of the title 'social worker' in 2005, so that it may not be used by anyone other than registered social workers.

A strong emphasis on responding to inequalities in health provision between poor and rich communities led to a stronger emphasis on health promotion and development. Following the Black Report (1980), neglected by the Conservative governments of the 1980s and early 1990s, the Acheson Report (1998) on health inequalities led to a substantial programme of change to achieve health promotion targets (Exworthy et al., 2003) and further work for the Treasury on a wide range of health promotion activities, acknowledging the interaction of health inequalities and poverty (Wanless Report, 2004).

Conclusion

Health and social care have developed alongside each other, connected and yet separate. Their development has been part of a wider public concern for responding to poverty, which has stretched from the public health pioneers and the Poor Law to the present concern for health inequalities and health promotion. Social care has also been inextricably linked with education, in its concern for children and adult personal development, and with social housing provision in its concern for healthy living. The twentieth century saw a progression of attempts to connect health and social care with concern for people in their own communities and the twenty-first sees a greater concern for service user and carer involvement in decisions that affect them and in planning and managing services. Complex service organisations and professions have developed, each with their own focus within a complex field of biological, psychological, social and spiritual knowledge. All this is an attempt to respond to the complexity and importance of human needs for health and social care.

REVIEW QUESTIONS

1   In what ways do health and social services share common origins?

2   Why do you think the legislation that, in effect, founded the NHS is important now?

3   What policy features do health and social care share and what is distinctive about each?

FURTHER READING

Busfield, J. (2000) *Health and Health Care in Modern Britain*, Oxford, Oxford University Press
   A good introduction to a range of issues about health and the healthcare services in the UK.

Jones, K. (2000) *The Making of Social Policy in Britain: From the Poor Law to New Labour*, London, Athlone
   A broad account of the history of social welfare and health in the context of a wider summary of the development of related services. It has a good balance between different services, but is strong on health and social care.

Payne, M. (2005) *The Origins of Social Work: Continuity and Change*, Basingstoke, Palgrave Macmillan
   A summary of the history of social work and social care and of issues about their role in current services.

RESOURCE FILE: Linking the Past and Present of Health and Social Care, in Part II Introduction
   You may like to use this to help you to connect some of the historical context referred to in this chapter with your experiences and those of the people with whom you work.

Resource file

Key healthcare policy changes in the twenty-first century

We introduce below five major areas of policy change and debate.

Primary Care Trusts

In the 1990s, health authorities were abolished and their commissioning functions transferred to Primary Care Trusts (PCTs). PCTs are free-standing statutory bodies in the NHS, designed to be responsible for delivering integrated healthcare services at a local level, alongside an enhanced community pharmacy service (DoH, Scottish Office, Welsh Office, 1996; NHS Executive, 1999). The PCTs carry out many tasks formerly carried out by health authorities, including commissioning (secondary care) health services, investing in primary and community care and developing health promotion and ill-health prevention programmes to improve the health of local people.

Questions about whether private funding should exist in the NHS

There continues to be active debate between those wanting to retain an NHS purely funded from public funds and supporters of the government's private finance initiatives (PFIs), which were launched to raise funding from the private sector in order to undertake large projects, such as building new hospitals. At the same time, the government has introduced treatment centres run by independent bodies to carry out thousands of routine cataract, hip and knee operations for the NHS. The controversy is whether these will make the NHS more efficient, or will simply 'cherry-pick' the most lucrative, high-volume, less complex work, destabilising the NHS in the process.

Management: questions about whether it is fit for purpose

The McKinsey Report on fitness for purpose of the management structure in the Department of Health was carried out in the winter of 2005–6. Although McKinsey's findings were not published in a report, perhaps as a consequence, changes in management were made, including cutting the 28 strategic health authorities (SHAs) by almost two-thirds and reducing the number of PCTs by half and bringing their boundaries more into harmony with local authority adult care services.

Performance: measures attempting to improve quality of services

The performance of NHS Trusts was assessed by the Healthcare Commission using a system of 'star ratings' until April 2005, when it was replaced under section 46 of the Health and Social Care (Community Health and Standards) Act 2003, following *Standards for Better Healthcare* (DoH, 2004a), which set out 24 minimum standards for the quality of care in all healthcare organisations and provided a framework for continuous improvement. This fits into a broader government agenda to improve public services. The local government White Paper (Department for Communities and Local Government, 2006, p. 18) sets out to provide a single performance framework for all the work done by local authorities and health services, in about 200 national indicators covering public health, health protection, disease prevention, mental health and all aspects of social care.

Measures to improve citizen participation in healthcare performance

There are policy moves towards strengthening section 11 of the Health and Social Care Act 2001, thereby increasing opportunities for people to be informed about the performance of their health services and contribute to decisions about policies and staff pay (Department for Communities and Local Government, 2006, p. 16). Since 2001 there has been rapid shift from the creation and implementation of patient and public involvement structures to LINKs (see also Patient and Public Involvement Team, 2006).

Many of the above areas of debate and change are reflected in the 2006 White Paper *Our Health, Our Care, Our Say* (DoH, 2006a). The White Paper sets out a strategy for delivering:

- greater emphasis on prevention and less on illness
- shifting spending from large hospitals to smaller community hospitals and other units such as more walk-in centres, closer to local communities
- improved NHS and local authorities working together to provide better joined-up and integrated health and social care services
- democratised services with improved service user, carer and patient choice and say.

Among the detailed changes are the following, many planned by 2008:

- a new NHS 'life check' assessing lifestyle risks, actions to take and referrals where necessary
- the guarantee of registration at local GP practice
- supporting self-care with increased investment in the 'expert patient programme'
- an 'information prescription' which enables people to take better long-term care of themselves
- a 'personal health and social care plan' contributing to a person's integrated health and social care record
- improved support, including respite arrangements, for carers
- extended direct payments and piloting individual budgets for social care.

The White Paper is an attempt to promote partnerships between NHS bodies and local government departments such as those responsible for adult care and children's services, to achieve what the government calls 'joined-up' thinking and practice. (See Resource File: Health Promotion (3) Understanding Health, at the end of Chapter 38.)

FURTHER READING

Department for Communities and Local Government (2006) *Strong and Prosperous Communities: The Local Government White Paper*, Vol. II, Cm 6939-II, London, TSO, www.communities.gov.uk

DoH (2004) *Standards for Better Healthcare*, London, DoH

DoH (2006) *Our Health, Our Care, Our Say: A New Direction for Community Services*, White Paper, Cm 6737, London, TSO

DoH, Scottish Office, Welsh Office (1996) *Choice and Opportunity: Primary Care: The Future*, London, TSO

Health and Social Care Act 2001

Health and Social Care (Community Health and Standards) Act 2003

NHS Executive (1999) *Primary Care Trusts: Establishing Better Services*, London, NHS Executive

Resource file

Key social care policy proposals in the twenty-first century

In 2005 the government published a strategy for the next 10–15 years, resources to be met from existing funds (DoH, 2005). The aim is for the NHS (providing health) and local authorities (providing social care) to work together to enable people to maintain their independence. This will be achieved by giving people increased choice and control over how their needs are met. Carers' needs and roles will be valued, with wider resources from the local voluntary and community sector feeding into care packages.

People will be enabled to take more control of their own lives. This will be achieved partly by striking the right balance between protecting people and enabling them to manage their own risks and partly by extending direct payments and introducing individual budgets for social care for people with a disability, assessed as needing social care support.

The single assessment process, care programme approach and person-centred planning could be extended to provide single assessments for people with complex needs.

Other important policy initiatives include the publication of statements of minimum standards for services, such as for older people (DoH, 2001a) and also the White Paper on the future of services for people with learning disabilities (DoH, 2001b).

FURTHER READING

DoH (2001) *National Service Framework for Older People*, London, DoH

DoH (2001) *Valuing People: A New Strategy for Learning Disabilities in the 21st Century*, White Paper, Cm 5068, London, HMSO

DoH (2005) *Independence, Well-being and Choice: Our Vision for the Future of Social Care for Adults in England*, White Paper, Cm 6499, London, TSO

Resource file

Key childcare policy changes in the twenty-first century

All major policy initiatives are linked with the report and follow-up reports under the heading of *Every Child Matters* (DfES, 2004a, 2004b). The Green Paper (DfES, 1998) on childcare, produced six years previously, is also significant, as is the 10-year strategy for childcare (HM Treasury, DfES, DTI, DWP, 2004).

This strategy initiated Sure Start for children and families needing additional support and resources and was updated in 2004. The aim of the strategy was to make sure that affordable, good quality childcare was delivered to children aged 0–14 in every neighbourhood.

There were three elements in the strategy – quality, affordability and availability:

Improving the *quality* of childcare:

- Introducing Early Excellence Centres in at least 25 places offering models of good childcare
- Introducing new standards for early education and childcare
- Creating new qualifications and training for childcare workers
- Daycare settings to be led by trained professionals
- Improving support for parents and informal carers
- Reforming regulation and inspection.

Making childcare more *affordable*:

- Introducing a new child tax credit, part of the new working families tax credit
- Introducing help with childcare costs, including more free places
- Extending paid maternity leave for mothers and fathers.

Increasing the *availability* of childcare:

- Out of school childcare for all children aged 3–14 by 2010
- Increasing the number of childcare places the local authority has a duty to provide
- Improving information about available childcare and support.

FURTHER READING

Brannen, J. (2003) 'Some Thoughts on Rethinking Children's Care', in J. Brannen and P. Moss (eds) *Rethinking Children's Care*, Buckingham, Open University Press

DfES (1998) *Meeting the Childcare Challenge: A Framework and Consultation Document*, Green Paper, Cm 3959, London, TSO

DfES (2004) *Every Child Matters: Next Steps*, London, DfES

DfES (2004) *Every Child Matters: Change for Children in Social Care*, London, DfES

Hayden, C., Goddard, J., Gorin, S. and Van Der Spek, N. (1999) *State Child Care: Looking after Children?* London, Jessica Kingsley

HM Treasury (2003) *Every Child Matters*, Green Paper, Cm 5860, London, TSO

HM Treasury, DfES, DTI, DWP (2004) *Choice for Parents, the Best Start for Children: a 10-year Strategy for Childcare*, London, TSO

Resource file

Demographic changes

- In 2001, the census showed 4.4 million people over 75 in the UK, of which 2.8 million were women over 75 and 1.6 million were men, almost half that number.[2]
- Between 2003 and 2031, the population of the UK is anticipated to increase from 59.6 million to 65.7 million, most of this growth being in England.[1]
- By 2031, 23 per cent of this population are likely to be aged 65 and over.[1]
- Currently, 10.5 million people are aged 50–65, 8 million are aged 65–84 and 1 million are 85 plus – a total of nearly 20 million. By 2051, the figures will be 12.1 million aged 50–64, 13 million aged 65–84 and 4 million aged 85 or over.[1]

Factors contributing to these changes include:[1]

- Decreasing mortality rates
- Decreasing birth rates
- Large numbers of people born during the 'baby boom' years of the 1950s and 1960s reaching retirement age
- An expected 3.6 million younger adults migrating.

As regards this ageing population:

- The highest life expectancies are in the southeast of England and the lowest in the northwest and west of England and in Scotland.[2]
- 1 in 5 men aged 65–84 live alone and 2 in 5 women.[2]
- 400,000 older people live in residential homes.[3]

Higher life expectancies will have the advantage of enabling more families to have two generations living and more older partners to care for each other. Against this, however, younger people may be less willing or able, because of work and other family commitments, to care informally for older relatives.[4]

At the beginning of the twentieth century, retirement was almost unknown, but at the end it was common.

Between 1900 and 2000, the typical working life shrank from 14 to late sixties – around 50 years – to around 40 years.[4]

Lower fertility and mortality rates over the last decades of the twentieth century have been linked with a reduction in the size of the typical household and more people living alone. The general rise in people living alone does not mean families are less important. People have more ways of keeping in touch, by phone and the internet (email) and travel by car and public transport is common.[4]

Foreign born people in the population doubled between 1951 and 2001 and the numbers of people in British minority ethnic groups increased. Family patterns are different. For instance, less older Asian women live alone.[4]

FURTHER READING

1 Government Actuary's Department (GAD) (2003) *Principal Projections* referred to in http://www.dwp.gov.uk/opportunity_age/section_one.asp accessed 25.06.06

2 www.cloreduffield.org.uk/word/older%20people%20literature%20review_31%july_o6.doc

3 Office of Fair Trading (2005) *Care Homes for Older People in the UK*, London, OFT

4 'Population Trends' *National Statistics* (Autumn, 2006) p. 100 www.statistics.gov.uk/downloads/theme_population/PT125_main_part3.pdf

4 Sociological Contexts for Practice

NEIL THOMPSON

By the end of this chapter, you should:

■ HAVE a basic understanding of what we mean by 'sociological perspectives'

■ UNDERSTAND the relevance of discrimination to health and social care

■ GRASP what is meant by domestic violence and abuse.

This chapter explores the importance of sociological contexts for practice. It provides a brief outline of sociological perspectives on health and social care, with particular regard to social divisions (how society is divided into particular sectors), discrimination (how some groups are treated less favourably than others), oppression (the detrimental and dehumanising effects of discrimination) and abusive and violent relationships (the ways in which some people can mistreat others). These are all significant issues in health and social care, and it is important to pay attention to them. This chapter therefore offers an overview of how some key sociological issues have a bearing on health and social care practices and thus provides a foundation for further study and understanding.

Why Sociological Perspectives?

Sociology is the study of society, and is therefore concerned with such important questions as:

1. What is social cohesion based on?
2. How do social conflicts arise?
3. How does social change take place?

4. What influence do social factors have on individuals and families?

It is the fourth question that is of particular interest to us in this chapter. This is because social factors can be seen to play a major role in shaping the life experience of people in receipt of health and social care services, especially in relation to discrimination, oppression, abuse and violence, as we shall see below.

Some people see sociology as a broad subject related to society at large and therefore assume that it has little or nothing to do with the experiences of specific individuals and families. However, this is a misunderstanding and oversimplification of what sociology is all about. Sociology does indeed concern itself with wider social patterns, but these are not unconnected with the life experiences of individuals. Indeed, how each of us experiences the world will depend to a great extent on social factors. For example, each of us is influenced by 'social divisions', the different social categories (such as class, race/ethnicity, gender, age, sexuality and so on) that make such a difference to the opportunities (or 'life chances') we have, the access to power available to us and so on. Consider, for example, the difference between a rich white man and a poor black woman in terms of the life chances available to each of them. What this means is that life is not a level playing field – some people have advantages bestowed upon them because of their social position (that is, where they fit in to the complex web of social divisions), while others face disadvantage for the same reasons.

If we are to develop an adequate understanding of the perspective of the people we are trying to help, we need to have at least a basic understanding of their social background and the implications of this for how they are likely to experience their health and social care needs. This is an important part of working in partnership (Carnwell and Buchanan, 2004).

Social divisions are not the only way in which society influences individuals. For example, culture is important in shaping the assumptions we make about people and life more broadly, the language we use and the 'unwritten rules' we follow. The culture (or cultures) we belong to play an important role in constructing our identity – our sense of who we are. In fact, if we think about it carefully, we can identify many ways in which social issues have a significant bearing on individual experience. Again, this is an important part of seeing the situation from the point of view of patients or service users as a foundation for partnership working.

Adopting a sociological perspective should not be seen as a matter of rejecting or neglecting personal or psychological issues. Rather, it is a case of trying to broaden and deepen our understanding of these important issues by developing a fuller appreciation of the *sociological* factors that are also a central part of the situations we encounter.

Tackling Discrimination

What is Discrimination?

Literally, to discriminate means to identify a difference and, as such, is not necessarily a problem. In fact, it can be a helpful thing to do and certainly something we need to be able to do as part of our general life skills. However, in its legal or moral sense, it is used to mean discrimination *against* an individual, group or category of people. That is, it refers to the process of identifying a difference (for example a gender difference) and treating people unfairly because of that difference (for example excluding women from certain activities or making unfair assumptions about them: 'Women are not decisive enough to be good managers').

Very often the consequence of discrimination is oppression, that is, certain people will be treated in a degrading or inhuman way as a result of the process of being discriminated against. In other words, discrimination is not only unfair and thus morally objectionable, it can also be oppressive and have a detrimental effect on people's health and wellbeing. It is therefore a serious issue (or set of issues) worthy of close attention.

Why Discrimination is Important in Health and Social Care

There are two main ways in which discrimination is significant in health and social care. First, there is the question of understanding the people we are trying to help. We need to have an understanding of how discrimination may play a part in their lives, for example how an older person may have experienced age discrimination (see S. Thompson, 2005) or a disabled person may have been subject to disability-related discrimination or 'disablism' (Oliver and Sapey, 2006). An assessment of an individual's health and social care needs will need to take account of such sociological factors as racism, sexism and disablism and how these may have contributed to the current circumstances and/or may have a bearing on what needs to be done.

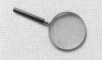

Practice study

Margaret

Margaret was very surprised to learn that a complaint had been made against her. In working with the Patel family, she had tried hard to treat them the same as she would have treated any other family, white or black. She was therefore puzzled when she found out that the family had expressed concerns that she was not taking account of their cultural background and needs. She discussed the situation with her line manager, who tried to explain to her that 'treating everybody the same' was not a good strategy when it comes to promoting equality. He explained to her that it was important to look at how issues like race and culture had to be taken into consideration and not glossed over. Following an extensive discussion, she began to realise how naive she had been in trying to treat everybody the same.

Second, there is the question of how we make sure that our own actions (or inactions) do not contribute to discrimination and oppression. For example, we must make sure that we do not rely on discriminatory stereotypes (that older people are hard of hearing or that disabled people are not capable of making decisions for themselves, perhaps). Wherever possible, we should be doing all we reasonably can to prevent discrimination arising and challenge it when it does arise (see below).

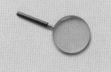

Tim

Tim was anxious about attending the equality and diversity course, as he was concerned that it would be 'a lot of political correctness nonsense'. However, it turned out to be quite different. He came away from the course with a much better understanding of discrimination and how it is rooted in the way society works rather than just in the minds of certain bigoted individuals. The course helped him to realise that he needed to develop a broader, more sociological perspective on these matters. He recognised that he had been thinking in narrow, individualistic terms and had failed to see the big picture. He came to realise that there were many ways in which he could play a part in preventing or tackling discrimination, but that this would involve thinking more broadly about the social context of people's lives.

How we can Prevent or Challenge Discrimination

A key part of preventing or challenging discrimination is awareness. This is because discrimination is not simply a matter of personal prejudice on the part of some people. The reality is more complicated than this, insofar as discrimination can also be 'institutionalised', that is, it can be built into systems and structures and can also be part of cultural patterns and assumptions (see the discussion of PCS – personal, cultural and structural – analysis in Thompson, 2006). Discrimination is a sociological matter as well as a psychological one.

Given that discrimination is not simply the result of prejudice, we need to recognise that discrimination can arise even where no one is intending to discriminate, that is, it can be unintentional (see Practice study on George, below). We must therefore accept that our concern should be with outcomes, not simply intentions. We cannot rely on such notions as: 'I'm not prejudiced, so discrimination is not an issue for me.' People with no specific prejudices could nonetheless be involved in discriminating against certain others as a result of the wider social processes involved.

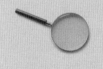

George

In a seminar on anti-racism, George made the point that, in his service, they dealt with people from such a wide range of ethnic backgrounds that they could not hope to address everyone's cultural needs. 'It's not racism', he said, 'it's just the way it is.' The seminar leader gently challenged this point by saying that, if people from ethnic minorities do not have their needs met to the same level as white people, then that amounts to racism. She went on to say: 'I can accept that it is not *deliberate* or *personal* racism, but if the lack of resources produces an unfair outcome for black people, then the result is racial discrimination – indeed, this is a good example of what is meant by institutional racism.' This gave George much food for thought and made him aware that there was a lot more to issues of discrimination than he had previously realised.

Violence and Abuse

It is unfortunately the case that violence and abuse feature in our society far more than we would like them to. While family values are actively promoted and the family is seen as a source of love, help and protection, it also has to be recognised that families can be the location of:

- *Domestic violence:* A large number of women are subject to violence from their partners, and many men also experience such problems. This is in large part a reflection of the significance of gender differentiation, that is, men and women are brought up (or 'socialised', to use the technical term) to adopt gender-specific roles. Part of this process is an emphasis on men seeking positions of power and dominance, while women are encouraged to focus on nurturing others.
- *Child abuse:* Physical, sexual and emotional abuse as well as neglect are sadly far more prevalent than the general public usually realise. These are deeply ingrained problems in our society. Although there are important psychological issues here, we should also note the sociological dimension, for example in terms of social expectations about the role of children in society and how they are to be treated.
- *Abuse of vulnerable adults:* Older people and people with learning disabilities can be particularly vulnerable to abuse. It is only fairly recently that we have started to appreciate the extent and seriousness of these problems. Again, there are significant sociological issues here in terms of power relations and how they can be abused (see Chapter 9).

How we can Prevent Violence and Abuse

There are long-established child protection procedures for responding to child abuse concerns (see Chapter 10) and more recently we have seen the establishment of 'POVA' procedures – Protection of Vulnerable Adults. It is therefore important that you should be aware of your responsibilities under these procedures. If you have not been informed of your responsibilities, you are strongly advised to seek advice from a senior colleague about this.

Responding to domestic violence has yet to be formalised in this way. However, even formalised procedures do not guarantee that people will be protected from harm, although they are likely to reduce the risks of harm occurring (see Chapter 11). A key issue is being aware of the possibilities and not adopting a complacent attitude that assumes that such problems are unlikely to be occurring. There are many cases on record of abuse persisting over time because people who were suspicious did not report their concerns as a result of rather naively assuming that 'Things like that wouldn't happen round here.'

What we should do if Violence or Abuse has taken Place

In the case of abuse, the appropriate procedures should make it clear what steps need to be taken (hence the need for you to be aware of the procedures, as indicated above). A central theme of those procedures will be the need to report any concerns to the appropriate authorities. The same can be said to apply in relation to domestic violence. It is important to get the balance right between the two unhelpful extremes of sweeping the matter under the carpet by not reporting our concerns and overstepping our duties by getting overinvolved – such complex matters have to be handled sensitively and carefully on a multidisciplinary basis.

Practice study

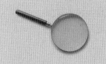

Suhita

Suhita had been working with Lisa, aged 12, for some months and was getting on very well with her. However, she was surprised when Lisa suddenly became quite withdrawn and out of sorts, quite unlike her former self. Suhita was puzzled by this and tried to talk to Lisa about it. However, the more she tried, the more withdrawn Lisa became. She reported the matter to her line manager who asked her to consider the possibility that Lisa might have been abused. Suhita was quite taken aback by this at first, but the more closely she looked at the situation, the more she realised that Lisa was showing signs of having been sexually abused. Suhita was quite disgusted by this and found it hard to accept that anyone could treat a child in this way. Fortunately, though, her line manager gave her a lot of support in helping her come to terms with the fact that violence and abuse are part of our society, whether we like it or not. This was a hard lesson for Suhita to learn but nonetheless an important one.

Conclusion

There is a long-standing tradition in health and social care of paying close attention to individual matters. While this is not a problem in itself, it needs to be balanced by an emphasis on the social context of practice. That is, while everyone we seek to help is indeed a unique individual in their own right, they are also individuals *in a social context*. To do justice to the complexities of our work, we need to make sure that we have at least a basic understanding of both the specific individual whose needs we are trying to meet and the wider social context which has such an important bearing on how each individual experiences his or her life.

These important social influences include:

- *Social divisions:* Each of us belongs to different 'sectors' of society, such as class, race or ethnicity, gender and so on. This shapes how we experience the world and how other people relate to us; for example a person's gender is a key factor in how people relate to him or her. Consider your own gender identity: how significant is this in terms of how people relate to you? How different would it be if your gender identity were to change?
- *Discrimination:* It is commonly the case that people can be treated unfairly on the basis of one or more social differences (the 'social divisions' mentioned above). Such discrimination can arise from personal prejudice, but it is just as likely (if

not more so) to arise because of wider sociological factors, such as cultural assumptions and stereotypes and structural patterns of inequality.

■ *Violence and abuse:* These arise in large part as a result of the abuse of power, which in turn can be seen as a reflection of patterns of social relationships. They are not simply psychological matters, as there are important sociological dimensions that also play a part.

As mentioned earlier, adopting a sociological approach is not a matter of rejecting or neglecting personal or psychological issues, but rather trying to broaden and deepen our understanding of such issues by developing a fuller appreciation of the *sociological* factors that are also a key part of the equation.

REVIEW QUESTIONS

1 How do social divisions (such as class, race, gender, age, disability, sexual orientation or religion) have an impact on your work?

2 In what ways might the people you are trying to help be discriminated against?

3 How might you learn more about how to prevent and tackle discrimination?

4 What are your responsibilities in relation to domestic violence or other forms of abuse? What dangers are involved in failing to consider the sociological dimensions of health and social care?

FURTHER READING

Corby, B. (2000) *Child Protection: Towards a Knowledge Base* (2nd edn) Maidenhead, Open University Press
Deals with child abuse issues.

Giddens, A. (2006) *Sociology* (5th edn) Cambridge, Polity Press
Of several good general introductions to sociology, I particularly like this one.

Martin, J. (2007) *Safeguarding Adults*, Lyme Regis, Russell House
Addresses the protection of vulnerable adults.

Mullender, A. and Hague, G. (2003) *Is Anyone Listening?: Putting the Views of Survivors of Domestic Violence into Policy and Practice*, London, Routledge
A helpful text on domestic violence.

Thompson, N. (2006) *Anti-Discriminatory Practice* (4th edn) Basingstoke, Palgrave Macmillan
A clear and helpful introduction relating to tackling discrimination and oppression.

Resource file

Equality and non-discriminatory practice

Inequalities in health

In 1980, the DHSS published a major report by Sir Douglas Black, which traced the deeply entrenched patterns of inequalities in health provision and the health of people across Britain (Black, 1980). It high-lighted the fact that better off people enjoyed longer lives and a healthier lifestyle, and there are pronounced differences in the quality of key health services such as maternity and postnatal care between different parts of Britain (Whitehead, 1992). Twenty years later, Sir Donald Acheson's review for the government of these inequalities in health found many still persist, often based on how poor people are, the quality of their housing and their access to services (Acheson, 1998).

Anti-discriminatory practice

Anti-discriminatory practice attempts to overcome discrimination on any basis. Equality-based practice includes rights-based approaches, such as human rights (Human Rights Act 1998) and children's rights (Children Act 1989). These rely on laws to achieve justice and eliminate unfair and unequal treatment of people. Bullying and harassment policies must cover age, to comply with age discrimination legislation.

Summary of relevant legislation

▪ Equal Pay Act 1970
Provides people of either sex equal contractual benefits in the same work.

▪ Sex Discrimination Act 1975
Forbids discrimination on the grounds of sex or marriage; but it isn't unlawful to discriminate against a person because he or she is not married.

▪ Race Relations Act 1976
Forbids distinction on the grounds of race, colour, ethnic origin or nationality and citizenship. The Race Relations (Amendment) Act 2000 extended the law to include public functions and requires public authorities to promote race equality.

▪ Disability Discrimination Act 1995
Forbids discrimination against disabled people.

▪ Employment Equality (Sexual Orientation) Regulations 2003
Protect people in work and training from direct and indirect discrimination, harassment or victimisation, in respect of their sexual orientation.

▪ Employment Equality (Religion or Belief) Regulations 2003
Protect people from direct or indirect discrimination, harassment or victimisation, in respect of their religion or beliefs.

▪ Human Rights Act 1998
Protects no less than 16 aspects of people's rights – from the right to live a life free from torture to the right not to be discriminated against – making it possible for their cases to be dealt with in courts in the UK.

▪ Equality Act 2006
Dissolved the Equal Opportunities Commission (EOC), the Commission for Racial Equality (CRE) and the Disability Rights Commission (DRC) and in their place set up the Commission for Equality and Human Rights (CEHR). From autumn 2007, the CEHR has the goal of eliminating prejudice on the grounds of age, disability, gender, race, sexual orientation, religion or beliefs. It is the central point for advice and guidance on all equality and human rights issues in Britain.

FURTHER READING

Acheson, Sir Donald (1998) *Independent Inquiry into Inequalities in Health*, London, TSO

Black, Sir Douglas (1980) *Inequalities in Health*, London, DHSS

Butler, F. (2006) *Rights for Real: Older People, Human Rights and the CEHR*, London, Age Concern, www.ageconcern.org.uk

Doyal, L. (ed.) (1998) *Women and Health Services: An Agenda for Change*, Buckingham, Open University Press

Millam, R. (2002) *Anti-discriminatory Practice: A Guide for Workers in Child Care and Education*, London, Continuum

Thompson, N. (2003) *Promoting Equality: Challenging Discrimination and Oppression* (2nd edn) Basingstoke, Palgrave Macmillan

Whitehead, M. (1992) *Inequalities in Health: The Black Report and the Health Divide*, Harmondsworth, Penguin

5 The Context of Values for Health and Social Care

BERNARD MOSS

Introducing Values

Picture the scene. You are driving home on a dark, wet night and on a country lane your car breaks down. Fortunately you have your mobile phone with you and have soon contacted a rescue service. They promise to be with you in 15 minutes.

Scenario 1

It is 25 minutes later and there is no sight of the rescue service. You are about to ring again when the van roars into view. The mechanic has obviously had a bad day. He emerges with a scowl on his face, curtly asks what is wrong and delves under the bonnet to mess around. From time to time he orders you brusquely to 'turn her over', and eventually your car bursts back into life. He slams the bonnet lid down, thrusts a document under your nose to sign, and without further ado speeds off. You drive home safely.

Scenario 2

You have been waiting for 15 minutes with still no sign of the rescue service. Suddenly your mobile rings and you are informed that the van should be with you a little later than they had hoped, due to a more complicated repair on the previous call-out. Ten minutes later the van arrives, the mechanic introduces himself to you by name, apologises for the delay and explains why this has happened. He asks if you are all right, and says that it can be frightening to be all alone in a dark lane. He asks you to explain the problem and then gets under the bonnet to fiddle around. From time to time, he asks you 'to start the engine up for me, please', and eventually the engine starts up. He grins and says something about the distributor which you don't fully understand, so he explains it in simple terms while asking you to sign the documentation. He then offers to follow you until you reach the main road to check that all is well, which he does. You drive home safely.

These two scenarios are not intended to be customer training materials for roadside rescue teams, although they could easily serve that purpose. Rather, they are intended to illustrate how values can affect practice. It will be argued in this chapter that in all types of people-work, the value base is all-important, and plays a major part in how services are both delivered and received. Best practice will always strive to ensure that the values underpinning the service being offered are kept centre stage in the worker's own approach to what needs to be done.

Let's return to the anxious scene at the roadside. What is at issue here is not whether the mechanic diagnosed the fault correctly and put it right, thereby enabling you to get home safely, as in both scenarios this was achieved without difficulty. The issue is *how* the mechanic treated you and behaved towards you. Ultimately, this is an example not just of customer care, but of how certain values affected how you were treated. In the first scenario, the values of the mechanic were centred on him, how he was feeling (stressed, too much being asked of him, resentful perhaps, problems outside work 'getting to him') and how soon he could do the job and get home. This made you feel that you were an inconvenience, and certainly not a valued customer without whom the mechanic's wages would not be paid.

By contrast, in the second scenario, you were put centre stage, the mechanic took your feelings and needs into account so that you were treated respectfully. You received an explanation for the delay, you were involved in the process and great care was taken to ensure that the problem did not recur.

In both scenarios your repair was successful and you got home safely. But in all other aspects, the experiences were as different as chalk and cheese. The mechanic whose actions put you (how you were feeling and what you needed) at the centre of his concerns was working from a value base which stressed the importance of the individual as a valued customer, for whom satisfaction with how you were treated was as important as completing the repair efficiently.

In both scenarios you would have felt relieved that the car was now repaired and that you got home safely, but in terms of how you felt you had been treated, you will have had two very contrasting experiences.

People-work Values

We have started with this common, everyday example because in people-work generally it is often felt by those who are beginning their training, or contemplating going into some aspect of people-work (or the helping professions as they are sometimes called), that this whole topic of values is difficult to understand. Nor do they always realise the importance of values to the work they will be doing. If you put yourself in the shoes of someone who has come, let's say, to the nurse, dietician, chiropodist or counsellor at the local health centre for help, how you are treated by that person will be every bit as important as the quality of the information they may give you. The same holds true even if you directly are not receiving these services. If it were one of your parents, a relative or one of your children, you would want them to receive just as much appropriate attention from the professional worker as you would for yourself. Or, to return to our roadside analogy, you would want them to experience scenario two, and feel valued as individuals and treated with dignity and respect.

Already we have begun to draw out what some of the core values of people-work are: treating people with dignity and respect are two of them. As our discussion develops we will uncover more, but for the moment we need to draw a distinction between our individual personal values and the values which our employing organisation holds. If this distinction is not immediately clear to you, let us return for a final time to our mechanic at the roadside. We would hope that that organisation had a value base which insisted that each mechanic treated people in the way we described for scenario two. This would mean that, whatever the mechanic himself felt, he would be bound by the values of his organisation to treat people (the customers) accordingly. Scenario one illustrated what happens when an individual bases his or her behaviour on a set of individual values which may (or, of course, may not) be at odds with those of the organisation.

Let us give an example of how this might happen in people-work. An individual worker may feel (for whatever reason) that gay relationships are wrong, or even sinful. That will be bound to influence how they treat gay people who come to them for help, unless they have carefully scrutinised themselves to ensure that they work strictly within the code of conduct of their agency, which will insist that everyone receives a fair service, irrespective of issues such as sexual orientation. For this worker, then, his or her individual value base will be challenged by the value base of the organisation, and unless they can operate honestly within this framework, they should not be employed there.

Where our Values Come From

Our individual value base will have been derived from a number of sources, and if we are honest, we may not be fully aware of them until we are challenged in some way (as in the example just cited of gay relationships). This has led Woodbridge and Fulwood (2004) to talk about the 'squeaky wheel' principle. Normally a bicycle runs smoothly without sound; only when a squeaky wheel attracts our attention do we wonder what the problem is, and think about applying some oil. So too with values; sometimes, these authors argue, 'we notice values only when they cause problems, e.g. when they conflict' (p. 26). Most of the time we take our values for granted; only when we are brought up with a jolt by something or someone which challenges our values do we pause to think about them.

The most common indirect sources of our values will be: our parents; the groups, political party or communities to which we belong, especially if we are actively involved in some way; various cultural influences; and finally religious traditions, whether or not we actively belong to a faith community. We may subscribe to the value put forward in the classic text on the nursing process by Yura and Walsh (1988, p. 96) that 'the family is the primary unit for human need fulfillment of the person'. However, this is a particular view of the centrality of the family in meeting people's needs, which is not shared equally and universally in all cultures and countries. Simply by meeting and interacting with different cultural and ethnic groups we will find our values and opinions have been influenced by them. Two writers have expressed this very clearly. Cree (1995, cited in Beckett and Maynard, 2005, p. 50) observes that:

> Social work values and practice are rooted in traditions which derived from Christian, or Judaeo-Christian discourse. Although expressed today in language which has deliberately forgone its Christian tone, social work is built on assumptions about individual subjectivity, community and service to others which have a strong continuing presence in Christian discourse.

To this we must also now add a Muslim perspective, which although still numerically a minority, is having an increasingly powerful impact on the values debate in the UK and throughout the world.

The second quotation is from Patel et al. (1998) who remind us of the multicultural, multifaith context of people-work, and talk about the impact of religious discourse and values on all of us, whether or not we actively subscribe to a faith community. They say:

> Everyone is influenced by religion and religious practices whether they are believers, agnostics or atheists ... Ever the invisible presence in modern social work, its place should be recognised and taken account of in the work of the profession. (p. ii)

None of this should suggest, however, that *all* our values come from these indirect sources. All of us will have made certain decisions about our lives and what values we want to live by. Sometimes these will be in direct contrast to what we were brought up to believe. Powerful influences may have caused us to rethink previous assumptions. We may have joined, or moved away from, a faith community and the values it espouses. We may have joined a political party or movement. All these actions will help to determine the values we hold.

The message from this section, then, is that the value base for each of us is a combination of chosen and inherited values. It will be this combination that makes up the world-view we have chosen, that is, the way we look at and understand the world and our place in it. We all seek to uncover a sense of meaning in our lives and in the world so that we can try to make sense of what happens. It is this search that characterises the contemporary understanding of spirituality, whether or not it is religiously faith-based (Moss, 2005). We are, indeed, what we believe.

From a people-work point of view, the crucial thing is that we become fully aware of the values we hold, and the impact these have on our outlook and behaviour.

Wider Perspectives

We suggested earlier that someone entering a caring profession needs to be keenly aware of the values that organisation holds, which set the benchmark for the way its employees behave towards each other, and especially towards those who use their services. From a people-work perspective, there have been a number of important contributions that have been highly influential in creating a contemporary value base for people-work.

We have mentioned religious contributions to this debate, and the important place given in many faith communities of treating all people with dignity and respect. From a philosophical perspective, the work of Immanuel Kant stressed the importance of never treating human beings 'solely as a means but always also as an end', which is a value base underpinning all people-work. In other words, people's values consist of who they *are*, not what they do or how they contribute to society. (For a helpful discussion of this and other philosophical perspectives, see Beckett and Maynard, 2005, Ch. 2.)

When dealing with people who come to us for help, some basic values were laid down by practitioners whose expertise lay in the field of counselling. Rogers (1961), for example, laid great store in the importance of active listening, where the person being counselled was helped to feel completely the focus of attention. Biestek (1961) and Egan (1998) both explored the value and importance of acceptance, and what the listener needs to do in order to offer really helpful (and therapeutic) attention. (For a good introduction to these values, see N. Thompson, 2005).

It is fair to say, however, that the emphasis for all these writers, as far as the value base is concerned, has been the individual and the problems that caused them discomfort, at times needing therapeutic counselling help. These individual values (if we may call them thus) were later placed into a much wider societal context which has become of great importance for contemporary people-work.

In the later half of the twentieth century, a greater awareness developed of the societal context of people's difficulties. We began to be more aware not only of how society is structured, but of the impact this has on people's lives. How you fare in society depends not so much on your talents and abilities, but where you are located. So, if you were black, you stood far less chance of receiving fair and equal treatment than if you were white. Women similarly needed to struggle to gain equality in terms of status, employment and pay. And disabled people, returning home after the Second World War, found they were often discarded by society because they were deemed unable to make a useful contribution. It was against that background that some of the major themes – or isms – were highlighted: racism, sexism, classism, disablism, heterosexism. These powerful societal forces discriminated against people on the basis of their 'race', gender, class, 'ability' and sexual orientation, by implying that they were, by definition, second-class citizens.

The impact of these insights on people-work was profound. For one thing, it challenged the assumption, inherent in some counselling approaches, that the main task of people-work was to help people to adjust to the 'status quo'. But if the status quo was profoundly unjust and had contributed significantly to the person's problems, this clearly was unsatisfactory and, moreover, immoral.

Thus we found the equal opportunity movement of the former Greater London Council introducing equal opportunities policies for all organisations in its area who wished to receive contracts for services. The needs of minority groups and those who were at the rough end of discrimination and oppression had to be taken seriously; no longer could they be ignored. Major legislation was introduced tackling many of the issues that had been identified, and in the forefront of people-work practice another major value base was introduced: anti-discriminatory practice.

Anti-discriminatory Practice

Without doubt anti-discriminatory practice has become one of the most important ingredients in the value base of the professional people-worker. It is explored in more detail in Chapter 4, but for our purposes it is crucial to underline its central values. Its starting point is the injustice in society, and the ways in which discrimination and oppressive attitudes serve to disadvantage sections of society for no other reason than they are black, female, disabled, working class or gay (this list is by no means exhaustive). People-workers need to both understand how this works and then ensure that their practice takes these issues into account, not least by challenging the very factors that disadvantage those with whom they are working.

Thompson (2006) offers one of the best introductions to this important theme. He argues that discrimination and oppression work at three levels – the personal, the cultural and the structural level. This has come to be known as the PCS analysis, and you are strongly encouragesd to read more about this, as it is so central to the contemporary value base of people-work.

One good example of this was the report into the behaviour of the Metropolitan Police following the death of Stephen Lawrence in 1993. The inquiry found evidence of institutional racism in the Metropolitan Police (Macpherson Report, 1999), which meant that racist attitudes were not confined to some individual officers (P), or to groups of officers in certain areas (C), but were somehow ingrained into the very fabric of the organisation as a whole, leading to widespread racism throughout (S).

This affected not only promotion opportunities and career structures, but generally how black and ethnic minority groups in the community were both seen and treated by the police.

The above example is not intended to single out the police. One of the fundamental tenets of the PCS analysis is that *all* organisations are prone to this sort of institutional discrimination, and that this applies not just to racism, but to all the other major 'isms' we have identified. Sensitive people-workers, therefore, need to have these wider considerations at the forefront of their consciousness if they are to undertake work that is really effective, rather than applying a temporary cosmetic sticking plaster to an injury that is far more deep-seated than they acknowledge.

The most recent development has been an articulation of the value base of celebrating diversity exemplified in the establishment of the Commission for Equality and Human Rights (CEHR). Perhaps this signals a move away from viewing society as problem-ridden, towards appreciating its richness and diversity as something to celebrate, an enrichment by which everyone stands to benefit.

The Changing Role of People-work

These important developments in the value base of people-work have had profound implications on professional practice. Depending on which aspect of people-work you enter, you will find professional codes of conduct that have been designed not only to articulate the value base of the organisation, but also to guide workers on how to implement them in what are often complex situations. The Nursing and Midwifery Council's Code of Conduct (NMC, 2004) and the General Social Care Council's Codes of Practice (GSCC, 2002) are good examples of this. Workers will be faced with challenges to identify where the problem lies – is it with the individual, or should it rest with society? Should the worker be trying to improve the individual's health and wellbeing, change the individual's lifestyle or seek radical change in society?

It should come as no surprise that there are no easy answers to these practice dilemmas. Some decisions we take will be compromises and some will reflect the powerful influence that discrimination has, and will only offer a modest tinkering with the system to achieve a slight improvement for those who seek our help. Sometimes our role will have a societal protection element to it, when we take decisions to protect society from the behaviour of those who would harm or abuse others. On occasion we will be positioned side by side as an advocate and seek to tackle injustice 'head on'.

This is both the challenge and the glory of people-work that will be facing you as you complete your training at both theoretical and practical levels. In the end, the most important thing you will bring to people-work will not be the knowledge you have gained and continue to update (vital though that is), but the person who you are, and how you regard and treat those with whom you work. (Remember the roadside mechanic?) And the key 'ingredient' in this will be that powerful mix of personal and organisational values which will (we hope) help others to look back on their professional encounter with you with a sense of gratitude and respect.

Conclusion

This chapter has introduced you to values as a central aspect of health and social care work. We have discussed the origins of values and the relationship between our personal and practice-based values. Finally, we have examined some of the difficulties in practice that are related to our values.

REVIEW QUESTIONS

1   What have been the influences on your own value base?

2   In what ways do you think there may be a clash between your personal values and the values of the organisation you hope to work for?

FURTHER READING

Beckett, C. and Maynard, A. (2005) *Values and Ethics in Social Work: An Introduction*, London, Sage

Fulford, B., Dickenson, D. and Murray, T.H. (eds) (2002) *Healthcare Ethics and Human Values*, Oxford, Blackwell

GSCC (General Social Care Council) (2002) *Code of Practice for Social Care Workers and Code of Practice for Employers of Social Care Workers*, London, GSCC

Harris, J. (2004) *The Value of Life: An Introduction to Medical Ethics*, London, Routledge

Moss, B. (2007) *Values*, Lyme Regis, Russell House

NMC (Nursing and Midwifery Council) (2004) *The NMC Code of Professional Conduct: Standards for Conduct, Performance and Ethics*, London, NMC, www.nmc-uk.org

Pierson, J. and Thomas, M. (2002) *Collins Dictionary of Social Work*, Glasgow, HarperCollins Contains a value base entry in Chapter 5.

Thompson, I.E., Melia, K.M., Boyd, K.M. and Horsburgh, D. (2000) *Nursing Ethics* (5th edn) Edinburgh, Churchill Livingstone

Thompson, N. (2005) *Understanding Social Work: Preparing for Practice* (2nd edn) Basingstoke, Palgrave Macmillan, Chapter 1, 'What are Values?'

Thompson, N. (2006) *Anti-discriminatory Practice* (4th edn) Basingstoke, Palgrave Macmillan Contains material on values.

Resource file

Ethical tensions in practice

It is not possible to begin a book on health and social care with a clear-cut statement of values and ethics to which all practitioners and members of the public will subscribe. Values – statements of belief – are not absolute, but are socially constructed. That is, they differ according to where we are living and/or our cultural affiliations, that is, what sets of beliefs we profess. A doctor or care worker in China may be less likely than an English one to promote the value of empowering the individual person above valuing the continuance of family traditions and beliefs.

Just as values are constructed differently in different parts of the world, so too are statements of ethics.

Ethical statements are statements of 'how we should act'. They usually have moral assumptions embedded in them. Statements of professional ethics often are inseparable from personal beliefs. Some areas of health and social care are particularly debatable, that is, they raise special tensions and dilemmas in practice because there is controversy about whether or not practice should be conducted in a particular fashion. These tensions are reflected in government policy. The Human Fertilisation and Embryology Authority (HFEA), a statutory body created under the Human Fertilisation and Embryology Act 1991, is responsible for:

- keeping patients, the public, professionals and government informed
- licensing and monitoring UK clinics offering IVF (in vitro fertilisation) and DI (donor insemination) treatments
- monitoring research into human embryos
- regulating the storage of human sperm, eggs and embryos
- overseeing the safety and appropriateness of fertility and embryo treatment and research.

In 2003, a government White Paper (DoH, 2003d) set out how genetic techniques could benefit people and announced a £50 million three-year implementation plan. In 2006, the government initiated a review of the plan and there were indications that some areas would be reined in. Specifically, the HFEA turned down research proposals to create hybrid embryos or chimeras (so-called therapeutic cloning, see below) from human and animal material (cows and rabbits) to use in research into conditions such as motor neurone disease, Parkinson's disease and Alzheimer's disease.

Eugenics

Eugenics is the study of hereditary (genetically transmitted) improvement of the human species by selective breeding, that is, eliminating genes judged to be bad or harmful.

The routine scanning of fetuses when women are pregnant makes it possible to identify conditions such as Down syndrome and an increasing number of other characteristics. Where the fetus displays a severe impairment, the parent/s may be counselled about a premature termination.

Discuss with a colleague which of the following you would consider justifies a termination:

- Down syndrome
- Twins, triplets or quadruplets
- Not the preferred sex.

Genetic manipulation of disabled people

In the USA, nine-year-old Ashley, at the request of her parents, has had growth restrictive surgery and continuing hormone treatment to ensure that she will not grow any further. Ashley has disabilities which mean her mental age will remain at around three months and her physical movements are severely restricted. Because she does not walk, wherever she is placed, she tends to remain all day, although she does appear to respond to music, which she seems to enjoy, by moving her limbs with pleasure. The parents maintain that the treatment is intended to improve their daughter's quality of life, because she will be less likely to develop bed sores. Critics maintain that such treatment is to keep the child small for the convenience of the care-giver. Advocates for the rights of people with disabilities maintain that children have the right not to have their growth impaired and to develop as adults. Some people argue that this treatment opens the way for eugenic policies.

Genetic cloning

Leading stem cell scientists want to use eggs from humans, cows and rabbits to create chimeras or hybrid human–animal embryos in vitro. Genetic manipulation may involve cloning two cells, using embryonic stem cells, removing the genetic information from the egg and replacing the nucleus of cell with animal material. However, scientists claim this will help to find out how to cure diseases such as motor neurone disease, Alzheimer's and Parkinson's.

Assisted death

There is a strenuous debate about whether in certain circumstances people should be allowed to end their own lives, for instance when they are suffering from an incurable disease and their quality of life has been reduced to the point where they no longer want to live. An associated issue is whether people should be allowed to make a living will, stipulating the conditions in which the means to support their life, such as artificial breathing or intravenous (through a vein) feeding, would be turned off. Terms such as euthanasia, mercy killing and physician-assisted dying are often used. Partners and relatives may be involved in assisted suicide. In some countries such as Britain, assisted suicide remains illegal, but in countries such as Switzerland, it is legal.

If a person asked you to cooperate in an assisted suicide, how would you respond? If you cooperated, would you be prepared to face criminal prosecution and a possible charge of murder?

Activity 5.1

1. Spend a few minutes jotting down on a piece of paper those aspects of health and social care about which you feel strongly.
2. Pair with a colleague who has done the same task and each work through your list explaining your personal views and professional stance to the other.
3. Are any items on your list matters on which you are immovable?
4. Do you hold any beliefs about what you would or would not do in your practice over which you would resign rather than back down?
5. Do you hold any beliefs over which you would never back down, regardless of the threats made to you?

Be warned. This activity has the power to arouse strong emotions.

FURTHER READING

Banks, S. (2004) *Ethics, Accountability and the Social Professions*, Basingstoke, Palgrave Macmillan

Chadwick, R. and Levitt, M. (eds) (1998) *Ethical Issues in Community Health Care*, London, Arnold

DoH (2003) *Our Inheritance, Our Future: Realising the Potential of Genetics in the NHS*, White Paper, Cm 5791-II, London, TSO

Doxiadis, S. (ed.) (1987) *Ethical Dilemmas in Health Promotion*, Chichester, John Wiley
   A useful collection covering mainly health promotion issues in developed countries.

WEBSITES: www.euthanasia.com
                   www.ves.org.uk; www.dignityindying.org.uk
                   The Voluntary Euthanasia Society (VES) has changed its name to Dignity in Dying.

6 Physical Basis for Health and Wellbeing

ROBERT ADAMS

Learning outcomes

By the end of this chapter, you should be able to:

- ■ DESCRIBE the main features of the normal functioning of the human body
- ■ UNDERSTAND the physical basis for people's health and wellbeing
- ■ APPRECIATE the relevance of a knowledge of physiology to health and social care.

This chapter should be read in conjunction with Chapter 25.

Physiology is the study of the functioning of a biological system. We begin this brief tour of the physical basis of human activity with the fundamentals of how our bodies are shaped by cells, genes, tissues and organs. As we visit each aspect, we indicate some of the main diseases and conditions affecting them.

Cells, Genes, Tissues and Bodies

The major systems of the body such as the digestive and nervous systems have organs such as the stomach and brain doing essential tasks. These organs are made up of tissues. A tissue is a group of cells. Each cell has a nucleus containing the chromosomes composed of deoxyribonucleic acid (DNA). The genes housing the genetic information shaping the characteristics of the body are composed of strands of DNA.

Over time, cells divide many times, which is partly how the body grows and repairs itself. There is a limit, though, to the number of times a cell can divide. As cells age, 'mistakes' can occur in the process of cell division and these are what we refer to as *mutations*. These mutations can be a sign that a gene or chromosome has changed. If such changes occur on a significant scale, cancers can grow, a process which is more common as the cells and the person grow older.

Genes are located in chromosomes and DNA is in the nucleus of the cells. DNA contains the blueprint or formula which makes the body grow in a particular way. DNA not only contains 'innocent' information such as eye and hair colouring, height and other physical characteristics, but can also contain information about various conditions or diseases to which the person may be prone. Research into DNA and illnesses is proceeding apace and month by month there are new developments in the search to find links between the genetic information and a person's susceptibility to some of the major conditions – multiple sclerosis (MS), Parkinson's disease and many different cancers.

A *genetic disorder* is one which a person has inherited through her or his genes. A *congenital disorder* is one which is noted at birth. Thus, a congenital disorder could have either resulted from a genetic factor or come about through some condition that developed through the pregnancy or the birth itself.

One of the major debates is about whether children and young people are more likely to develop certain behavioural problems because of genetics or the way they are brought up, or socialised. This is one aspect of the so-called *nature–nurture* debate (see Resource File: Child Development: The Nature versus Nurture Debate, at the end of Chapter 8). The identification of certain genes as linked with some illnesses and conditions has brought about the possibility of treating or preventing them by implanting unaffected genetic material into the person's body, or even growing entire organs such as a new bladder and transplanting this. This is often referred to as *gene therapy*.

There are more than 200 different types of cell in the human body. Some of these are more generalised, with the potential to develop into a variety of more specialised cells. These generalised cells are called *stem cells*. Many of these stem cells can regenerate certain tissues in the body when they become damaged through accident or illness. Research is proceeding apace to find out the extent to which transplants of stem cells into a person can bring about the possibility of them repairing certain serious genetic disorders, making it possible to intervene to 'cure' failures in many of the body's major organs. It may also be possible to halt or even reverse certain conditions such as those causing muscles, limbs and even brain cells to degenerate. Attempts are being made, for example, to find a cure for Alzheimer's disease (a form of dementia, see below).

The Endocrine System

The endocrine system consists of exocrine and endocrine glands. Exocrine glands such as sweat and salivary glands produce secretions outside the internal blood and tissue fluids of the body, so are not carried round the body systematically. Endocrine glands carry out similarly essential functions within the body's circulation systems and include:

- the *pituitary gland*: produces hormones such as the growth hormone
- the *thyroid gland:* regulates the body's metabolism
- the *adrenal glands:* regulate the heartbeat, enlarge the lungs, divert blood to the muscles so that the body can react to an emergency, for example by running
- the *pancreas:* produces insulin which regulates the conversion of soluble blood sugar – glucose – into insoluble glycogen which is stored in the liver. Diabetes can follow when the production of insulin is not adequate.

The Blood and Cardiovascular System

The expression 'lifeblood' is close to the truth. Blood is necessary to sustain life and a wound which causes a large loss of blood is life-threatening. Blood contains two main components: blood cells and the plasma in which they float. There are two kinds of blood cells: red and white, the former carrying oxygen from the lungs to tissues and carbon dioxide back to the lungs, the latter fighting to protect the body against infections and diseases. If a wound causes blood to flow, the blood cells stick together forming a clot, enabling the body to repair the wound.

The blood is pumped around the body by the most important organ in the cardio-vascular system, the heart. It consists of two pumps, one of which pumps blood to the lungs to be filled with oxygen (oxygenated) and to have the carbon dioxide cleaned out of it (excreted), the other pumping blood round the body. The blood flows around the body pushed by the pulses, or heartbeats, from the heart, passing oxygen into the body as it flows through arteries and on its return journey flowing through veins. If you see a person who has a cut to an artery, the blood will possibly be pulsing out, bright red, due to the oxygen it contains. If the cut is to a vein, the blood may ooze and will have a bluish tinge. A cut to a major artery, for example the femoral artery supplying the leg through the thigh, can be fatal because of the pace of blood flow. **You can save a person's life by learning how to stem the bleeding** by applying an improvised *tourniquet*, such as a pad of folded cloth, or using pressure from the thumbs until the blood stops pulsing out. Every quarter-hour or so until medical help arrives, the pressure should be released to enable the blood to flow around the affected limb, otherwise the tissues will be so starved of oxygen that they will start to die and gangrene will set in.

Sometimes the largest of a person's arteries, the coronary arteries, the first two leaving the heart, will become diseased. This is called coronary heart disease and is the most common cause of death in Western countries. One common cause is blocking of the arteries by fatty substances composed of cholesterol. Some substances based on cholesterol are useful to the body, others are harmful. If there is a lot of harmful cholesterol, it is more likely the person will develop one or more blood clots in the artery, known as a thrombosis. The proneness of people to a build-up of choles-terol can contribute to high blood pressure. This can be controlled by drugs taken regularly, although some of the stronger drugs have side effects. Sometimes the clogged arteries are narrowed so much that when the person tries to climb the stairs, walk faster or carry a heavy object, they experience a tightening in the chest and severe pain. This may be angina, which, in effect, is the body's way of warning the person to slow down, when hopefully the pain will disappear. It may be possible through surgery (angioplasty) to introduce a sleeve through the inside of the artery, using local anaesthetic, which will widen the artery and relieve the condition.

The other way of improving the health of the cardiovascular system is not through drugs or surgery, but by avoiding becoming overweight, adopting a healthy diet – low fat, low salt and plenty of vegetables and fruit – and taking regular exercise which strengthens the heart muscles and lowers blood pressure.

Health and social care work with older, vulnerable and physically impaired people often involves stimulating them to exercise, thus preventing them from becoming more passive, dependent and depressed and consequently lethargic and inactive.

Activity 6.1

Spend 10 minutes writing down the physical complications that can arise from allowing people to stay immobile for long periods.

Many complications can occur through immobility, including pressure sores, constipation, thrombosis and congestion of the lungs. If the muscles of the arms and legs are not used regularly, they will waste and the person will become unsteady and lacking in confidence when walking. Inertia can become a vicious circle, with the person resorting more and more to a wheelchair or asking others to carry out errands rather than making the physical effort to remain independent. Since the late 1990s, there has been increasing concern about possible links between immobility on long-haul plane flights and deep vein thrombosis (DVT), although the poor quality of the air on these flights has also been called into question as a possible factor. People confined to a chair or bed in a residential or daycare setting will need to practise deep breathing and exercise their ankles and feet regularly, to avoid a blood clot in the veins returning blood to the heart.

The Liver

This is the largest solid organ and gland in the body. It performs more than 500 complex biochemical functions, including receiving and passing on blood and cleansing many toxic substances from the body. If it fails, the person may suffer hepatitis, cirrhosis or jaundice. The liver makes many essential substances for the body, including proteins that contribute, for example, to blood clotting and bile acids that are needed for the body to digest fat and absorb vitamins. If a person drinks alcohol regularly, the liver cells will not be able to secrete properly and fat will start to accumulate in them. This will cause the liver to become fatty and the cells will start to die, a process called cirrhosis. If the person is persuaded to stop drinking regularly at this stage, the cirrhosis can be reversed. Once the tissues become fibrous, the cirrhosis is irreversible.

The liver also cleans many impurities, including substances not made by the body, such as drugs, out of the blood. If the liver becomes diseased and starts to fail, these can be left in the blood, creating more damage.

The Nervous System

This is a network for the communication of perception, the processing of information and regulation of responses within the body. The transmission of information through the nerves is by electrical impulses and chemical transmitters. The *central nervous system* (CNS) consists of the brain and the spinal column and the *peripheral nervous system* (PNS) consists of the rest of the nervous tissue. The brain is the most complex structure in the body and is composed of grey matter (mostly nerve cells) and white matter (mostly nerve fibres). The different parts of the brain are each associated with different functions: thinking, remembering, hearing, seeing and so on.

The entire nervous system is composed of billions of nerve cells called *neurones*, carrying out different specialised tasks such as governing movement, in other words *motor neurones*. The condition where the motor neurones progressively die is called motor neurone disease. *Sensory neurones* carry the signals from all five senses to the area of the brain known as the sensory cortex, which enables us to make sense of what we see, hear, touch, smell and taste.

Neurones are unable to divide to repair damage, so, on the whole, destruction of parts of the brain or spinal column is usually irreversible, although there are some remarkable examples of recovery of functions after severe injuries. Alzheimer's disease is an example of a degenerative condition of the brain, a symptom of which is wholesale destruction of the neurones, which unfortunately is still irreversible, despite efforts to find treatments which will halt or even slow its progress.

The two parts of the nervous system are *autonomic* and *voluntary*. The autonomic nervous system functions independently of control by the person and consists of the sympathetic nervous system, which responds to danger by preparing the body to defend itself or run away, and the parasympathetic nervous system, which slows the heartrate and breathing rate (the metabolic rate) down. During sleep, the metabolic rate slows and a certain level of regular sleep (and, some would say, dreaming) is necessary to maintain mental and physical health, although the precise level varies between individuals.

The Skin

Skin covers the outer surface of the body as we know, but its characteristics are less well known. Its several protective layers comprise two main ones – the outer *epidermis* and underneath it the *dermis*. Together these comprise the largest organ, totalling almost a tenth of the weight of the body. Skin stretches like elastic and is also waterproof. The cells of the skin are constantly dying, being shed and regenerating. As we grow older, the condition of our skin deteriorates. It loses elasticity, develops wrinkles and takes longer to heal. In a serious injury such as a burn, the deeper dermis is destroyed and thus the protective barrier against infection; in extensive severe burns, the body may lose large quantities of fluid. Unless damaged skin from a burn is removed quickly and a substitute skin replaces it, burns can take a long time to heal and, where extensive, can be life-threatening.

The Lymphatic System

Non-medical practitioners do not need to know much about the lymphatic system, which has its own drainage vessels containing tissue. There are some similarities between the way the lymphatic system and blood circulation work. Lymph nodes full of white blood cells are present in different parts of the body. When the body is fighting infections, the lymph nodes are very active, attacking the invading microbes. Lymph nodes can become swollen in certain diseases, including some cancers.

The Respiratory System

The respiratory system includes the nose, mouth, trachea (windpipe), lungs and diaphragm. It ensures the body can inhale (breathe in) air and extract from it the oxygen needed to maintain life, before exhaling (breathing out) again. The average adult's lungs contain about 600 million tiny, honeycombed, air-filled alveoli (bags) surrounded by minute capillaries through which arterial blood flows, soaking up oxygen, while blood from the veins discharges carbon dioxide into other nearby alveoli.

The Digestive System

The digestive system is the part of the body which digests food and drink and excretes the waste matter from that digestion. It includes the oesophagus, which connects the mouth to the stomach, the stomach which connects to the duodenum linked with the small intestine (6–8 metres long) and large intestine (about 1.5 metres long) and the wider passage of the colon from which bowel movements propel waste through the rectum to the anus.

The elements of nutrition are dealt with in Chapter 21. Digestion involves mixing food, first with saliva then with stomach acids and enzymes that digest protein, thereby breaking it down chemically into usable, smaller molecules. Digestion is also helped by the gall bladder, which stores fat created by the liver until it is needed. The pancreas produces the hormone insulin, which maintains low blood glucose levels, and also enzymes that contribute to digestion.

Urinary System

The body extracts nutrients from the food we eat in order to maintain day-to-day activities, leaving waste products in the blood and the bowel. The urinary system works alongside the skin, lungs and intestines to secrete these waste products and consists of the two kidneys and the bladder, which manage the storage and excretion of 2–3 litres of urine daily from the body of an average adult. Urine travels from the kidneys to the bladder along two tubes called ureters, which perform muscular contractions to force the liquid along. The bladder is rather like a balloon and can expand and contract greatly. Muscles at its opening called sphincters help to prevent urine leaking. For details of what can go wrong in the urinary system, see Chapter 25.

Infection and Immunity

The body may acquire immunity through previous minor infections, vaccination or innoculation, or it may possess natural immunity. *Vaccination* involves introducing a small amount of the toxin causing the disease, creating an immune reaction in the immune system and, hopefully, avoids the person having to suffer the condition. *Innoculation* involves introducing a substance with the known power to prevent the disease. The skin also acts as a barrier to infection. Other forms of protection consist of mucous membranes in the mouth, inside the eyelids and in the genital tracts. Mucus, saliva and tears also ward off infection by acting to digest bacterial material. The entire respiratory (breathing) system is protected, beginning with tiny hairs and mucus in the nose and a mucous lining in the throat. Sneezing and coughing also help to expel infected material from the breathing tubes.

Allergic reactions occur when the immune system does not recognise an innocent substance and is stimulated to produce an immunological response.

Inflammation

Inflammation is recognised through redness and swelling of the tissue, heat, pain and inability to move it freely. Damage to tissue, such as through a blow or cut, may lead to inflammation, which also may be caused by swellings such as through rheumatoid arthritis. Inflammation may result also from immune reactions, such as to pollen in hay fever. Inflammation can be painful, but is part of the normal process of healing.

Thermoregulation

The higher the metabolic rate of organs in the body, the more heat they produce. The *metabolic rate* is a term describing the rate at which cells stimulated by the thyroid gland in the neck use glucose, fatty acids and oxygen to produce more energy. An overproduction of the thyroid hormone will cause the person to feel hot and lose weight.

The body loses excess heat through three physical processes: *convection, conduction* and *radiation*. Convection consists of air being warmed near the surface of the body and moving away to be replaced by cooler air which in turn is warmed. Conduction involves heat passing from the warmer body to colder objects by direct contact, as, for instance when the person takes a cold shower and stands in the bathroom afterwards, dripping wet and lets evaporation cool the body down. Radiation involves the skin emitting radiant heat from its surface, which it does very readily, for instance when a man takes off his shirt in an effort to cool down. A person loses less heat through radiation when dressed than when undressed.

These physical characteristics become extremely important when working with young children, older people, or people whose physical impairments lead them to spend long periods in a seat or wheelchair. Normal body temperature is about 36.4–37°C, but for some individuals this can vary from 36°C to 37.5°C. Vulnerable children and adults may lose heat if in a cold environment and this may be worse if they are exposed to wet weather as well.

Hypothermia can result if the body temperature falls below 35°C. In this situation, it is important to keep the person awake, otherwise the body temperature may plummet still further. It is important to avoid the mistake of giving alcohol to a person suspected of hypothermia, because this gives the illusion of feeling warmer, but at the expense of allowing more heat to leave the body, this actually accelerating the hypothermia.

Hyperthermia can set in once the body temperature rises above 38–40°C, for example if the person is exposed to the sun on a hot summer's day and is unable to take off clothes or seek the shade. Dehydration may exaggerate the effects of hyperthermia, because the person is unable to sweat efficiently. It is important to keep taking fluids when in hot conditions. Because the arms and legs have large surface areas, putting clothes on them or taking them off can regulate the body temperature very effectively. Hyperthermia is one symptom of an infection which the body is fighting off, involving the immune system working more efficiently at a higher temperature.

Conclusion

This chapter has reviewed briefly the physical basis for health and social care work. It is impossible to deal with specialised aspects, many of which have entire shelves of books and journals devoted to them. Below are some suggestions for more detailed reading, should you want information on a particular aspect.

REVIEW
QUESTIONS

1 What is the difference between a genetic and a congenital disorder?

2 What is DNA?

3 What is a stem cell?

4 What are the most effective ways of improving health and preventing heart disease?

5 What are the three physical processes by which the body loses heat?

6 What is hyperthermia?

7 Can you name seven major 'systems' of the body?

FURTHER
READING

Campbell, J. (2003) *Campbell's Physiology Notes for Nurses*, London, Whurr

Hubbard, J.L. (1987) *Physiology for Health Care Students*, Edinburgh, Churchill Livingstone

McGeown, J.G. (2002) *Physiology: A Clinical Core Text of Human Physiology with Self-assessment*, Edinburgh, Churchill Livingstone

Martini, F. (2001) *Fundamentals of Anatomy and Physiology* (5th edn) Upper Saddle River, NJ, Prentice Hall

Rutishauswer, S. (1994) *Physiology and Anatomy: A Basis for Nursing and Health Care*, Edinburgh, Churchill Livingstone

Schmidt Prezbindowski, K. (1997) *Introduction to the Human Body* (4th edn) Harlow, Addison Wesley

CHAPTER

7

Psychological Basis for Health and Wellbeing

ROBERT ADAMS

By the end of this chapter, you should be able to:

■ SPECIFY the main features of psychology

■ DISCUSS the main psychological theories relating to health and wellbeing

■ EXAMINE the ways practitioners draw on psychological theories in health and social care work.

This chapter deals with the factors affecting a person's character and personality, as well as how the individual relates to other people, in the family, at work or in settings such as the hospital ward, sheltered housing or day centre. It is a fallacy that psychological ideas and research only deal with individuals. Clinical psychologists may focus on the individual, but may also take into account the relationships between that individual and other family members. Social psychologists study how small groups of people interact and their ideas have influenced how group therapists work and how professionals understand and work with family groups and many other groups.

What is Psychology and What Does it Contribute?

Psychology deals with the mental life of people – their thoughts, feelings, wishes, motives and memories – and how these relate to their actions. It is a discipline which we draw on to help to understand why people behave in particular ways and, with less certainty, to help us to predict how they might behave in the future.

Psychological theories attempt to understand and explain how people think, feel and behave and are extremely varied and complex. We select a few here of direct relevance to health and social care work with people. These include psychodynamic, personality trait, humanistic, cognitive-behavioural and eclectic theories.

Psychodynamic Theories

These derive largely from psychoanalysts and therapists such as Freud (1933), Jung (Progoff, 1953), Klein (1997), Winnicott (1991) and Bowlby (1991). *Psychodynamic* perspectives generally emphasise the links between how people behave and their inner thoughts and feelings. *Psychoanalytic* perspectives are more specifically derived from the theories of Freud and focus on finding the connections assumed to exist between people's behaviour, thoughts and feelings and their unconscious mental processes. Sigmund Freud (1933) saw the human mind as divided into conscious and unconscious and the personality into three components: *id* (the inherited 'instinctive' components such as the sex drive), *ego* (the 'I' component), and *superego* (the conscience, curbing the id's drives for immediate gratification). Therapists using psychoanalytic ideas try to reconcile the different components of the personality, working with the consciousness, the small directly accessible portion of the personality, to try to gain access through dreams and free association to the person's unconscious mind. Whether or not therapists accept specifically Freudian theories, they may still work on the basis of developing treatments for problem areas, such as some people's tendency to hide behind defence mechanisms to avoid facing the reality of their need to change. Psychoanalytic and psychodynamic theorists have the strength of highlighting that people's motives for their actions are often deep-rooted in previous, even infant or childhood, traumas and other experiences. Their weaknesses include a tendency to pathologise human behaviour and a lack of rigour in therapy, which may lead to some people using a therapist on a long-term basis, almost as though they need a permanent personal trainer to maintain their mental health.

Personality Trait Theories

Personality trait theories are linked with personality test approaches and are represented by Eysenck (1963), who was convinced of the reliability of testing people to categorise them into types of personality and then predict how they are likely to behave. He distinguished extraverts from introverts: the former tending to be outgoing, sociable, easy-going, optimistic, aggressive and quick to turn to anger; the latter tending to be shy, cautious, not aggressive, pessimistic and slow to rouse to anger. These are ideals, or extremes, and Eysenck suggested that most people's personalities reflect a mixture of these two types. Eysenck has been criticised for relying too much on a rigid, test-based categorisation of people, reducing complex aspects to simplistic stereotypes.

Humanistic Theories

Humanistic psychological ideas could be regarded as a reaction to some of the more obviously scientific approaches based on personality measurement and the observation of behaviour. Humanistic ideas derived from existential philosophy have influenced humanistic approaches to helping people. One of the key terms signalling these approaches is 'person-centred'. Carl Rogers (1951) developed the notion of the client as the expert, which has echoes in the current emphasis in the NHS on 'the expert patient'. Rogers emphasised the importance of the person fulfilling personal potential and many of his ideas are reflected in the importance given to empowering the person receiving services nowadays, prioritising choice and maximising human potential.

Cognitive-behavioural Theories

Cognitive-behavioural approaches derive from behaviourist psychologists such as B.F. Skinner and learning theorists such as Albert Bandura. Skinner (1953) developed methods of changing behaviour based on rewarding desired behaviour and punishing undesired behaviour, thereby hopefully reinforcing the former and extinguishing the latter. Bandura's (1986) learning theories worked on the basis not of punishing undesirable behaviour but simply waiting for the desired behaviour to happen and rewarding it. Cognitive-behavioural therapy (CBT) draws on the scientific approach of behaviourism as well as highlighting personal awareness which is central to cognitive psychology (see Chapter 42).

Eclectic Approaches

There are a number of so-called eclectic approaches which do not fit easily into one category, for which the work of George Kelly is a good example. Kelly (1955) developed 'personal construct theory' around the basic proposition that a person acts on the basis of anticipating events and constructing personal and social realities on the basis of judgements which he or she continually revises in the light of experience (Kelly, 1970a, p. 9). Kelly's theory has three advantages:

1. Over personality measurement, in that it allows flexibility in the ways that people continually revise their beliefs on the basis of experience.
2. In advocating that people act rather tentatively and experimentally on the basis of constructs (assumptions, questions and hypotheses) which they revise in the light of experience, personal construct theory has the advantage of making a link with psychological theorists who believe in the experimental approach (Kelly, 1970b, pp. 257–9).
3. Over many other psychological theories, in that in focusing on how people construct their reality, it provides a direct link with sociological theories on the construction of reality.

Applications of Psychology

There are many different applications of psychology. Here we deal with three of particular interest to health and social care workers: firstly, clinical psychology and other therapeutic applications, including counselling and psychotherapy; secondly, developmental psychology, which deals with how people change through the life course (see also Chapters 8 and 17); and thirdly, social psychology, which is concerned with how small groups, including therapy or family groups, interact.

Clinical Psychology, Mental Health Treatments and Counselling

Applications of psychological theories are many, not least in different methods of work drawn on by practitioners in health and social care. Psychological insights inform a range of techniques, from assessment and diagnosis, through advice-giving and informing to counselling, psychotherapy and psychoanalysis. This last item is not really part of everyday practice, but is the preserve of the specialist psychoanalyst and we exclude it from this chapter. The other techniques require varying levels of education and training on the part of the practitioner and psychology contributes a good deal to them, probably more than any other discipline.

Assessing personality and personal characteristics

Many different measures have been devised to try to capture the complexity of people's personalities in questionnaires, interview schedules and many other means. Schemes have been devised to categorise personalities into different types and to use these to predict how prone the individual may be to difficulties such as delinquency or mental health problems. Some of the measures have emphasised intellect, such as intelligence tests, while others have concentrated more upon emotions.

Psychological origins of physical illnesses

Some psychologists and psychiatrists advocate so-called 'psychosomatic' factors leading to the origins of physical illnesses, including psychosomatic conditions such as asthma, colitis and hypertension.

Counselling and advice-giving

Counselling (see Chapter 45) is a form of helping that focuses on enabling people to identify, clarify and, perhaps, tackle their problems. Thus, counselling is a kind of self-help therapy, which enables people to empower themselves.

Treating mental health problems

A great variety of psychologically based treatments have been developed which aim to tackle people's mental health problems. These range from physical treatments such as surgery and electroconvulsive therapy (ECT) at one extreme, through the use of drugs to various 'talking' treatments such as psychoanalysis and psychotherapy. These include psychodynamic (see Chapter 43), cognitive-behavioural (see Chapter 42) and social and cultural approaches (see Chapter 44).

Developmental Psychology

There are different dimensions of human development – biological, social, emotional and cognitive – and psychology has made a major contribution in this area (see Chapter 8). Children's cognitive development has been studied extensively by psychologists. The most important debate opened up by this work is about whether children have their development primarily shaped by factors outside their control, whether within their biological makeup or by external – family or environmental – influences, or whether they have 'agency', the power to choose to act purposefully, or, as Bloom and Tinker (2001) say, with 'intentionality' (see Resource File: Child Development: The Nature versus Nurture Debate, at the end of Chapter 8).

Attachment and loss

Particular contributions have been made by psychology to the understanding of how babies and young children develop bonds with significant adults in their lives. The term 'attachment' is used to refer to this process and a huge amount of debate and research has surrounded this area since the 1950s. Links have been made by these researchers between the patterns of attachment that people experience when infants and young children and when they are older, as, for instance, when people are dying or experience bereavement (although these experiences, unfortunately, are not restricted to older people) (see Resource File: Attachment and Loss: Death and Bereavement, at the end of Chapter 28).

Attachment does not take place in a social vacuum. Culture affects attachment. It could be said that Western societies promote independence, while some Eastern countries such as Japan, certainly until the latter half of the twentieth century, have promoted interdependence. These differences are complex and the frequency and distance of movement made possible by modern means of travel and 'virtual' travel via the internet and other, including mass, media complicate the many variables involved, making research difficult and generalisation almost impossible.

Parenting styles differ and great consideration has been given by researchers to the consequences for the child, in terms of future traumas or delinquency for example, of particularly inconsistent or violent parenting. A related issue, of great relevance to society in the twenty-first century, is to what extent a child brought up by one parent, or two same-sex adults, is better or worse off than a child reared by a hetero-sexual couple. Also, the question as to whether there is a unique quality in the so-called 'blood bond' between parent and child is very relevant to adults wishing to foster or adopt a child.

Social Psychology

Social skills and social interaction

Social psychologists have made a major contribution to understanding how people interact and developing social skills training. Michael Argyle (1969) has developed a motor skill model to explain how to use the acquisition of social skills to understand how social behaviour takes place. The principle of this is that as people are talking and behaving, they are responding to cues from each other all the time, taking action to reduce or increase the physical distance between each other, and responding to remarks by increasing or decreasing the pace and intensity of their replies, depending on how they feel about what the other person is saying and doing. This is a way of understanding that takes account of both planned and unplanned social behaviour, as well as giving scope for body language along with the actual talk to be included in the equation. The motor skill model also extends to the motives, goals and plans of the people interacting, allowing for each person's goals to affect and be affected by the other (Argyle, 1972).

Social skills training (SST) has been used in work, educational and therapeutic settings. Work-based training 'on the job' is used in a great many settings, using role playing linked with detailed instructions on particular tasks in work with people, followed by feedback from the trainer and repeated practice, more feedback and so on (Argyle, 1988). Training groups (T groups) have been used to train people in social skills. SST has been developed also in therapeutic work, such as in mental health, with abusers of alcohol and drugs and with offenders, to build their confidence and assertiveness and enable them to manage their stress.

Groupwork

A major industry has grown up since the mid-twentieth century around the application of various social psychological ideas about group dynamics and the interaction of people within groups. The main applications of this are in the following:

- Group-based tests for the recruitment and selection of personnel
- Group-based management leadership training in industry and the uniformed services, especially the armed forces, police and penal agencies
- Group therapies for people with problems (see Chapters 32 and 43).

Understanding organisations

Many psychologists have studied the behaviour and interaction of individuals and groups in organisations, in many instances led, no doubt, by the desire to enhance the running of manufacturing organisations such as factories as well as service-based organisations such as hotels, thereby enhancing profits.

Much effort and resources have been devoted to the study of how different ways of organising and managing the work of work-based organisations affect their efficiency. The styles of managers have been studied with the aim of determining which leadership styles are most effective.

Some theories about how organisations function best have focused more on the organisation as a closed system, its internal arrangements – the hierarchy, the roles of staff, how the power is distributed and how decisions are made – while others have viewed the organisation more as an open system that relates to other systems and thus have concentrated on the relationships between different organisations and professions, how they communicate, interact and influence each other and how well they work together. Much attention has been devoted by social psychologists to studying how people work in teams within organisations and the learning from this is relevant to effective health and social care (Chapter 47).

Understanding institutions

Just as people's emotions and behaviour are affected by the organisation in which they work, so they are influenced by the institution in which some people live. Institutions vary in their so-called 'totality', that is, the extent to which they are cut off from the outside world. Examples of extreme total institutions are Trappist monasteries (where the monks are isolated and do not speak for long periods), top security prisons and special hospitals. Parts of institutions can take on a more total character than their parent establishment, for example locked wards in mental hospitals, and although social psychologists have spent much time studying life in institutions, the most important author to begin reading about this is the anthropologist and sociologist Erving Goffman (1961).

Attempts to create therapeutic communities

At the other extreme from institutions, there have been attempts since the nineteenth century to establish utopian or 'ideal' communities, from New Lanark established by Robert Owen in the early 1800s to Titus Salt's Saltaire near Bradford. So-called 'therapeutic communities' were set up in the twentieth century to counteract what were seen as the negative characteristics of total institutions and reinforce positive aspects of interaction between people. (See Chapter 54 on residential establishments and Resource File: Theories and Models of Residential Care, at the end of Chapter 54.)

Conclusion

This chapter has reviewed the main theories and ideas in psychology on which professionals in health and social care tend to draw. Illustrations have been given of some applications in practice. There is a great wealth of books and articles on the aspects discussed and any good library will contain a good choice of items on each of these.

REVIEW QUESTIONS

1 Can you distinguish between clinical, developmental and social psychology?

2 Can you give an example of an area of work in one of these areas to which psychologists have made a contribution?

3 What is social skills training?

4 To which types of groupwork have psychologists contributed?

FURTHER READING

Argyle, M. (1994) *The Psychology of Interpersonal Behaviour* (5th edn) Harmondsworth, Penguin

Hjelle, L.A. and Ziegler, D.J. (1992) *Personality Theories: Basic Assumptions, Research and Applications*, New York, McGraw-Hill

Journal of Health Psychology

Marks, D.F., Evans, M., Willig, B., Sykes, C.M. and Woodall, C. (2005) *Health Psychology: Theory, Research and Practice* (2nd edn) London, Sage

Ogden, J. (2000) *Health Psychology: A Textbook* (3rd edn) Buckingham, Open University Press

Rungapadiachy, D.M. (1999) *Interpersonal Communication and Psychology for Health Care Professionals*, Edinburgh, Butterworth Heinemann

Human Growth and Development

CHAPTER

8

JULIETTE OKO and MAGGIE JACKSON

By the end of this chapter, you should have:

■ SURVEYED different 'common-sense' perspectives on how we develop, grow and change over the life course

■ REFLECTED on more formal 'academic' ways of understanding human development.

Researchers have developed a variety of different explanations or theories about human growth and development which can be used to help us make sense of how people develop and grow up. How can we understand these? Firstly, we ask you to consider your personal experiences and identify significant events that you feel have impacted on you. In providing an explanation about our situation, we begin to move from a personal or informal understanding towards a more formal understanding that enables us to make links with formal theories of human growth and development. This view is echoed by Gitterman (2004, p. 101) who says:

> As educators we must provide the conditions which facilitate opportunities for students to bridge personal experiences and styles with facts, concepts and theories.

In this chapter we shall try to build this bridge between formal theories and concepts and your experiences as the reader. To start with, we need to distinguish between *informal theories* and *formal theories*. Informal theories or explanations are those we use in everyday life to make sense of the world – they can also be called *common-sense views*.

So the first step is to make explicit those common-sense views or informal theories (stories) we use to make sense of the world and to show that these informal theories fit in with more formal frameworks of theory.

The next step in this process is to ask you to draw a 'life snake'. This is a device whereby you can record key moments from your life. Figure 8.1 shows the life snake of John Bailey, a 42-year-old white man of Irish descent.

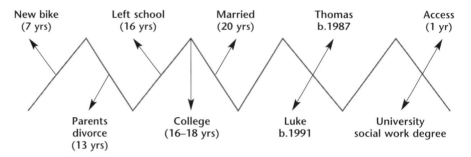

Figure 8.1 The life snake of John Bailey

When discussing his life snake, John makes the following remarks:

> I remember getting a big new bike when I was 7 – it was red and blue and I was really excited and pleased that my parents had bought it for me – I'd wanted a big bike for ages, but my Mum wasn't keen … but I remember learning to ride it and showing off to Mum and Dad that I could ride it, and how pleased they were! When I was 11 years old my parents separated – my Dad met someone – and when I was 13, my parents divorced. I saw my Dad quite regularly, weekends mainly. I didn't like my parents separating, because in those days it was still quite unusual, and I felt quite conscious about it, but I didn't tell anyone how I felt. I left school at 16 and went to college to do catering, which was quite enjoyable actually – it impressed Louise when I met her – a bloke who could cook! I met her at a disco when I was 19, and we got married the next year. We've been married for 22 years now, which I think nowadays is quite an achievement, but we both believe very strongly in marriage and that it's important for the boys to see that it is possible for marriage to last and be happy. A couple of years ago I began to get itchy feet, I was fed up working in the catering trade … I also do football training with young lads and really enjoy the banter and that I'm doing something useful, and I started to think more about youth work and the importance of boys having positive role models and using their time creatively. I made some enquiries at the local college and felt social work would be a good career move, but needed to go back to college to get an Access qualification. Me and Louise talked it over, about the cost and me returning to study and last year I started my Access and applied to university to do the social work degree. I was really surprised but pleased when I got offered a place! It made the effort and the work all the more worthwhile.

John's comments are useful in helping us understand the benefit of a life snake. It represents in a pictorial way the events you feel are significant in your life, and in asking you to talk (if you wish) about your experiences, it reveal feelings, for example John's excitement at a new bike and feeling self-conscious about his parents' separation. It also reveals John's beliefs about marriage and the importance of family and his motivation for getting involved in social work. The life snake is a useful tool for beginning to develop our self-awareness and reflective skills, as we can see a range of different factors that have impacted on us and shaped who we have become. This provides the basis for beginning to look at theories of human growth and development, since these theories provide us with an explanation and a framework for helping us to understand why and how these factors impact on us in the way they do.

Theories of Human Growth and Development

Now let us examine some of the main theories. There are four main groups of theory of human growth and development – biological, psychological (divided into psychodynamic and behavioural perspectives) and social/environmental. We shall briefly outline these four perspectives, and we shall relate these theories to John's life snake. The purpose of this analysis is to indicate how we can begin to look at the informal stories people tell about themselves and how these relate to more formal theories, which can then be used to begin to pick out significant and relevant information to help plan future interventions. By making connections to the relevant theories, we can frame our assessment and try to work out what further questions we need to ask.

Biological Theories

Biological perspectives on human growth and development advocate that it is our biology that determines our behaviour (Piaget and Inhelder, 1969; see also Resource File: Child Development: The Nature versus Nurture Debate, at the end of the chapter). Thus it is our genes and instincts that drive us; we are biologically determined and essentially have very little control over how we develop, having character traits that predispose us to act and respond more or less in a particular way. Typically, we might consider this explanation to consider a medical model of understanding how people develop through their life course.

In looking at John's commentary, we may want to know why John's mother was reluctant to let her son have a big bike – did she feel John was not old enough for the bike and therefore unable to ride it? Was John developmentally delayed? A biological perspective may provide an explanation for John's excitement at having a 'big bike'; perhaps it would allow us to look for clues about muscular development and poor coordination, which may have prevented John from engaging in physical activities as a young child. We note, however, that in later life John engages in football training and so if there had been any physical difficulties in his early life, we might want to consider the relevance of him being physically active at present, and what significance this has for him in terms of his own sense of self and that of his children.

Psychodynamic Theories

Psychodynamic perspectives are reflected in the work of Freud, Erickson and Bowlby (discussed in Beckett, 2002). These approaches seek to understand human behaviour and development as a result of a psychological impact. They focus on feelings and emotions – from this perspective, the explanation is located internally, much as a biological perspective is; however, psychodynamic perspectives argue that feelings and emotions stem from close interpersonal relationships, most often located in the individual's family of origin or early childhood experiences.

When we consider John, if we took a psychodynamic approach, we may want to explore more fully the relationship he had with his parents. Firstly, it is John's comments about his mother's concern about him riding a big bike that might point to an anxious mother and a consideration of the relationship that developed between her and her son; and secondly, John's relationship with his father, following his parents' separation. We may also want to consider his early childhood experiences and how they may have framed his view about marriage and the relationship he has with his children. Typically, here we would consider the importance of 'attachment theory', first put forward by John Bowlby. This talks about the importance of the quality of the relationship between the primary caretaker and the young child and how this has a significant impact on all subsequent relationships. The converse side to attachment is loss and we see here that John talks about the distress and shame he felt when his parents divorced and the importance to him of his long marriage to his wife. This may not be indicative of a secure attachment but of anxiety of being abandoned – but may lead us to explore these issues further with John.

Behavioural Theories

Among behavioural theories, Skinner uses 'operant conditioning' and Bandura uses 'social learning theory' as ways of explaining how people learn behaviour in the course of development (discussed in Berger, 2004).

This approach argues that behaviour is primarily learnt – it is not particularly concerned with internal processes, that is, the 'why', but instead focuses on observable behaviour or responses. It is rather like the environmental perspective in that it is outcome-oriented rather than process-directed like the psychodynamic perspective. Those who favour such an approach seek to understand how behaviour is learnt. Behavioural perspectives suggest that since behaviour is learnt, it can also be unlearnt and their techniques have been used in social work with a range of different service users, for example drug and alcohol service users, people with learning disabilities and those experiencing neurotic disorders, and work with offenders. Thus behaviour can be learnt through observation, modelling and imitation.

In John's commentary we can see evidence that perhaps this is John's view; he talks of wanting his boys 'to see' (observation) that marriages can last, and the importance he attaches to modelling in his youth work with young men. Behaviour can also be encouraged through positive reinforcement, for instance by the use of praise, particularly with children, or with a reward system, and unwanted behaviour discouraged by consistent negative reinforcement, for example ignoring certain behaviours, the withdrawal of a treat, or punishment. There are also behavioural approaches that emphasise cognitive processes; thus our beliefs or feelings about particular events or people can affect our behaviour, and these feelings will need to be challenged in order to change behaviour. The fact that John describes himself as wanting to be a role model for the children with whom he comes into contact may also give us some clues about John's beliefs and values.

Environmental Theories

Environmental theories include systemic theories, ecological theories and post-modern theories (Bronfenbrenner, 1979; Payne, 2005b). Environmental or social explanations about growth and development focus on the individual's social environment and how this can impact on our development. This approach seeks to understand people's development as most significantly influenced by their social environment, such as familial relationships (the micro-level); the local community and the individual's relationship within it, such as school, the workplace, or religious or political affiliation (the mid-level) and the widest, macro-level, which takes into consideration more formal social factors such as socioeconomic status, gender and sexual identity, and cultural and ethnic identity for example. These factors are taken into consideration in forming a judgement about how much one's development has been influenced by environmental issues.

In John's case, we might be interested to learn more about his Irish background – was this significant for him? Was religion a significant factor in his upbringing? He mentions being reluctant to talk about how he felt when his parents separated – does John feel that as a boy he was expected not to talk about his emotions? How does John feel his upbringing has influenced his view on family life? We might speculate here about the notions of manhood or being manly that may have impacted on John's early life. He comments on the fact that he is able to cook and that, as far as he is concerned, this is not usually seen as a manly attribute. We also note that he left school at the age of 16 and married relatively early. Social background may have played a significant part in these choices and may have shaped his view of himself, perhaps indicated by his comment about his surprise at being offered a place on the social work course – maybe he has taken on board messages about university not being 'for the likes of him'.

Conclusion

In this chapter we have seen briefly how the 'life snake' has two main benefits. Firstly, it can be used to develop our self-awareness of the issues we consider relevant and how these may have shaped our view of the world around us (and to help develop our understanding of how we view the world.) Secondly, it shows how key events can give us clues about what may be of importance in the life of an individual and may still have an impact on our current life. It points towards a way of theorising someone's life – but is not intended to give us all the answers.

We may also see, like John, that when we begin to consider this, we inadvertently start to provide explanations about our life history, and this is the beginning of us recognising that we already have an informal understanding of the events that have shaped our development. Without necessarily knowing it, John identified several perspectives of human growth and development to explain significant events. As we identify these perspectives, we move from an informal understanding to a more formal understanding of the theories that are necessary to begin to help us understand how people develop and grow, and the realisation of how events and feelings can significantly impact on us and shape who we become. Of course, this is only the beginning; in having a theoretical framework for helping us to understand and explain behaviour and development, we also need to have the tools and skills that are required for working with service users.

It is perhaps the most important function of the teaching that we are not attempting to teach a truth about the way the world is by introducing theories but rather to show you that

> what makes theories worth reading and discussing is not the assumption that they mirror reality but that they serve as suggestions or estimations. They help us arrange our minds. (Stott and Bowman, 1996, p. 172)

The aim of this chapter about human development is not to argue that there is one valid interpretation, nor to be able to choose the correct model for any given situation, but rather to acquire the skills of evaluating the relative strengths and weaknesses of different alternatives (Roer-Strier, 2005, p. 314). This should help us to develop our critical thinking, rather than uncritically trying to offer a bag of tricks into which you can dip to find a suitable theoretical explanation to fit and so match to it the 'proper' intervention. The next major step in promoting thinking about theories and the understanding of how they can be relevant is to invite you to come up with your own examples, to test out your knowledge. Even with very basic information, as illustrated with the life snake, you can begin to arrange your thinking and making assumptions, or trying to justify your thinking, by reference to general theories about human development.

The main aim of this method is to prompt you to ask 'why might that be the case' and then to try to connect the answers to theoretical perspectives which may or may not justify those initial assumptions. You should be able to use the material in this chapter to ask questions about how people develop, grow up and grow older, the ways people may assume, or tell us, this happens and our own experiences of reflecting on these processes. It is clear we can examine our experiences and those of other people we read about and revise them in the light of our changing understanding of theories about human growth and development. We should expect that this process of constant evaluation and re-evaluation never ends. We should feel a sense of achievement at being able to incorporate this into our developing view of ourselves as critical practitioners.

REVIEW QUESTIONS

1 What four main groups of theories about growing up can you identify?

2 What are the main points of comparison and contrast between any two of these theories?

FURTHER READING

Biological theories

Davey, B. (ed.) (2001) *Birth to old Age: Health in Transition*, Milton Keynes, Open University Press

Behavioural theories and psychodynamic theories

Beckett, C. (2002) *Human Growth and Development*, London, Sage

Berger, K.S. (2004) *The Developing Person across the Lifespan* (6th edn) New York, Worth

Psychodynamic theories

Bronfenbrenner, U. (1979) *The Ecology of Human Development*, Cambridge, MA, Harvard University Press

Environmental theories

Winston, R. (2003) *Human Instinct*, London, BBC

Winston, R. (2004) *The Human Mind*, London, BBC

Resource file

Child development: The nature versus nurture debate

For many years debates have continued about whether people's current thoughts, feelings and actions are shaped more by their physical, physiological, genetic makeup (nature) than by their upbringing, including parenting, neighbourhood, cultural and environmental factors (nurture). Researchers and practitioners continue to argue whether genetic factors (nature) are more important than environmental (nurture) factors in contributing to the development of the child.

The predominant view of development is in terms of biological and physiological processes, as Piaget (1963) views it, divided into sensorimotor, pre-operational (aged 2–4), intuitive (aged 4–7), concrete operational (aged 7–11), formal operational (aged 12 and over). Piaget creates several substages, describing how the child mentally constructs physical or mental actions, assimilates new experiences and accommodes, that is, modifies, his or her existing ways of constructing the world to adjust to new experiences or generate new constructions.

An important area of research and debate has been children's *language development*. Three important perspectives on understanding how children develop language are those based on *biological, social learning* and *social constructionist* assumptions:

1. Chomsky (1968), a linguist, takes the biological perspective, arguing that people are born with a genetic linguistic inheritance, or a biologically programmed language acquisition device (LAD), so language is innate and this inherited store is triggered by external environmental factors, rather than being learned according to (for example Skinner's) behaviourist assumptions (see Chapter 42).

2. Among the social learning theorists, there have been two important streams of ideas: those of Piaget (he and Chomsky were opposed) and Vigotsky (he and Piaget were opposed):

   ■ Piaget did not believe that language influences cognitive development (how we perceive, think and feel), rather the reverse of this; children's language reflects their thoughts and was one way of expressing them.

   ■ Vygotsky (1978) believed that language plays an important part in children's communication and cognitive development.

3. Some more recent researchers, notably Lois Bloom (Bloom and Tinker, 2001), argue that none of these

perspectives are satisfactory because they take 'agency' – the power to act on their own behalf – away from the child, on the basis that either the biological makeup of the child or other wider, social factors are responsible for how the child learns language. These researchers argue that children are 'intentional', that is, actively able to 'construct' their world on the basis of the meanings they give to what they feel, think, say and do.

Development of personality or proneness to illness

The multiple factors leading to a particular personality or illness cannot be reduced to a single cause. Only in a minority of cases can a single 'cause' be held completely responsible for a particular outcome. The belief that this is so is called *determinism* and it is preferable to work on the basis of *probabilities* and the *risk* of an outcome, rather than the certainty that it will come about. Two examples – both extreme views from the nature and nurture camps – are as follows. The nature view is that a particular man's *genetic inheritance* is entirely responsible for his tendency towards criminal activity as a boy and his record of violence towards women as an adult, leading to him serving a life sentence for murder. The nurture view is that a particular woman's personality traits, her pattern of depression, mental illness and eventual suicide were entirely due to *environmental* factors, such as the family she was born into, the family's social circumstances and the way she was brought up.

One of the main ways in which researchers attempt to discover whether nature or nurture is the key to understanding people's personality traits, proneness to certain physical disorders and mental health problems is the study of twins and adopted children. Situations where twin babies born from a single egg (monozygotic twins) are brought up in one household or are adopted at birth provide researchers with ideal experimental conditions to study the relative significance of nature and nurture.

Professor Sir Michael Rutter, an authority on child development and child psychopathology, has evaluated the substantial body of research on both sides of the nature–nurture debate and has reached a balanced view. The use of statistical techniques to quantify different behavioural and genetic factors has limitations. One way of overcoming these is to assess whether the weight of research findings in studies conducted using many different methods is towards similar conclusions. Using this approach, we can conclude that 'there are substantial genetic and environmental effects on almost all types of behaviour and all forms of psychopathology or mental disorder' (Rutter, 2006, p. 60).

However, we cannot determine in quantitative terms without all reasonable doubt the causal effects of a particular genetic or environmental factor on the behaviour of a person or their subsequent pattern of mental illness or health. Rutter concludes that:

> there is not, and cannot be, any absolute value for the strength of genetic influences on a trait, no matter how accurately the trait is measured or how carefully the genetic effect is assessed. (Rutter, 2006, p. 60)

The relative importance of genetic and environmental factors is such that neither determines absolutely a particular outcome in terms of behaviour or mental illness. Although genetic influences are significant, for instance in shaping proneness to autism, attention deficit disorder and dyslexia (Rutter, 2006, pp. 168–9), the interaction with them of particular environmental factors in particular circumstances is also crucial in shaping a specific outcome (Rutter, 2006, p. 207).

Rutter's work is by no means the last word on this debate about nature and nurture. Genetic screening and manipulation are rapidly developing fields with implications for research and practice. A key area for future research is the implications for personality, behaviour and psychopathology of the interplay between genes and environmental factors.

FURTHER READING

Bloom, L. and Tinker, E. (2001) The Intentionality Model and Language Acquisition: Engagement, Effort and the Essential Tension in Development, *Monographs of the Society for Research in Child Development*, **66**(4) Serial No. 267

Piaget, J. and Inhelder, B. (1969) *The Psychology of the Child*, London, Routledge

Piattelli-Palmarini, M. (ed.) (1980) *Language and Learning: The Debate between J. Piaget and N. Chomsky*, Cambridge, MA, Harvard University Press
This is about Chomsky's writing and work. He is a controversial academic with strong, left-wing political views.

Rutter, M. (2006) *Genes and Behaviour: Nature–Nurture Interplay Explained*, Oxford, Blackwell
Offers a careful explanation of the main arguments.

Vigotsky, L.S. (1978) *The Development of Higher Psychological Processes*, Cambridge, MA, Harvard University Press
Explains his social development theory.

Part II

Knowledge for Practice

Part III
Knowledge for Practice

Introduction

Part III of this book aims to show how knowledge and well-established good practice, related to research findings where necessary, underpin key areas of practice.
There is a good deal of discussion about what is called 'evidence-based practice'
(EBP). The increasing popularity of evidence-based practice has come about for
three main reasons:

- the search for improved standards of practice

- the search for professional credibility by professions and aspiring professionals

- the widespread concern of politicians and managers to provide and deliver quality
  services at a known and even standard across different geographical areas. It is
  sometimes stated that this will avoid what is called the 'postcode lottery' of the
  quality of services being uneven and varying according to where you live.

Evidence-based practice is fully accepted by some but controversial with others. In
general, research of a more traditional, experimental kind tends to appeal more to
managers and practitioners in areas such as medicine, where research of this type is
more straightforward to organise. The effects on sickness rates and death rates of
specific operations or treatments are easier to measure than the impact on older
people who are infirm and depressed of moving them from their own homes to
daycare or residential homes. The fact is that a relatively small proportion of
research studies in social care, as opposed to healthcare, match up to the rigorous
requirements of traditional experimental researchers. In order to back up and justify
evidence-based practice, the quality of the research evidence has to be verified, by
being able to answer 'yes' to three questions:

- where the evidence came from: Was the source a reputable piece of research?

- the soundness of the evidence: Is the research verified as valid and reliable?

- the relevance of the evidence: Does it help to improve practice?

What we can do in this part of the book is achieve the more modest goal of
reviewing the knowledge base in key areas of practice. This can provide a basis for
discussing issues, including the more controversial aspects, as and when the occasion
arises. Often, we find it is at least as important to debate these issues, as to argue
about why, in so many areas of practice, there is insufficient research to point conclu-
sively towards a preferred method of practice.

It is necessary to retain our criticality when we read research. Hopefully, the research is done well, but it is a general guide to practice and not to be applied to our situation without careful thought. The key to developing skilled evidence-based practice is to make links between what we know about research into this or that aspect and the particular circumstances we are facing, deciding what is and is not relevant, before we decide what to do.

FURTHER READING

Dawes, M., Davies, P., Gray, A., Mant, J., Seers, K. and Snowball, R. (2000) *Evidence-based Practice: A Primer for Health Care Professionals*, London, Churchill Livingstone

Muir Gray, J.A. (1997) *Evidence-Based Healthcare*, Edinburgh, Churchill Livingstone

Newman, T., Moseley, A., Tierney, S. and Ellis, A. (2005) *Evidence-based Social Work: A Guide for the Perplexed*, Lyme Regis, Russell House

---

9 Safeguarding Adults

ROBERT ADAMS

This chapter deals with the linked issues of adult abuse and measures to tackle it. Increasing public and professional concern about the abuse of vulnerable adults has received impetus from the repeated exposure of child abuse scandals, as well as from a growing awareness of violence against women.

Adult Abuse: Ignored and Overlooked

From the 1960s, there has been a succession of exposures and inquiry reports into abuse, particularly of people with learning disabilities and mental health problems (Buckinghamshire County Council, 1998; Camden and Islington NHS Trust, 1999; Commission for Health Improvement, 2003). Until the 1990s, adult abuse was not tackled because:

- It was overshadowed by the attention paid to child abuse (Stevenson, 1996).
- The variety of settings in which adult abuse occurs and types of abuse did not create a single issue to focus on. Abuse can involve older people, disabled people

and people with mental illnesses. It can take place in a day or residential setting or at home by relatives and other carers for older people, disabled people and people with mental illnesses.

■ Abuse of adults tends to be underreported, for several reasons: people experiencing it may be vulnerable through age, disability or mental illness; abusers may intimidate their victims into silence; abused people may judge that it is pointless to complain or, if in an institution, may feel they have nobody to tell.

What we Mean by Abuse

As important as the above, of course, is that much abuse is not recognised as abusive. To be hurtful and harmful, abuse does not have to constitute a sexual attack or leave bruises on the body. Unfortunately, elder abuse has no legal standing and no standard UK definition (House of Commons Health Committee, 2004). According to the Department of Health, 'Abuse is a violation of an individual's human and civil rights by any other person or persons' (DoH and Home Office, 2000, p. 9). Types of abuse include *neglect* and *acts of omission* and *physical, psychological* (including *emotional*), *sexual, financial*, as well as *institutional* (providing inadequate facilities in a day centre or unjust and stigmatising regimes in a residential setting) abuse, or *discriminatory* abuse involving sexism, racism, harassment and discrimination based on disability. Many of these are underresearched. For instance, we do not know why staff abuse older people in hospitals and people with disabilities in residential settings, or why overmedication of antipsychotic drugs for people with dementia may be used to control them (House of Commons Health Committee, 2004, p. 18, para. 50).

Common symptoms of abuse by staff or carers include depression, distress or agitation when the person comes near; and signs include bruises, burns, fractures, unexplained incontinence, sexually transmitted diseases, and bruising of thighs and genital areas. Signs of neglect include loss of weight, hypothermia, dehydration and persistent infections. On its own, one of these signs should not be used to predict abuse. A good assessment will include systematic attempts to corroborate the evidence from more than one direction, that is, looking for at least two, and preferably more, signs. We should always talk to the person on their own where we cannot be overheard, in their main, first language, to find out their views.

We should be careful about how we define *vulnerability*, in case we imply that some people's weaknesses bring on the abuse. Government guidance (DoH and Home Office, 2000, pp. 8–9) defines a vulnerable person as a person

> in need of community care services by reason of mental or other disability, age or illness; and who is or may be unable to take care of him or herself, or unable to protect him or herself against significant harm or exploitation.

The House of Commons Health Committee (2004) widens this beyond people who use care services and we should bear in mind that able-bodied people may be vulnerable, simply by virtue of where they live or whether, for example, they are perceived by predatory offenders as potential targets for theft exploitation.

Annual statistics from Cambridgeshire (Cambridgeshire County Council, 2006) of 364 cases of adult abuse reported to adult support services from April 2005 to March 2006 show the following:

- Proved abuse   167
- Proved not abuse   56
- Still being investigated   24
- Inconclusive   117 (these require ongoing monitoring).

Of the proved abuse cases, the overwhelming majority were older people (120), followed by learning disability (24), mental health (13), physical disability (9) and sensory services (1).

Abuse by Carers

In health and social care, one of the more difficult aspects of abuse to expose is the abuse of people by their informal carers – usually close family relatives – or carers employed by them – often called personal assistants. Every form of service to vulnerable adults – including personal assistants supplied to service users and carers using direct payments – has the potential for abuse.

How does abuse by carers arise? Superficially, it appears that people who are more dependent create more responsibility and, potentially, stress for their carers. However, the investigation into serious abuse of people with learning disabilities at Budock hospital, Cornwall in 2006 (Healthcare Commission (HC) and Commission for Social Care Inspection (CSCI), 2006) prompted an England-wide investigation of learning disabilities services, in the light of other allegations of abuse in Norfolk and south London. A joint press release on 5 July 2006 by the heads of the HC and CSCI notes:

> Instances of abuse can be symptomatic of services that have been neglected for too long. They are the most serious signs of a problem, but our concerns are much broader. We detect a widespread lack of understanding about the rights and needs of people with learning disabilities.

Despite a lack of evidence about whether education and training of workers helps to reduce or prevent abuse, there are concerns about the lack of registration and adequate training of health and social care staff (House of Commons Health Committee, 2004, p. 27, para. 93). This reinforces arguments for abuse victims to receive the support of an independent advocate, rather than for this role to be undertaken by relatives and/or carers.

Madden (2005) points out that despite the fact that direct payment service users will have access to staff checking systems via the Criminal Records Bureau (CRB) and the Protection of Vulnerable Adults list does not mean they will be informed, supported and assertive enough to raise their concerns about the personal assistants they employ.

Madden highlights the complexities of the situation, arising partly from the fact that direct payments are intended to be an empowering measure. He says:

This is not to argue that service users managing direct payments should have to undertake checks on the staff they employ – that would surely prolong the view that vulnerable people cannot think for themselves. It may well be true that if people are in control of their lives and the support they need, they may be less likely to find themselves in abusive situations. But, as yet, there is no research evidence to substantiate this – just because service users are to be given more choice over their care does not automatically guarantee their safety. (Madden, 2005, p. 22)

Much abuse is by carers and because the true incidence of this is partly a matter for conjecture, its causes are also somewhat uncertain. Theories about why abuse by carers occurs include the lack of support and training for them, the negative impact on their work, leisure and family life, their problems in coping with difficult behaviour from the person they care for, and the increased stress on them in cases where the person they care for becomes increasingly dependent. Circumstances in which the carer does the caring out of a sense of duty also increase the risk of abuse by the carer.

Conventionally, accounts of abuse focus on the cases where individuals have been subjected to abuse. However, abuse does not have to be sexual or physical to be harmful to vulnerable adults.

Practice study

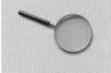

Maggie

Take the case of Maggie, a 24-year-old woman with a learning disability, who has hinted that a previous carer has taken charge of her money and not given some of it back. The worker takes on the task of advocate for her, contributing to safeguarding her by making sure she has direct access to the services she wants (under the Disability Discrimination Act 1995). Under the Mental Capacity Act 2005, Maggie is also protected through working with an officer appointed by the Court of Protection through the Public Guardianship Office. An independent mental capacity advocate (IMCA) is provided for her under the Act.

Institutional abuse of adults sometimes occurs. There is evidence of adults being abused in mental health settings (Williams and Keating, 1999, pp. 130–51), older people being abused in residential care (Glendenning, 1999, pp. 173–90) and people with learning disabilities being abused (Brown, 1999, pp. 81–109).

It is difficult to estimate the incidence of abuse of adults in the care sector, since many of the victims, by definition, are vulnerable and, we might anticipate, are less likely to complain. An analysis of calls to Elder Abuse Response – the national helpline of Action on Elder Abuse founded in 1993 – showed that during the two years 1997–99, 1421 calls were received, two-thirds from older people or their relatives, two-fifths reporting psychological abuse, one-fifth each reporting physical and financial abuse, one-tenth neglect and 2 per cent sexual abuse. Three times as many women as men were reported as being abused, over a quarter identifying a worker as the abuser, most being care workers and nurses the next largest group. Most of the calls concerned abuse in people's homes (Jenkins et al., 2000, pp. 4–5). Of 3,000 calls received in 2006, a quarter concerned a total of more than £2 million coerced or stolen from older people (www.timesonline.co.uk/article/0,,2-2573782,00.html).

The fact that the overwhelming majority of murders are by spouses or partners, coupled with evidence of domestic violence and child and adult abuse, is evidence that the family can be a particularly violent institution. The accumulated emotional burden and financial stresses of one person caring for another, dependent and possibly very vulnerable, close relative in a household over a considerable period of time can increase the likelihood of abuse. However, Pillemer (1986) states that this is not a causal factor.

Family Violence

Family violence extends beyond violence between men and women and can include any family member. A key area of abuse by adults against adults involves acts of violence against women. The growth of the women's movement since the 1960s has contributed to a growing awareness of criminal violence against women. The majority of offenders are adult males, but a proportion of violent acts are carried out by females and young people. Physical violence is at one extreme, but emotional pressure is an abuse of power and can be just as abusive and distressing. For many years, so-called 'domestic violence' was ignored or denied as a serious personal and social problem. Nowadays, it is widely recognised as criminal violence in the home. Labelling it thus is recognition that it is not just a domestic matter but equivalent to other crimes in society, a social problem with serious, long-term consequences both for victims, other household members and the health of society as a whole.

The prevention of violence against women is dependent on identifying the factors causing the violence, a task made more difficult by the complexity of the many causative factors identified by researchers (Harway and O'Neil, 1999, pp. 5–11). Among many possible preventive measures, some embodied in the Domestic Violence, Crime and Victims Act 2004, the following are particularly important: educating girls and young women into cooperating and supporting each other; empowering women to prevent them being trapped in abusive households; and using cognitive-behavioural approaches to help couples to understand how emotional and physical violence arises and how to avoid it.

Practice study

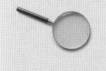

Ava

Ava is a support and advocacy worker with women who have experienced criminal violence in the home from their partners. Her role is to raise awareness of this violence, offer services to women and their children and contribute to protecting them. The range of issues she works with includes:

- enabling women to deal positively with violence
- helping women who have left home to find fresh accommodation
- building the confidence of women who feel they are victims of violence
- enabling families to tackle the effects of abuse.

Approaches to Adult Protection

In England, multiagency codes of practice aiming to tackle and prevent abuse of vulnerable adults developed in the light of the publication of the official guidance *No Secrets* (DoH and Home Office, 2000). In Wales, similar developments occurred following the publication of guidance (National Assembly for Wales and Home Office, 2000). In England, the publication of *No Secrets* was followed by guidance on the protection of vulnerable adults (DoH, 2001g), through developing a register of people judged as potential abusers – the POVA (Protection of Vulnerable Adults) arrangements. Four years later the Association of Directors of Social Services (ADSS) published its own guidance for safeguarding adults (ADSS, 2005). By 2006, the CSCI took responsibility for promoting the safety of adults receiving a service it regulates.

Protection of Vulnerable Adults (POVA)

The Protection of Vulnerable Adults (POVA) scheme was introduced in England and Wales in a phased programme from 2004, as required in the Care Standards Act 2000. This created a list of people considered unsuitable to work with vulnerable adults in England and Wales. People considered harmful to vulnerable adults could be referred by registered providers of care for inclusion on the list. These providers also could ask for checks against the POVA list as part of an application for a CRB disclosure regarding people applying for jobs in care work. National minimum standards were introduced for residential care (DoH, 2000b). Some imaginative initiatives developed, for example the learning disability pilot scheme based in a crisis centre on Tyneside. There, women with learning difficulties were able to access a mainstream sexual abuse or rape counselling service (Bartlett, 2005, p. 41).

Under the POVA procedures, 'safeguarding adults' partnerships have been set up from 2005 in each CSCI area. Alerts may be triggered by inspectors, sometimes when inspecting or investigating a complaint. Safeguarding inspectors will deal with any safeguarding adults matters arising from this. Where there are concerns about the fitness of the manager of an establishment, a registered person, or service or a breach of the Care Standards Act 2000, the CSCI could be the main investigating agency. A safeguarding plan should be produced through a case conference, normally reviewed within six months.

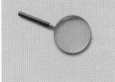

Practice study

Malek

The following example follows the guidelines for good practice developed by the ADSS (2005, pp. 41–9), based on the *No Secrets* government initiative (DoH and Home Office, 2000), which led to most local authorities appointing a lead officer in adult protection work.

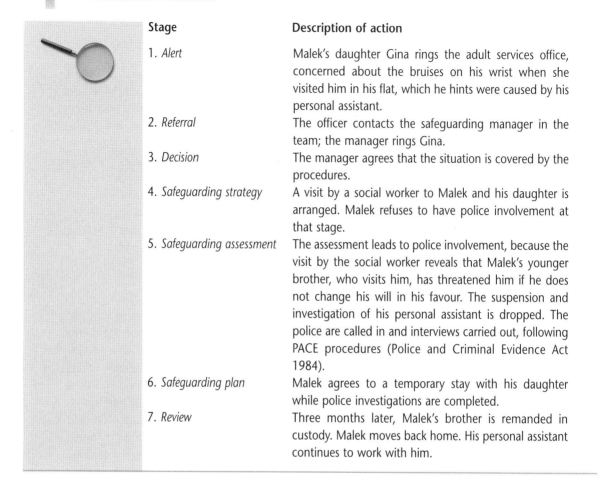

Stage	Description of action
1. *Alert*	Malek's daughter Gina rings the adult services office, concerned about the bruises on his wrist when she visited him in his flat, which he hints were caused by his personal assistant.
2. *Referral*	The officer contacts the safeguarding manager in the team; the manager rings Gina.
3. *Decision*	The manager agrees that the situation is covered by the procedures.
4. *Safeguarding strategy*	A visit by a social worker to Malek and his daughter is arranged. Malek refuses to have police involvement at that stage.
5. *Safeguarding assessment*	The assessment leads to police involvement, because the visit by the social worker reveals that Malek's younger brother, who visits him, has threatened him if he does not change his will in his favour. The suspension and investigation of his personal assistant is dropped. The police are called in and interviews carried out, following PACE procedures (Police and Criminal Evidence Act 1984).
6. *Safeguarding plan*	Malek agrees to a temporary stay with his daughter while police investigations are completed.
7. *Review*	Three months later, Malek's brother is remanded in custody. Malek moves back home. His personal assistant continues to work with him.

Safeguarding adults should form part of the agency's mainstream policies, including values. There are four main values linked with the protection of vulnerable adults: independence and self-determination; choice; rights; and fulfilment. It is one thing to list these, but quite another to apply them in a complex situation. Many issues arise in adult protection work that cannot be 'solved' by a quick-fix formula. For example, in different faith communities there may be a diversity of attitudes to abuse and protection and a worker who challenges family customs with regard to caring for adults may be accused of intervening in a racist way. There may be a tendency for workers either to overintervene or underintervene by not being conversant with legislation and practice guidance. The best way forward is to engage in long-term work with people in faith communities to explore the diversity of views and practices and become familiar with cultures and beliefs.

Clearly, the recognition of abuse is an early stage on the path towards preventing future abuse (Clarke and Ogg, 1994) and some areas such as financial abuse will be helped by legislation, such as the Mental Capacity Act 2005. However, it is essential that practitioners are familiar with the nature and signs of abuse, understand the complexities of current legislation, know how to carry out current agency guidance in line with POVA and PACE procedures, appreciate how to deal with risk assessment in relation to adult abuse, and work effectively with other practitioners, including those from other agencies and professions.

Conclusion

This brief survey of adult abuse and protection has shown the range of types of abuse and the settings in which they occur. We have explored some of the difficulties preventing the true extent of abuse being exposed. On the positive side, we have given some indications of policy and practice initiatives aiming to safeguard adults, including indications of how to prevent abuse occurring. You may need all your confidence and assertiveness to complain or 'blow the whistle' when you encounter abusive practice (see Resource File: Making a Complaint/Whistleblowing, at the end of Chapter 36).

REVIEW QUESTIONS

1 Can you name at least seven main types of abuse of vulnerable adults?

2 What does research indicate as to the main cause of abuse?

3 What policies are being implemented to safeguard vulnerable adults?

FURTHER READING

Essential practice guidance

ADSS (Association of Directors of Social Services) (2005) *Safeguarding Adults: A National Framework of Standards for Good Practice and Outcomes in Adult Protection Work*, London, ADSS

DoH and Home Office (2000) *No Secrets: Guidance on Developing and Implementing Multi-agency Policies and Procedures to Protect Vulnerable Adults from Abuse*, London, TSO

DoH (2006) *The Protection of Vulnerable Adults Scheme in England and Wales for Adult Placement Schemes, Domiciliary Care Agencies and Care Homes: A Practical Guide*, London, DoH

Other reading

AIMS for Adult Protection (1998) *The Alerter's Guide*, Brighton, Pavilion Publishing

Biggs, S., Phillipson, C. and Kingston, P. (1995) *Elder Abuse in Perspective*, Buckingham, Open University Press

Brammer, A. and Biggs, S. (1998) 'Defining Elder Abuse', *Journal of Social Welfare and Family Law*, **20**(3): 285–304

Clough, R. (ed.) (1996) *The Abuse of Care in Residential Institutions*, London, Whiting & Birch

Domestic Violence, Crime and Victims Act 2004

Journal of Adult Protection
    This contains many practice-based articles.

Lockley, P. (1999) *Counselling Women in Violent Relationships*, London, Free Association Books

McCreadie, C. (1996) *Elder Abuse: Update on Research*, London, Age Concern/Institute of Gerontology, King's College

O'Callaghan, A. and Murphy, G. (2003) 'The Impact of Abuse on Men and Women with Severe Learning Disabilities and their Families', *British Journal of Learning Disabilities*, **31**: 175–80

Pritchard, J. (ed.) (2001) *Good Practice with Vulnerable Adults*, London, Jessica Kingsley

Stanley, N., Manthorpe, J. and Penhale, B. (eds) (1999) *Institutional Abuse: Perspectives across the Life Course*, London, Routledge

Stevenson, O. (1996) *Elder Protection in the Community: What We Can Learn from Child Protection*, London, Age Concern/Kings College

RESOURCE FILE: Making a Complaint/Whistleblowing, at the end of Chapter 36

WEBSITES:　　　www.respond.org.uk
　　　　　　　　www.elderabuse.org.uk
　　　　　　　　www.jrf.org.uk/knowledge/findinfs/

Protecting Children

LIZ DAVIES

Learning outcomes

By the end of this chapter, you should be able to:

■ UNDERSTAND the policy context of child protection

■ KNOW how child protection procedures work

■ BE AWARE OF what direct work with abused children may entail.

It is an adult responsibility to protect children. The Resource File: Child Protection Policy, at the end of this chapter, indicates how child protection policy has shifted over the past 50 years and defines what we mean by child abuse. The Children Act (CA) 2004 places a duty on local authorities to ensure that every child has the support they need to 'stay safe' (CA 2004). The main principle of the Children Act 1989 is the paramountcy of the child's welfare, which underpins all other aspects of legislation with regard to children. The United Nations Convention on the Rights of the Child (UNCRC) stated that 'government should make sure that children and young people are protected from abuse, neglect and harm by the people looking after them' (UNCRC, Article 19; CA 1989).

It is only by all agencies working together according to national guidance (DfES, 2006a) and local procedures (ALG, 2003) that children gain protection and it is the responsibility of the Local Safeguarding Children Board to ensure that all professionals in their area train together, share common guidance, reach agreement on protocols and learn the lessons raised by child abuse inquiries.

It may seem obvious that a child's welfare is the first consideration but in fact this is often lost in the context of adult agendas. Childism, oppression of children, is not as recognised as other concepts of discrimination such as racism or sexism. Children may slip through the protective net laid down in law and policy or may be excluded completely from the protective systems.

Shortcomings in Policy and Practice

We start this chapter by listing 11 shortcomings in policy and practice with an initial, critical comment, each of which would repay more detailed examination. They are as follows:

1. Children are increasingly defined as presenting a risk to society. This criminalisation of children diverts professional attention away from them as possible victims of child abuse. The age of criminal responsibility is low – 10 years (this being the age at which children become liable for prosecution through the courts), and increasingly children are being locked in prison for longer periods of time for less serious crimes and are even kept in isolation cells – 28 children have died in prison since 1990 (www.howardleague.org; Goldson and Coles, 2005). The Children Act 1989 applies to children in custody but once in prison they are often out of sight of the professional social workers.

2. The numbers of children who go missing are not recorded. A police investigation based at Heathrow airport found that, within a three-month period, 28 unaccompanied minors were missing and not found (Biehal et al., 2003; Metropolitan Police, 2003) and a report in 2007 showed 48 trafficked children were missing from care in the north of England (Lewis, 2007). Other children run away and are sometimes described as throwaways as one-fifth of them have not even been reported missing by their parents or carers (Children's Society, 2004). Missing children may be victims of trafficking for sexual or domestic exploitation, used in abusive images or sold on the international adoption market. There is only one safe house for children in the UK.

3. Children asked about child abuse describe bullying, particularly racial bullying, as very serious abuse and yet this is not recognised as a category of abuse. One charity states that 5 per cent of children referred to them have tried to commit suicide (www.bullying.co.uk).

4. Common assault of a child is subject to the legal defence of the parent or carer using 'reasonable chastisement' (CA 2004, s. 58). Childcare organisations campaigned unsuccessfully for this clause to be abolished, arguing that children deserve the same protection under the law as adults. Children have said that they consider physical punishment of any kind to be harmful (Willow and Hyder, 1998).

5. More than 2,000 children, including babies, are detained in immigration detention centres every year. They have not committed any crime but are locked up behind high fences and there are concerns about their access to healthcare and education. Detentions last from 7 to 268 days (www.noplaceforachild.org).

6. By exempting itself from the UN Protocol to the Convention on the Rights of the Child (2004), the UK reserves the right for young people of 16 years and above in the armed forces to take part in hostilities. There is a lack of clarity as to whether

the Children Act 1989 applies to young soldiers (http://193.194.138.190/html/menu2/6/crc/treaties/opac.htm).

7. Dr Falkov studied cases of children who had died from abuse where a parent had a mental illness and found that the professional focus was commonly on the adult rather than the children (Falkov, 1996).

8. Female genital mutilation is a crime in the UK and yet there have been no prosecutions since 1985. This form of abuse may not always be investigated because professionals are reluctant to intervene in 'cultural' issues. A culturally sensitive response is required but the paramountcy principle must apply (Dustin and Davies, 2007).

9. Police operations such as Operation Ore and Wonderland locate thousands of abusive images of children – each image showing a crime against a child – yet the scale of the crime is such that few of the child victims are traced (www.sundayherald.com/print30756).

10. Sometimes children are mistakenly perceived as responsible for abusive situations. Professionals must respect children's wishes and feelings but not if these are inconsistent with promoting the child's welfare. If a child wishes to be a 'sex worker' or live with a known child sex abuser, these situations are clearly not in the child's best interests despite their wishes and protective action must be implemented

11. Research by Women's Aid found that, within a 10-year period, 29 children in 13 families had died during contact visits with an abusive parent. It was said that children caught within conflictual parental relationships are not being protected by effective courts and professional decision-making (www.womensaid.org.uk).

An Overview of Policy

Since 1945 and the death of Dennis O'Neill who was beaten to death by his foster carer (Monckton, 1945), there have been numerous child abuse inquiries (DHSS, 1982), some focusing on individual children who died from abuse, such as Maria Colwell (Secretary of State for Social Services, 1974), Jasmine Beckford (Blom-Cooper, 1985), Kimberley Carlisle (London Borough of Greenwich, 1987), Tyra Henry (London Borough of Lambeth, 1987) and Victoria Climbié (Laming, 2003), some addressing the abuse of children within institutions, such as the Pindown Inquiry in Staffordshire (Levy and Kahan, 1991) and the Waterhouse Inquiry in North Wales (Waterhouse, 2000) and others about sexual and organised abuse such as those in Cleveland (Butler Sloss, 1988) and the Orkneys (Clyde, 1992; Batty 2003; Corby 2005). These have provided all the information professionals need about how to protect children from abuse.

Why then do about a hundred children every year die from abuse by those entrusted with their care? Comprehensive legislation, policy and practice guidance is firmly in place but the problem inevitably lies in effective implementation. Children up to the age of 18 years old, or who are the subject of multiagency child protection planning through formal processes, are usually safeguarded. Children die from abuse or suffer serious harm mainly when these procedures are not in place. They may not have come to the attention of the statutory agencies or, having been referred, may not have been defined as children in need of protection. Lack of professional compliance with statutory requirements commonly lies in defective systems rather than individual responsibility (Reder et al., 1993).

Time and again the inquiries referred to above have emphasised the allocation of complex cases to inexperienced, untrained, unsupervised staff with unrealistic case-loads working within chaotic work environments. Underlying this situation is the serious public misperception that protecting children is simple common sense. Few public resources are allocated to the protection of children who, as they do not vote, have no political voice.

Since 2000, childcare policy has emphasised the assessment of children in need to promote children's welfare (CA 1989, s. 17; DoH, 2000a). Initial assessments of seven days may be followed by a more in-depth core assessment. There has been less emphasis on implementing proactive child protection investigations under the duties stated in section 47 (CA 1989) and *Working Together to Safeguard Children* (DfES, 2006a), which require statutory authorities to investigate when they have reasonable cause to suspect a child is suffering, or is likely to suffer, significant harm. Child abuse inquiries fit uneasily within static timescales and although assessment informs investigation, the process requires different skills (Munro, 2002). Victoria Climbié, who died from many serious injuries inflicted by her carers, was defined as a child in need requiring a family support response because of housing and refugee issues rather than as a child needing protection and section 47 (CA 1989) was not implemented (Laming, 2003, 6.217).

It is only through debate and analysis that professionals working together mainly within formal structures such as conferences reach decisions about when the threshold of 'significant harm' has been reached. The Children Act definition of significant harm refers to the criteria of ill-treatment and impairment of health and development (CA 1989, s. 31). Emails and telephone calls are no replacement for sitting around a table in discussion to assess risk, plan enquiries and consider intervention.

Professionals working together may hypothesise about the cause of an injury or the interpretation of a child's statement or behaviour but this hypothesis must be rigorously tested. Knowledge of research findings as well as reflection derived from supervision will assist judgement. Decisions must be constantly subject to review and re-evaluation because there is often reluctance to revisit decisions reached at the initial stages of investigation.

Protecting Children in Practice

Assessment, investigation and intervention are highly complex tasks. There is a need for the skills of a detective – the ability to question, challenge and critique – and to be prepared to think the unthinkable because the acts of harm committed against children are often beyond comprehension. Children may be harmed through unintentional acts, but those who intentionally abuse children may be deceitful towards professionals and an enquiring mind is essential as is an awareness of the blocks to effective intervention. Professional dangerousness is the process by which professionals unwittingly collude with abusive adults and increase the dangerous dynamics in the family. Typically, they may withdraw from a family because they themselves are afraid of the abusive adult or they falsely convince themselves that all is well in the child's world because they emotionally avoid the horror of the abuse.

Activity 10.1

1. Think about what criteria you might use in differentiating between a section 17 child in need assessment (Children Act 1989) and a section 47 child protection investigation (Children Act 1989). Section 17 requires the local authority to safeguard and promote the welfare of children in need in their area. Section 47 requires the local authority to investigate where there is reasonable cause to suspect that a child is suffering, or is likely to suffer, significant harm. The investigation should include an assessment of the child's needs, including the risk of abuse, the need for protection and the ability of the family to meet the needs of the child.
2. Consider what influenced you in the selection of these criteria.

Here are my reflections. In one case, a child may be left at home alone. How are you going to decide whether this is a case of serious neglect or of no concern at all? It is a matter for multiagency judgement whether:

- a crime of serious neglect has been committed
- child protection or child in need procedures apply
- there is no need for intervention at all.

Perhaps you based your decision on your:

- experience as a child or a parent or from your observation of and interaction with children
- professional experience of a particular case
- cultural or religious perspective on family life
- knowledge of the law and child protection policy and practice guidance
- knowledge of lessons learnt from child abuse inquiries and serious case reviews (Part 8 or serious case reviews take place where a serious incident, such as a child's death, occurs. They check whether lessons can be learnt, what will change as a result and how multiagency joint working will improve, DoH, 1999b, 1999c – see Chapter 33)
- understanding of the concept of neglect
- knowledge base of the subject from research findings.

You might consider the following:

- age and vulnerability of the child, for example physical and learning disability, language and/or communication difficulties

- attitude and circumstances of the parent/carer
- child's view of being left alone
- impact of cultural norms
- previous history of the family
- home environment – warmth, light, food, shelter, locked rooms, safety
- child's access to emergency services or support
- child's responsibilities, for example as a carer for younger children
- exposure to dangerous adults.

A child left home alone will be a prime target of abusers and to intervene effectively at an early stage may prevent this downward spiral into even more serious forms of child abuse and may reduce the pool of vulnerable children available to exploitation by child sex abusers.

Implementing Child Protection Procedures

From the moment a referral is received, the relevant checks must be made. Inquires have shown that mistakes are made when information is incomplete. Key facts often lie buried in old files and undue emphasis is often placed on recent emotive information as opposed to substantive medical facts, children's and carer's statements, known criminal convictions or evidence from prior investigations. Within a section 47 investigation, checks may be made without parental or child consent in order to protect children – the 'need to know' principle is the basis for information-sharing. It is important to work openly with families and to gain consent wherever possible, but ultimately the need to act in the best interests of the child must be the deciding factor.

A strategy discussion between social services and the police will determine whether immediate action is needed to safeguard the child. In practice the vast majority of child protection investigations result in children remaining with their families, but, if necessary, the police can remove children from their parents using the police powers of protection or social workers may apply for an emergency protection order (Children Act 1989, ss. 44 and 48).

Safety is the first priority. It would be quite wrong to interview, examine a child or inform their parents of professional concerns if meanwhile the child was not safe. Even if a child is in hospital, it cannot be assumed that the child is safe as the parent could remove the child at any time. This is a matter for discussion between social workers and the police, with advice from professionals who know the child well such as health visitors, teachers and the GP and in consultation with the local authority solicitors.

Victoria Climbié spoke little when the social worker and police officer interviewed her in hospital to ask her about her injuries caused by a scald. There had already been much information available to professionals such as a history of unexplained and unusual old and recent injuries, a confused family history, evidence of neglect and a prior hospital admission, as well as concerning inconsistent explanations for the scald being either from a kettle, tap or cup. A section 47 investigation was clearly indicated as was legal action to ensure her safety. She should, prior to interview, have been assured of her safety.

A strategy meeting allows police and social workers to discuss the referral in detail and to meet with other professionals who have knowledge of the child and/or circumstances of the referral. This is a meeting for professionals only. The meeting decides whether section 47 inquiries are necessary and which agency should conduct them. In cases of sexual abuse, or serious physical abuse and neglect, police and social workers investigate jointly but sometimes it is agreed that a social worker can investigate 'single agency', for example in cases of emotional abuse or a lower level of neglect. In historic abuse cases, where an adult discloses having been abused as a child, the police will usually investigate unless, following enquiries, it becomes clear that children are currently at risk.

At the strategy meeting it will be decided how an investigation will proceed and whether there is a need for a paediatric assessment or a formal child interview. If criminal proceedings are being considered, then the police will take the lead. The meeting will need to assess the risks to any other children in the household or in contact with the alleged perpetrator, and decisions will be made about sharing information with the parents and carers and who is best placed to conduct the interviews. The family's need for interpreters or intermediaries will be addressed as will the need for specialist advice relating to disability issues, religion or culture.

Accurate recording is a key part of the jigsaw that needs to be in place for safeguarding children. In the Victoria Climbié case, professionals at the strategy meetings made many decisions but did not identify who should complete the tasks, there were no stated timescales, and the majority of the important decisions were never acted on. Clarity in decision-making is essential.

As each stage of the investigation proceeds, there may be a series of strategy meetings, constantly allowing evaluation of the information obtained and assessment of the risk to the child. Thorough investigation may take many weeks. If the case is to progress to a child protection conference, this must take place within 15 days of the decision being agreed (DfES, 2006a, 5.81). This is the main forum for sharing information and assessing risk to the child. Parents and carers are invited unless there is a valid reason for excluding them, such as if they are subject to criminal proceedings or are known to be violent. It is a matter of judgement as to whether children should attend. Their views must be available to the conference – through drawing, writing or recording and some will want to present their views in person.

A decision will be made about whether or not the child needs a child protection plan to be safe. This is a local register of children where there are unresolved child protection issues. There must have been an incident of actual or likely significant harm to the child or, on the basis of research findings, such harm may be predicted. There must also be a continuing risk of harm, decided according to four categories of abuse – physical, sexual, neglect and emotional. Of course all forms of abuse include emotional abuse and so this is only used when it is the sole or main category.

A key worker has a statutory duty to coordinate the child protection plan, ensure that information is shared and the plan implemented. A core group of key professionals and parents meet frequently to implement the plan and a review conference is held three months later and then six-monthly. If the children are not being protected by the plan, then a strategy meeting is convened to reassess the situation and consideration will be given to any legal safeguards required.

Some forms of abuse require more complex multiagency responses. Abuse of children within organised crime networks such as child trafficking for domestic or sexual exploitation or the use of children for abusive images demand a senior level strategy meeting convened by the local authority child protection manager following specific guidance relevant to the organised abuse of children (DfES, 2006, 6.8).

Multiagency child protection procedures focus primarily on the child and family but there must also be a focus on the perpetrators of crimes against children, with the aim of changing the behaviour of the abusive adult or removing them from access to the child. The Multi Agency Protection Panel is the local forum which focuses on adults who pose a risk to children (and vulnerable adults) in the community. Since 1997, this panel is responsible for monitoring convicted sex abusers whose names are on the sex offender register. All professionals must refer adults to this panel if they are thought to pose a risk to children so that protection strategies can be put in place (DfES, 2006a, 12.12).

When professionals disagree about what should be done to protect a child, this must be resolved if children are not to slip through the net. Differences must be addressed through the Local Safeguarding Children Board, which has multiple responsibilities for the protection of children within each locality.

Direct Work with Children

Very few children ever speak about suffering abuse until they reach adulthood. Children who do tell are often met with denial and disbelief by adults and then it is common for them to retract their statements. Retractions actually may indicate that pressure has been placed on the child to remain silent and protect the abuser. Child abuse only exists because it is in a context of secrecy and silence. Abusers rely on the child not telling and other adults not reporting.

To learn more about children's perspectives on child abuse, the very best way is to listen to survivors. Phil Frampton, in his book *Golly in the Cupboard* (2003), provides a wealth of information about a child's experience of abuse within the care system. It is also important to learn from survivors groups such as the National Association of People Abused in Childhood (NAPAC).

Although there are specialists who work therapeutically with children – child psychiatrists, psychologists, psychotherapists and play therapists – it is very important for both health and social care workers to gain basic skills in communication with children. The specialists will always provide consultancy and support. In order to gain a child's perspective, materials such as toys, drawing materials and resource books are essential.

The *Anti-colouring Book* (Striker, 2004) enables the social worker to enter into the child's world by facilitating the child's view without prejudging or imposing professional responses. If there is high suspicion of child sexual abuse or physical harm but with no forensic evidence or disclosure from the child, *My Body My Book* (Peake and Rouf, 1989) provides an excellent resource for work with the child to assess the child's perception of Yes and No touches. This book does not introduce concepts of abuse or contaminate the evidence of the child.

Storytelling allows children to gain healing without any professional interpretation. Davis (1990) provides stories for children addressing a wide range of circumstances. Someone close to the child such as a carer or teacher reads the story, enabling the child to absorb the message contained within it and then relate this message to their unique situation. The *Turning Points* training pack provides many useful basic tools for work with children (NSPCC, 1997). Such materials support recovery from abuse.

It is essential to break the cycle of abuse by listening to children and acting to protect them. In North Wales alone over 2,000 children had been abused within children's homes. Children in the care system became targets for abusers (DoH, 1998c). The importance of professionals being the voice for vulnerable children as whistleblowers was key to exposing the systems that allowed such abuse of vulnerable children to continue. More information about whistleblowing can be found through the charity Freedom to Care (www.ftc.co.uk).

Conclusion

The prevalence of child abuse is high (NSPCC, 2004, www.nspcc.org.uk.inform). Children who suffer abuse experience the impact throughout their lives. Seeking justice and effective protection for children is a demanding and challenging task. Legislation, policy, practice guidance and a vast knowledge base are in place to assist but each case raises new questions and it is only through professionals working together to combine skilled analysis that safe decisions are made and children's voices heard.

REVIEW
QUESTIONS

1   What are the main shortcomings of child protection policy?

2   What are the main legal duties and powers of the local authority under sections 17, 44 and 47 of the Children Act 1989 to protect children and meet their needs?

3   What are the main statutory meetings and groups for professionals working together to protect children?

FURTHER
READING

Bray, M. (1997) *Sexual Abuse: The Child's Voice – Poppies on the Rubbish Heap*, London, Jessica Kingsley

Davies, L. (2006) 'Responding to the Protection Needs of Traumatised and Sexually Abused Children', in A. Hosin (ed.) *Responses to Traumatised Children*, Part 2, Basingstoke, Palgrave Macmillan

Davies, L. (2007) *Protecting Children*, Gloucester, Akamas

DoH (1999) *Working Together to Safeguard Children: A Guide to Inter-agency Working to Safeguard and Promote the Welfare of Children*, London, TSO

Frampton, P. (2003) *Golly in the Cupboard*, Manchester, Tamic

Laming, L. (2003) *The Victoria Climbié Inquiry Summary Report*, Norwich, HMSO

Lewis, P. (2007) 'Missing 48 trafficked children taken into care', *Guardian*, 15 January, www.guardian.co.uk/immigration/story/0,,1990495,00.html

Munro, E. (2002) *Effective Child Protection*, London, Sage

Reder, P. and Duncan, S. (1999) *Lost Innocents: A Follow-up Study of Fatal Child Abuse*, Oxford, Routledge

Reder, P., Duncan, S. and Gray, M. (1993) *Beyond Blame: Child Abuse Tragedies Revisited*, London, Routledge

WEBSITE: www.nspcc.org.uk (NSPCC)

Resource file

Child protection policy

Child protection work carried out by local authorities shifted in the second half of the twentieth century away from preventive supervision towards the 'heavy end' of intervention in the lives, and treatment, of children deemed at risk of harm, or already harmed, through child abuse and neglect. The assessment of these children's child protection needs has become closely associated with risk assessment and the management of risk. Approaches to risk management tend to follow the following steps: identifying risks; analysing risks; tackling risks; and reviewing the effectiveness of the work done (Kavaler and Spiegel, 1997).

Risk assessment, risk management and childcare

Yet fear of risk increasingly dominates other decisions. We live in a society that tries to minimise risk. In public life, the spiralling cost of legal claims for compensation means that risks have to be reduced, whether they be the risk of rain on sports day, the risk that acrobats will fall or children injure themselves while being supervised by teachers on school outings. Every activity has to be subjected to risk analysis, irrespective of its potential benefit to the person.

Child abuse was rediscovered after the 1940s as a problem requiring diagnosis and medical-style treatment (Parton, 1985). The Children Act 1989 focused on whether the child was likely to suffer significant harm, rather than on the assessment of risks. However, by the 1990s, assessment of the child's needs was becoming inextricably linked with the dangers of harm to the child and child death in particular. The task of assessing the potential harm was associated with the necessity of assessing risk to children. The publication of a compilation of *Messages from Research* (DoH, 1995b) reinforced the intimate linking of assessment as to whether the child is deemed a child protection case with the notion of assessing and managing the risk to the child (Parton et al., 1997). In this sense, childcare work has prioritised fire fighting sources of present and future harm to the child, rather than being concerned with meeting the developmental needs of the child.

Tensions between prioritising risk and harm and meeting developmental needs

At the same time, in contrast with the above, the very mechanical approach to the comprehensive assessment of the child's needs, using a checklist of questions, was displaced in 2000, when the government introduced a more holistic framework for the assessment of the child's needs, based on assessing the needs of the whole child in terms of three domains:

1. the health, educational, emotional and behavioural stage of development the child has reached

2. the capacity of relatives, partners and carers to respond to the child's needs

3. the resources available in the family, neighbourhood and wider environment (DoH, 2000a, p. 17).

FURTHER READING

Parton, N. (1985) *The Politics of Child Abuse*, Basingstoke, Macmillan – now Palgrave Macmillan

Parton, N., Thorpe, D. and Wattam, C. (1997) *Child Protection: Risk and the Moral Order*, Basingstoke, Macmillan – now Palgrave Macmillan

11 Risk Management and Safe Practice

MARTIN PAGE

Risk and Safety: Policy Context and Meanings

This chapter helps the reader to understand sensitive issues in health and social care regarding risks to health and wellbeing, safety in practice and the management of both risk and safety in health and social care delivery. Management of risk and management of safety in practice are the duty of everyone who works in the health and social care sector, regardless of level. The NHS Reform and Health Care Professions Act 2002 (Chapter 17, Section 11: Duty of Quality) provides the right environment for enhanced safety for individuals in care. This is underpinned by the health and social care worker's *duty of care* towards the service user and hence why the profession operates in a state of constant upgrade and update.

Risk is an interesting word because it indicates the possibility of more than one outcome. One simple way of making an *assessment of risk* is by asking 'what happens if this activity does not go according to plan?' The question suggests two things:

1. There is a plan in the first place.
2. Before the plan is put into action, a range of *contingency plans* that accommodate different unexpected outcomes is drawn up.

Safety is just as interesting. The simplest definition will include the notion of avoiding harm. For the healthcare worker, *safety in practice* will also include avoiding harm while at work, but this raises two key questions:

1. Who is it that we should protect from harm?
2. How can that be done?

As with many aspects of health and social care, the answer is not straightforward, but it can be reduced to two groups of people:

- *Service users*, namely the 'clients' or patients of whatever service is given.
- *Service providers*, including the GP, the social worker, the community psychiatric nurse, the midwife, the occupational therapist, the care worker and all those who are engaged in organising and providing some of the care required by the service users.

Several different theoretical models can be used to good advantage in most caring environments. Here we look at three of them and modify them to suit our practice needs.

The first is Maslow's hierarchy of needs (Maslow, 1970), which suggests that a person will have a range of needs across the lifespan, but that some of these needs must be met every day (see also Chapter 30). These include the need for food, protection, warmth and shelter, often referred to as the 'basic needs' (see Figure 11.1).

Second, there is King's theory of goal attainment (King, 1981), which considers the personal and social systems, or dimensions, in which a person lives. These include the

- physical dimension
- intellectual dimension
- emotional dimension
- social dimension
- spiritual dimension.

The third model is offered by Brearley (1982). Brearley's model considers the probability of harm, hazards and dangers in a wide context, and this in turn provides a focus for planning to address such events. The model does this by asking a series of questions and using a 'strengths and weaknesses' table. These are the questions:

- What is the nature of the risk?
- How serious are the consequences of it happening, for the service user?
- What previous incidents, evidence or history of this risk are available?
- Does the risk analysis match the service user's situation?
- What time constraints are relevant to the risk analysis being carried out?

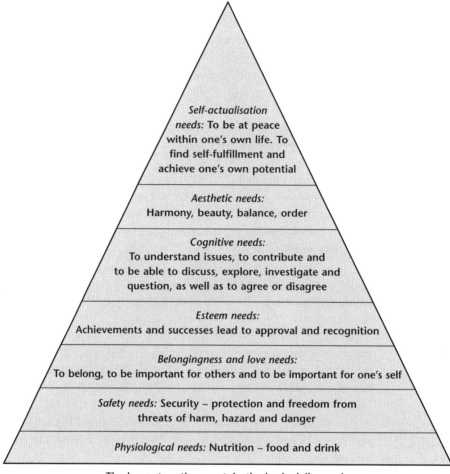

The lower two tiers contain the basic daily needs

Figure 11.1 Maslow's hierarchy of needs (Maslow 1970)

These three models interlock and work well together because they are based on common sense and are easy to remember. They also allow those who work to provide healthcare, social care and specialist care for vulnerable service users or patients to modify and adjust the important aspects so that they fit individual users' needs better.

Management of Risk and Safety

The management of risk and safety is, in part, the duty of everyone who is professionally involved in the delivery of healthcare and social care, irrespective of the level of seniority. It requires a complex assessment of a number of things:

■ care workers'/practitioners' training

- agency policy and adherence to current legislation
- good consulting/listening skills to help the care worker/practitioner understand the opinions, preferences and ideas of the service user or patient at an individual level (this is the prerequisite for an *empowering* service)
- good judgement based on knowledge of service users' needs when laid against the different services to be provided.

In practical terms, these ideals can be applied to practice by considering two elements:

1. a particular practice study
2. how to use the models of Maslow, King and Brearley, irrespective of the disciplinary background of the practitioner.

Practice study

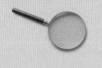

Alice

Following Alice's recent illness, the GP has asked for a multiagency team (led by occupational health) to visit because he was concerned that she had a range of needs that were not being met. Bear in mind that Alice's own opinions and wishes will be properly integrated in any care plan, but must be balanced against the agency's procedures on risk assessment and risk management.

Alice is a retired primary school teacher, in her late sixties. She divorced thirty years ago, and was given the custody of her autistic son. The son is now 35 years old, and three years ago was taken into a specialist care home, 45 miles away. Alice now lives alone in her bungalow, which is in the centre of a village, 15 miles from the nearest town. While the village has a GP, a pharmacy and a Co-op store, it does not have good public transport. There are only four buses per day, two in each direction to and from the nearest town. Her health problems include arthritis and osteoporosis.

Activity 11.1

Spend a few minutes writing notes on your assessment of Alice's needs, using our three models – Maslow, King and Brearley.

Here are my notes, as I reflect on Alice's needs, using each model in turn.

Maslow's Hierarchy of Needs

Maslow's hierarchy of needs predicts that Alice will have some basic needs that must be met every day, so we must identify what these would be and which agencies would be responsible for their delivery. For example, Maslow suggests that the *physiological and safety needs* are critical every day, which leads us to ask:

- Is Alice eating enough of the right foods? Is she getting sufficient fluids of the right kind? If not, then what can be done about it, and who has the responsibility for making sure that the right managers know the true situation?
- Is the bungalow warm and weatherproof, especially during the long winter nights? If not, what can be done, and by whom?
- Is the bungalow a secure and safe place in which to live? Are there any broken or damaged appliances? Is the furniture safe and clean? Does the lavatory flush properly? Are the various sinks, drains and bath maintained to a clean and safe standard? If not, who has the responsibility to ensure that the right manager knows the true situation?

King's Theory of Goal Attainment

I have used the easily remembered mnemonic 'PIESS' to call the following dimensions of health and wellbeing into the discussion: physical, intellectual, emotional, social and spiritual. With a little adjustment, this links directly with Maslow's safety needs. Both Maslow and King are concerned with ensuring safety. King's theory of goal attainment provides a useful list of questions that can be used in almost any health and social care circumstance. These questions include the following.

Physical risks

What are the risks to Alice of physical harm? Are there any damaged fixtures (like kitchen and bathroom units) or fittings (like carpets and curtains) that present a risk to her safety? Do all the facilities (like lights, electric and gas fires, the cooker, refrigerator and television) work properly? If not, what can be done and who has the responsibility to ensure that the right manager has a clear understanding of the true situation? It is clear that such questions are similar to those triggered by Maslow's hierarchy of needs.

Also under the heading of physical risks, consider the medication that Alice will be taking. Is the storage appropriate? Can Alice unscrew the tamper-proof caps on the containers? If not, what is the remedy and who has the responsibility to ensure that the right manager understands the true situation?

One way to identify the risks is to work through the day, starting with Alice getting up in the morning. Is that a risky activity for her? What about taking a morning bath or preparing breakfast? What daily tasks will be difficult for Alice to do? Work through the day and assess each task and each associated risk factor as it emerges. For example, holding a kitchen knife to peel potatoes when one has arthritis can be difficult. Washing and drying one's hair and getting dressed are also awkward things to accomplish with arthritic joints.

Intellectual risks

The risk is that Alice might suffer low moods if the stimulation at an intellectual level is withdrawn. Living in a rural area, it might be the community psychiatric nurse or the social worker who takes the lead role in addressing this need, but not exclusively so. Just about every agency that visits her will make a contribution to Alice's intellectual needs.

What do you think would be important for Alice? She had been in one profession for many years, which will have been intellectually stimulating for her. Conversations with parents and other teachers and working with young children would have been part of her daily routine. Now, living alone, how do you think her intellectual needs might be addressed? Do you think they need to be addressed at all, or could it be accepted that Alice is now retired, and no longer in need of intellectual stimulation? Are there any organisations to which Alice might apply for help? If so, what are they, and how can they be contacted? Most importantly, consider the choices that Alice has. Does she want help and if so, what exactly does Alice say she wants? Making one's own choices and decisions is a vital part of self-empowerment.

Emotional risks

In the same way that the person needs an intellectual stimulus to maintain a normal mood, so it follows that that person's emotional balance must be maintained. In Alice's case, a multiagency care plan could include questions like: How would you assess the need to mix with others of her own age group or to stay in communication with her son, and how would a journey to visit her son be arranged? You might wonder if a visit to see her son is a realistic option. Are there any public sector agencies that might help Alice to see her son on a regular basis? Think of the wider issues involved in emotional needs and see if it is possible to link these with intellectual needs in any way. For example, would writing to her son be useful for Alice? Would starting up a group specifically for other parents and siblings of autistic children help Alice, either emotionally or intellectually? Do any such groups exist? The aim is to avoid Alice suffering a low mood because of her lack of emotional expression. Once again, would Alice have any choices or decisions to make?

Social risks

Arthritis and osteoporosis might make Alice reluctant to walk far, and moving might be painful. Do you think Alice would be happy to socialise, knowing that the experience might be quite painful for her? Would having a social life mean that Alice would have to be mobile, or could it also be enjoyed without having to walk far? Can you find a way of linking the physical aspects of a social life with the intellectual and emotional aspects of life? For example, how does one aspect (say physical) affect another (say, emotional)? What are the risks to Alice of a social life that involves a moderate amount of travelling? If the risks are identified, is it possible to identify a plan that could mitigate the risk of harm and make it worthwhile for Alice? Or, having considered the risks of physical harm to Alice, would you say that it is too risky, and therefore Alice should have to live the rest of her life without the enjoyment of a social life? Does Alice have any choices? Can Alice make her own decisions about her social life?

Spiritual risks

It is common that one's first thoughts of *spiritual needs* include an assessment of a person's *religious belief*. Imogene King was clear in her definition of 'spiritual'. She included the ability of the individual to live a happy life, meet the various stresses of the day with confidence, and generally be of a positive disposition. In King's example, spirituality is more in line with 'keeping one's spirits up' than with religion.

The risk might be that Alice is not able to do very much for herself, and is reliant on others for help. Could this risk convert directly to loneliness? The ability to make one's own choices and decisions is empowering, and being empowered to make choices fulfils the basic need to feel important. To be empowered like this it is necessary for one to be in good spirits.

Consider how loneliness might impact upon Alice's physical, intellectual, emotional, social and spiritual needs. Give some thought to the effects of loneliness and find solutions to each negative point that you can list. What can be done to help someone avoid loneliness? Do you think that the vicar or rural chaplain could be useful for Alice? If so, what do you think they could do? The answers to these questions can be useful for the next model, and especially when devising the strengths and weaknesses table.

Brearley's Risk in Social Work

The third model of assessment can be used as a unifying questionnaire aimed at ensuring best practice as well as providing a thorough assessment of risk, safety and management planning. Brearley (1982) focuses on social work, but the model can be modified to be useful for all agencies that would be involved in Alice's situation. The questions in Brearley's model can be designed to help specify the risk, such as:

1. *What is the nature of the risk?* It might be that Alice is at risk of abuse or neglect.
2. *How serious are the consequences of it happening for the service user?* Is the multiagency approach robust and rigorous enough to distinguish the abuse from bad practice? Have there been any actual examples of abuse or neglect?
3. *What previous incidents, evidence or history of this risk are available?* Full details of past history of neglect or abuse must be recorded and action taken if appropriate.
4. *Does the risk analysis match the service user's situation?* The risk analysis should be specific to Alice. It is not appropriate to give a blanket analysis for all because each individual service user will have a unique range of needs. Different care staff and different (elderly) service users will create a different situation for assessment.
5. *What time constraints are relevant to the risk analysis being carried out?* Each risk analysis has a time frame. The analysis will age, and any changes to the care delivery package will alter the analysis parameters. For example, a change of key worker should automatically trigger a new analysis because the old one will not apply to the new key worker.

Table 11.1 Strengths and weaknesses approach to Alice's situation

	Strengths	Weaknesses
Q1	No abuse: Alice is happy	Possible complacency on occasion
Q2	Multiagency approach well practised. Good liaison between service user and health and social care workers	Communication between agencies might be at risk of occasional failure during public holidays
Q3	No history of allegations	Need to re-evaluate the risks to see that the analysis is properly focused
Q4	Risk analysis is dedicated to Alice in her current situation	If Alice's circumstances change, there will need to be a new analysis to address the changes within Alice's new situation
Q5	Time constraints are apt for Alice's situation	There may be an opportunity to delay a new risk analysis because of external influences such as staff shortages, annual holidays and so on

Table 11.1 answers the questions posed in Brearley's model. The strengths and weaknesses can be designed to incorporate questions and answers from all models. These will contribute directly to the contingency plans mentioned at the start of this chapter.

Conclusion

The three models can be seen to work together for Alice. By applying them as one coherent questionnaire, the professional health and social care worker can discover the real needs of Alice.

Risk management is done by maintaining a keen eye on the protocols and procedures of practice (doing your own job well and keeping abreast of improvements in practice) and by informing others of the ongoing and developing situation for every service user. This is sometimes reduced to 'case conference'-style meetings, but the health and social care staff should feel able to voice concerns at any time. In practical terms, it is the duty of everyone to discuss with leaders the current situation regarding the individual service user or patient and to make sure that the right manager is informed of the true situation.

The *empowerment* of a service user or patient involves giving him or her the freedom to make choices and decisions that could affect service delivery. In this practice study, it can be seen that Alice could make such choices and decisions for herself, providing she had all the relevant information. Herein lies the direct link between informing and empowering a service user or patient. The fact that Alice requires health and social support does not mean that she abdicates her authority to manage her own life.

Being given choices means that the service user or patient has the opportunity to think about what those choices actually mean from his or her own point of view, and it is in the practical aspects of decisions and choices that the solutions to the risks to safety lie.

REVIEW QUESTIONS

1 Can you name the three models of risk analysis and risk management by author?

2 What are the main components of each model?

3 Who, in practical terms, is responsible for protecting the service user or patient from harm?

FURTHER READING

Alaszewski, A., Alaszewski, H., Manthorpe, J. and Ayer, S. (1998) *Assessing and Managing Risk in Nursing Education and Practice: Supporting Vulnerable People in the Community*, London, English National Board for Nursing, Midwifery and Health Visiting

Health, Risk and Society

Heyman, B. (ed.) *Risk, Health and Healthcare: A Qualitative Approach*, London, Chapman & Hall

Kelly, S. and McKenna, H. (2004) 'Risks to Mental Health Patients Discharged into the Community', *Health, Risk and Society*, **6**: 377–85

Kemshall, H. and Pritchard, J. (eds) *Good Practice in Risk Assessment and Risk Management*, (2 vols) London, Jessica Kingsley

Marks, D., Murray, M., Evans, B., Willig, C., Woodhall, C. and Sykes, C. (2005) *Health Psychology: Theory, Research and Practice* (2nd edn) London, Sage
Although focused on medical health, Chapter 15 explores some key issues that are relevant to risk assessments in health and social care.

Thompson, N. (2001) *Anti-Discriminatory Practice* (3rd edn) Basingstoke, Palgrave – now Palgrave Macmillan, pp. 10–11
A short, well focused text that gives clarity to issues of empowerment from the view of social work.

Titterton, M. (2005) *Risk and Risk Taking in Health and Social Welfare*, London, Jessica Kingsley

Tulloch, J. and Lupton, D. (2003) *Risk in Everyday Life*, London, Sage, pp. 16–40
This text invites the reader to explore the notion of risk in a wide variety of contexts. It is a useful starting point for the subject of risk analysis.

Wilkinson, J.D. and Campbell, A.E. (1997) *Psychology in Counselling and Therapeutic Practice*, Chichester, John Wiley & Sons, pp. 2–4
This easy-to-read text illustrates four common theories upon which our basic assumptions on the sufferings of others are based. A valuable introductory text for anyone working in health and social care.

Managing Care in the Community

JENNIFER NEWTON

Learning outcomes

By the end of this chapter, you should be able to:

■ UNDERSTAND the basics of community care policy and practice

■ APPRECIATE what the government means by 'fairness' and 'need'.

This chapter deals with the wide range of services that have been developed for people whose health problems or disabilities mean they need support to enable them to live independently.

Community Care Services

In the not too distant past, there were few options for a disabled person or an older person becoming too frail to manage all their household chores and self-care tasks any more. Their relatives or close friends could help them out, or if they had the money, they could buy in some private help. With neither, charitable institutions or, more commonly, the workhouse may have been their only option. The residential care home, which came to replace many former workhouses after they were formally abolished in 1930, was not supplemented with a wide range of home care services until the closing decades of the twentieth century.

Community care today has expanded to include home care, occupational therapy, district nursing care, day activities, lunch clubs, meals on wheels, voluntary befriending, and a range of supported accommodation for people with a wide range of needs. It covers help with health, social care, income maintenance, and appropriate accommodation for people who cannot manage in their own homes without it. Providers of this care are increasingly within the voluntary or private sectors, but the health service and social work services continue to have a central role, particularly in assessment, care coordination and monitoring. Older people are the largest group in need of community care services, but other groups include younger adults with mental health problems, learning disability, physical disability, or chronic ill-health such as HIV/AIDS or multiple sclerosis.

Coordinating Care Services

One of the early issues for community care services was how best to coordinate such a range of provision. Margaret Thatcher was the Conservative prime minister who steered through the policy that resulted in the NHS and Community Care Act 1990. Her commitment to a market economy, privatisation and a reduced role for the state was emphasised with the shift in role for social services from the main providers of care into 'enabling' authorities, who were required to purchase the majority of service provision from the independent and voluntary sectors. The responsibility of the family as the main provider of community care was also re-emphasised.

To implement the NHS and Community Care Act, 'care management' guidance was issued to commissioning authorities, managers and practitioners, which specified a seven-stage process of assessment and care management. This changed the role of the field social worker from someone who worked with clients, providing direct support and referring people on to other services for particular types of help, to one of care coordination. The process begins with the publication of the range of services available, and who is eligible for them. After an initial assessment to clarify level and extent of need and urgency (stage 2), the care coordinator's role is then to assess need, plan with the client how best those needs could be met, then arrange that care, monitoring and periodically reviewing its adequacy and effectiveness. That is, they have moved from a 'care provider' role, to a 'care commissioning' or 'enabling' role.

Their individual accountability for the whole of the 'care package' of each of the people for whom they were designated 'care manager' or 'care coordinator' was a key change. Local authority social services departments and their health partners remained free to choose how to structure the workforce to deliver care management, however, and a range of collaborative arrangements and multidisciplinary teams developed. Many agreed at an early stage that nurses and occupational therapists could also take on the role of care coordinator. Problems of ensuring good collaboration and 'seamless' care continued in many areas, however, leading to ever greater integration of health and social care services, now often forming joint Care Trusts.

Targeting Resources

The second major concern for community care services has been to ensure the monies allocated are spent as cost-effectively as possible. Spending, particularly on residential and nursing home care, was growing at a rate that could not be sustained through the 1970s and 80s, and care management was to become a process to ration resources in the fairest way possible. Specifically, the monies were targeted on the people who most needed help, and the types of help they most needed.

The first task of local authorities implementing the 1990 NHS and Community Care Act in 1993 was therefore to set out their 'eligibility criteria', explaining what types and levels of need they would aim to meet. Only those people whose needs were assessed as being above the threshold set were eligible for care services paid from the care management budget. An early difficulty was that this threshold varied unacceptably between authorities, hence in 2003 the Department of Health issued a national set of criteria designed to reduce this variation called *Fair Access to Care Services* (DoH, 2003a). In addition, the power to charge for home care services, which is stated in law from 1983 (section 17 of the Health and Social Services and Social Security Adjudications Act), started to lead to charging in most authorities by the 1990s. Again this led to inequities, or a 'postcode lottery', and to guidance from the Department of Health to try to rectify the large differences between authorities in how much people were being charged (DoH, 2003b).

Under *Fair Access to Care Services*, people referred for help are assessed, and their needs designated as critical, substantial, moderate, or low. All authorities will meet critical needs, such as those of a 90-year-old woman who has osteoporosis, incontinence, difficulty in washing, and is isolated and depressed. Most authorities will also meet substantial need, such as those of an 80-year-old woman with chronic arthritis, early stage dementia, and needing some help with her finances, shopping and personal care, much of which has been provided by her daughter who is now moving abroad. While many authorities would initially also have met moderate needs, their rising costs have meant that more and more local authorities will rule these as ineligible, and almost no authorities will meet low needs. Hence, a 55-year-old man with physical disabilities resulting from a recent stroke whose relatives are only able to help him in the evenings will be unlikely to be eligible for help if he is able to manage his own personal care needs.

Activity 12.1

How fair is *Fair Access to Care Services?* Discuss the concepts of fairness and need. Read the case scenarios in the guidance document (DoH, 2003a, pp. 23–6), and the answer to questions Q3.12 and Q3.13.

You will see that needs are separated into *presenting needs*, only some of which may be *eligible needs*. The latter group are likely to include personal care tasks, the former, tasks such as gardening or letter-writing. This is because the rationing of spending is growing tighter and limiting the spending of public monies to meeting needs which, if not met, put the individual or others close to them at risk, including the risk of needing accommodating in a more expensive care setting.

Each person's needs should be determined on the basis of a comprehensive assessment undertaken by the care coordinator. To ensure that this assessment is person-centred, the level of information gathered is appropriate – given the complexity of need – duplication is avoided and best practice promoted, a single assessment process has been developed (see Chapter 30) for use with older people (DoH, 2001a). The principles underpinning this approach are currently being adapted for use across all adult care groups. This may involve obtaining assessments from others, such as a psychiatrist, GP or occupational therapist. The latter may advise on adaptations to the home that will improve safety or make tasks easier. The individual should receive a copy of the agreed needs, following which, they and their care coordinator should plan together how best to meet each of these.

For instance, Mrs Brown had had a problem with her arthritis for years, and had taken early retirement from the benefits office where she worked. Her knees in particular had been affecting her mobility, and the stiffness in her fingers meant it was hard to use the computer keyboard. She had lived alone since her husband died, and her only son had gone to live abroad with his family 20 years ago. By the time she was 70, the effect of the arthritis had become very disabling. She struggled to dress without assistance, cook, open lids or packets, or walk anywhere, even the local shops, and was becoming depressed at the bleak future she felt she faced. Even by the 1980s, the help that would have been available to her was still quite limited – meals on wheels three times a week maybe, a few hours and lunch at a day centre on the other two perhaps, some help with dressing and bathing at home from a district nurse, a home help once or twice a week. She would have had little prospect of finding help of any kind at the weekend. If the care needed had become this extensive, and she couldn't manage without it through the weekend, the usual decision was that a residential care option was required. Once the level of care needed increased, then a bed in a geriatric ward in hospital might have been the next stop.

Case Management Pilots

However, during the late 1980s, a number of UK pilot projects (see for example, Challis et al., 1988), based on innovative US research on *case management*, tried out some new options, giving the money that would have been spent on a care home to an individual *case manager* to buy help at home. This worker would have control over all the money needed for the range of services used by Mrs Brown. Instead of having to choose from the four or five services available, and only being offered help Monday to Friday, Mrs Brown could discuss with her case manager what she needed help with, and how she would like those needs to be met. Then, if the existing services were not appropriate, the case manager could purchase these. In the pilot studies (Challis et al., 1988), the help purchased was most commonly a home care assistant, or several, paid for from the care management budget.

The results of the evaluation of these pilots so impressed UK policy-makers that the approach rapidly became policy, the 1989 White Paper *Caring for People* specifying that 'proper assessment of need and good case management' was the 'cornerstone of high quality care' (DoH, 1989, p. 5). When the guidance was issued, the phrase became *care management* rather than case management, and while social workers and others then became 'care managers', the designated label by 2006 has become *care coordinator*.

These policy developments significantly change the power relationships between professionals and service users. We have moved from offering a fixed range of services (a *service-led approach* to care), offered at times and days that were decided as much because of the needs and convenience of the workforce as the needs of the service users, through a *needs-led approach*, to what is today now termed a *person-centred approach*. The needs-led concept refers both to the role the client plays in determining what help they need, but also to the way services are commissioned, which should now be based on these assessments, and not necessarily on the pattern of care offered in previous years.

Direct Payments

Today, the shift in control is moving even further towards the client, and since 1996, service users have had the right to control the money to buy in their own home care assistance and other similar services, through *direct payments* (see Chapter 14). Offered initially mainly to people with physical disabilities, further policy developments followed in 2000 to make these available to people aged over 65 years, parents of disabled children, and also to encourage take-up by people with learning disability or long-term mental illness. In a speech in April 2004 to the directors of social services, the then Health Minister Stephen Ladyman reiterated his commitment to this policy, linking it to the two key concepts of *person-centredness* and *social inclusion*. In particular, the values of the workforce should be moving away from seeing older people and disabled adults as in need of care and looking after, towards recognising their expectation to lead as full and active a life as possible, but needing help and support that enables them to do so (see Chapter 13).

Hence Mrs Brown can now directly employ a number of carers working different shifts, including night-time, weekends and public holidays, or she can opt to leave the care coordinator to organise this for her. The aim of her 'care package' is of course to enable her to stay in her own home as long as possible, and to avoid a need for residential care, nursing care and, above all, hospital care. Much policy development since the NHS and Community Care Act has been to strengthen the effectiveness of home care arrangements that prevent a need for these less desirable and more costly options. Local authorities have needed to respond by developing a range of intermediate care alternatives, often funded jointly with their health partner agencies, such as 'step down beds', to ensure swift discharge, hospital at home, crisis teams, intermediate care, all as temporary provision that minimises the need for time in hospital. For the longer term, when the person's own home is not suitable, a range of supported accommodation can be offered that tailors the level of support to the level of need, ensuring that only those who need round-the-clock care are accommodated in care homes.

Carers

Of course, most community care has always been provided by the family, and still is. But this role has been made more explicit in current policy, which encourages people to view the role of the state as to help the family to care, and to offer to provide direct care only when the family is unable or unwilling to do so.

Much discussion and policy has focused on how best to help informal carers to continue to care and maintain their own health, employment and wellbeing at the same time. While the resources to do so remain quite limited, there is at least clear guidance to enable social care staff to consider the needs of the carer and do what they can to help them. Under the Carers and Disabled Children Act 2000, local authorities have the power to offer a wide range of help, from driving lessons to holidays. Surveys of informal carers show that what is most needed is some respite, and monies have been made available for services to offer some types of carers breaks or respite care. However, help for carers remains largely a *power* that local authorities have, but not a *duty* (see Chapter 39 for more discussion of carers).

Activity 12.2

If you already cook all meals at home for your partner, your role may be as wife, husband or flatmate. When would you define your role as 'carer'?

In aiming to shift thinking by services towards helping people to help themselves, the *expert patient* programme (DoH, 2001d) is an exciting development. People with chronic ill-health are recognised as 'experts by experience', with much to offer by way of advice on self-care and management of difficulties to others with similar health problems. They then run or contribute towards an educational programme on living with particular chronic illnesses such as epilepsy, multiple sclerosis, asthma, schizophrenia, diabetes or arthritis.

People developing the problems faced by Mrs Brown can benefit, perhaps even before giving up work due to the disease, from a programme where those who have coped with arthritis for many years can share their expertise. This might include suggestions for pain relief, useful exercises to improve mobility, diet, effective medication, dealing with fatigue, useful aids and home adaptations, and accessing services. Linked to this initiative is also the power for frontline staff to offer training to informal carers on supporting relatives with particular types of chronic illness.

Issues

These initiatives are driven by the aim to develop 'person-centred' services, but also concerns for cost. These are in turn linked to the ageing population and the changes this brings, given the current retirement age of 65 for men and 60 for women, in the balance between the proportion of the population paying taxes and those dependent on taxpayers' money for their support.

For instance, the Office for National Statistics (ONS) population projections in 2004 were for a growth in the population of people of working age in the UK of 3.1 per cent by 2010, but a growth in people of retirement age of 9.3 per cent over the same period. Even with an increase in retirement age to 65 years for women, the dependency ratio is predicted to fall from 3.33 working people to each person of pensionable age in 2004, to 2.62 in 2031 (ONS, 2005). Retirement age, pensions and savings for old age are now high on the policy agenda for this reason. The shift to the individual person as responsible for his or her own care fits well with this imperative.

Of course, as more of us live longer, one particular problem is the development of dementia. This is by no means an inevitable consequence of old age, and most people will never develop the difficulties of memory loss and confusion that this brings. But the risk of someone developing dementia rises with age, so that 1 in 4 people over the age of 85 years will have become affected to the extent of limiting their capacity to look after themselves. Because of the risks associated with poor memory, such as a person forgetting they put some potatoes on to boil, to close the front door as they go out, how the shower works, or how to drive the car, they are a high priority for services.

Given the focus of services on those who need them most, the proportion of people in care homes and other services who have dementia has risen, but so too has the proportion of people receiving care packages at home who have dementia. The values and respect inherent in new policy must also be central to the help they are offered, and workers need understanding and sensitivity. Here, as in other areas of community care, the skilled worker must learn to balance a concern to foster independence with careful assessment of the risks involved. In this regard, a new range of technology is being introduced that is designed to assist, collectively referred to as *assistive technology* or *telecare*. This can provide a link via the telephone able to signal problems in, for example, temperature of the home, humidity, or the front door not having been closed.

Conclusion

Community care is developing rapidly. It needs a workforce that is caring, respectful and insightful, supported by systems and procedures that ensure cost-effective use of resources, good coordination between health and social care, and support for individuals and informal carers to lead lives that are as full and active as possible. Decisions should be led by the individual concerned, hence they need workers who provide as much information as possible to inform that choice.

REVIEW QUESTIONS

1 What is the difference between 'care' and 'support'?

2 Can you describe at least two of the aims of the NHS and Community Care Act 1990?

3 Why and how are resources being rationed?

4 What are the main differences between a service-led and a needs-led approach to community care?

FURTHER READING

Bornat, J., Johnson, J., Pereira, C., Pilgrim, D. and Williams, F. (1997) *Community Care: A Reader* (2nd edn) Basingstoke, Macmillan – now Palgrave Macmillan

DoH (1999) *Caring About Carers: A National Strategy for Carers*, London, DoH

DoH (2001) *National Service Framework for Older People*, London, TSO

Means, R., Richards, S. and Smith, R. (2003) *Community Care Policy and Practice* (3rd edn) Basingstoke, Palgrave Macmillan

Sharkey, P. (2006) *The Essentials of Community Care: A Guide for Practitioners* (2nd edn) Basingstoke, Palgrave Macmillan

RESOURCE FILE: Understanding Care and Caring, below

Resource file

Understanding care and caring

Policy shifts

In the 1990s, whereas community care was at the centre of care policy and practice, in the early twenty-first century, this has been replaced by *adult care*, *continuing care*, *domiciliary* (or *home*) care and *intermediate care*. The Commission for Social Care Inspection (CSCI) general report on home care services illustrates their richness and diversity (CSCI, 2006a).

Meanings of care

A practitioner told me that some women she identified as Caribbean like herself in her neighbourhood resist being called 'carers' because they regard caring as part of their family life. The fact that this book is built around a word that has everyday meanings and connotations as well as being the specialist word used by some carers to describe what they do for nothing, and by health and social care managers and practitioners to refer to their paid work, makes it extremely important to clarify what we mean by 'care'. Care can mean 'being careful'. When we leave people, we sometimes say 'Take care.' Caring can be an attitude or an adjective attached to a person: 'She's such a caring person.' Or it can be a description of a role at work: 'She is a care worker, the key worker caring for these residents.' This person may do the caring for these residents in a caring way, or may not care about them at all.

We can see already one of the problems with the word 'carer'. It has so much ambiguity and the potential for confusion and misunderstanding every time it is used. Here are some possible meanings of 'care' and 'carer':

■ unpaid, full-time care for a partner, parent or child
■ paid work as a carer

paid work in a job such as youth leader, teacher or minister of religion, in which many people have an expectation that part of the role will involve caring for other people.

For people who care informally and unpaid for a friend, neighbour, relative or partner, care is an experience that may be purely pleasurable or a complex mix of happiness, resentment, freedom to express one's feelings or an inability ever to mention what one thinks or feels. The carer may be well off or suffer extreme poverty, may not want to do anything other than care, or may feel that caring has destroyed forever the chance of personal or professional fulfilment, through a relationship or a career.

People who know the person as carer and/or doing care work may respond to him or her in different ways, with comments which he or she remembers, appreciates or resents. One carer, who organises a carers' group, said to me of my presence in the group, 'you're just a tourist', which was a dramatic way of highlighting the gulf between my role as an academic, 'visiting' the experience of carers, and their lives as carers, 24 hours a day, seven days a week.

Activity 12.3

Consider what care means to you in your own life:

1. Have you been a carer?
2. Have you done care work?
3. Have you had both to do?
4. What feelings do you have about your caring and/or your care work?

Social model of care

In *Options for Excellence* (DfES and DoH, 2006), a bold report projecting what the social care workforce will look like in the future, it is stated that the social care workforce will need to be:

- flexible
- multiskilled
- reflective
- practical
- solution-focused
- changing from a 'person-centred' to a 'relationship-centred' approach to practice (p. 75).

The report refers to the 'social model of care'. We can use the above statement about changing from person-centredness to a relationship-centred approach to expand slightly its statement of the possibility of moving to a social model of care which:

- places the work done with individuals in its wider context of the neighbourhood and local community
- assesses the needs of people in relation to their personal, family and community situation
- appraises not only the publicly funded services they may need but also the availability of informal, family, local neighbourhood and wider community supports available to them
- builds in safeguards and advocacy for people
- seeks to keep people independent, in control of their lives and continuing to be involved in the wider community
- encourages preventive approaches, that is, earlier interventions using additional supports to encourage individuals and families to develop their strategies for coping
- is strengths-based, that is, uses and builds on the strengths of individuals, families and communities
- promotes principles of non-discriminatory practice and social justice.

FURTHER READING

CSCI (2006) *An Overview of Home Care Services for Older People in England*, London, CSCI

DfES and DoH (2006) *Options for Excellence Final Report: Building the Social Care Workforce of the Future*, London, DoH

Fink, J. (ed.) (2004) *Care: Personal Lives and Social Policy*, Bristol, Policy Press/Open University

Working with Older People

SUE THOMPSON

You may already have experience of working in the care sector with older people, or maybe it is something you are planning to do in the future. Even if neither of these apply, it is unlikely that the issue of welfare provision for vulnerable older people will have passed you by completely, as it has long been a topic of debate among health and social care policy-makers and the general public too. What I want you to think about in this chapter is the danger that a focus on care and dependency may make us forget that each older person is an individual, with a unique past, but also a future – that is, life left to live and decisions to keep on making. While those you work with may be dependent in some respects, and for some periods of time, does it seem fair that it is their dependency that tends to define them? You may recall being dependent at some time in your life – perhaps you'd been ill or had an accident – but it was no doubt assumed that this would be temporary. After all, most of us need a little help at some time, and in some circumstances, but we wouldn't want to think that's how others see us from then on. Because of the potential for this to happen where older people are concerned, this chapter will look at two different models that underpin how we think about older people and their needs, and inform how social policy is developed in this field. The first of these is 'the care model' and the second 'the empowerment model'. By working through some practice examples, we will explore the tendency for the older people we work with to be thought of as a problem to be dealt with, rather than as people with problems, and think about how we can ensure that our practice does not reinforce the view that old age and dependency are one and the same thing.

Before looking at the two models and their implications for care provision, let us first think a bit more about why it is that older people are often depicted in negative terms – the wrinkled, confused, incompetent (and even incontinent) image we often see on television shows and greetings cards. Because ageism is so prevalent and powerful, it is something we need to think carefully about to ensure that our practice challenges rather than reinforces, it. So what is ageism?

Ageism

Ageism is a form of oppression that results in older people (and indeed children and young people) being treated unfairly purely on the grounds of age as an indicator of competence and worth. If we refer to the PCS framework described by Thompson (2006), we can see ageism operating at three levels:

- *Personal:* that is, in the attitudes and actions of individuals who think of older people as unimportant and therefore less deserving of respect.
- *Cultural:* negative stereotyping of older people is part of the dominant culture that most, if not all, of us will have been brought up in. This has the effect of pushing people to the margins of society and taking away their dignity. One of the processes through which ageism operates is that of 'internalised oppression', whereby older people are so used to hearing the message 'you are past it and no longer a useful member of society' that even they take it on board themselves.
- *Structural:* culture, in turn, is influenced by the ways in which society is organised or structured. For example, the workings of the economy have an effect on the role that older people are expected to play, such as to retire from work to allow younger (and supposedly better) workers to take their place.

The processes through which ageism operates are many and, within the confines of this short chapter, there is not the space to discuss all of them here. Some will feature in the discussions that follow and I would urge you to read more widely about this important subject (see the end of this chapter for suggestions for further reading).

The Care Model

In the *care model*, the emphasis is on providing care – on protecting a vulnerable person from harm. It is understandable that if you are working day in and day out with people who are dependent, it is difficult not to think of all older people in that way, especially given the ageist messages we are bombarded with through the media and so on. Fennell et al. (1988) usefully described this process as one of *welfarisation*, whereby old age itself is seen as a problem, rather than it being the case that some individuals, who also happen to be old, are in need of welfare support. While providing care and protection for those who need it is a necessary and desirable function of the welfare system, there is a danger that this can become *over*protection if it is carried out in a way that denies older people the right to live their lives as they choose, including taking risks that others may not think are in their best interests.

A tendency for older people to be seen as in need of looking after allows for processes such as *infantilisation* to flourish. This is where an older person is treated as if they were a child, and it is assumed that they will not object to being called by a given or pet name, rather than being accorded the respect of being asked how they would like to be addressed. I once witnessed the manager of a nursing home pat one elderly resident on the head and call her 'poppet'. I cannot comment on how the resident herself felt about this, but I would ask you to think about what that behaviour tells you about the manager's attitude to older people. She may have felt that it was her duty to protect and cosset someone she recognised as vulnerable and perhaps did not mean to act in a patronising, demeaning and therefore discriminatory way. This is a good example of how discrimination on the grounds of age does not have to be intentional, but the outcome is discriminatory nonetheless.

If, then, we necessarily equate old age with the need for care and protection, we reinforce the stereotypes of frailty and incompetence – it sets up a vicious circle in which one feeds into the other. So how do we break that circle? Let us now look at a model that does not deny the need for protection, but balances it with the need to promote other rights too.

The Empowerment Model

One of the key issues that underpins the *empowerment model* is the concept of partnership – the notion that we work *with* older people, rather than do things *to* them (contrary to the focus of the care model). As its name suggests, it is about power, more specifically about shifting the balance from having policy-makers and care providers calling the shots to a situation in which the role of care staff is to help facilitate an older person's lifestyle choices, rather than to assume that we know best. This is not to deny that staff have expertise in many fields, but rather to challenge the commonly held notion that older people don't. After all, who is the person most likely to have expertise in how he or she feels, what his or her hopes for the future are, what works best for them and so on? While the care model has a strong focus on protection, the empowerment model is one that emphasises rights, and that includes the right to take risks. This doesn't always sit easily with those who feel that their role is primarily one of protecting vulnerable people, and yet risk is something that is part and parcel of everyday life. For example, we all hear reports about how dangerous it is to take to the roads and yet most of us do so on a regular basis. We are alerted to risk in terms of lifestyle, diet and so on, but many choose to ignore it and would not take kindly to having these decisions made for us. And yet all too often decisions about risk are made for older people, as if they don't have the ability or right to make these choices for themselves (for empowerment, see Chapter 40).

There has only been space to explore these two models very briefly, but enough to suggest that attitudes and practices which are informed by an empowerment model are likely to provide more of a challenge to ageism than one which sees the relationship between carer and cared-for as one-way.

Practice study

Mrs James

Mrs James had been a heavy smoker all her life. Now aged 80, she had chronic breathing problems and knew only too well that her smoking habit was contributing to her poor health. Her carer was not happy to carry out her request to buy cigarettes for her as she wanted to encourage Mrs James to live a healthier lifestyle. When Mrs James discovered that her son had instructed the carer not to buy cigarettes for his mother, she was furious. She told them both that she had always been well aware of the consequences of smoking for her health but intended to carry on taking those risks anyway. The carer felt pulled in two directions. She shared the family's concerns but also felt that, as Mrs James was a free-thinking adult who made her own decisions in every other respect, she should assist her to live the life of her choosing, regardless of whether or not she approved of it. She thought about the man (aged 35) who she had met while working in a rehabilitation unit for disabled people. She had disapproved of his heavy smoking too, but realised that she had never even contemplated refusing to help him buy cigarettes.

- Is there a dilemma here for the carer in terms of rights and responsibilities?
- Do you think that the age of the two people might have made a difference to the carer's reactions? If so, why?
- In your experience, do older people often have other people's ideas about appropriate lifestyles imposed upon them? If so, can you think of any examples?
- From an empowerment perspective, how could the carer support Mrs James?

Towards Empowerment

There are many ways in which the denial of opportunity and choice in old age can be challenged. Reading around the subject and debating issues with colleagues, course tutors and, of course, older people themselves should help to keep the issues high in your consciousness as you continue with your studies. What follows is some food for thought.

Don't Take Things for Granted

In order to tackle a problem, you have to recognise its existence. Think carefully about what is going on around you. Are people being catered for differently, and less favourably, purely on the grounds of age and the assumptions made about it? Think about where the power lies in the provision of welfare services for older people. In your experience, is it commonplace for dependent older people to have decisions made for them? User involvement in education, training, policy-making and service delivery is much higher on the agenda than it once was but, while the political rhetoric promotes participation as a core value, the response can sometimes be a tokenistic one, rather than one which really strives to assist older people to live the life they want to, but need some assistance with. Anti-ageist practice is not just a personal responsibility – you can play a part in promoting change at an organisational level by discussing these matters with colleagues and managers. By getting these issues onto the agenda for discussion, you will encourage critical awareness in others too.

Not Just Old

As we age we often change, but much about us stays the same. Being old does not negate what has gone before, such as our social position, whether we have been subject to racism, sexism, disablism – or whatever. Ageist ideology promotes the idea that once someone is defined as 'old', then this blanket definition, and a 'one-size-fits-all' approach to welfare provision, will suffice. But the reality is that, in terms of prestige and life chances, it will still matter whether that person is black or white, rich or poor, gay or straight, disabled or able-bodied and so on. The potential for discrimination on such grounds as gender, ethnicity, religion and sexuality not only continues to exist, but is added to by the potential for discrimination on the grounds of age too. A damaging consequence of conceptualising older people as 'just old' is that negative experiences of discrimination go unrecognised and potentially helpful forms of intervention are not offered to them.

Practice study

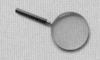

Mr Singh

On the morning that 77-year-old Mr Singh was due to have a surgical procedure performed, he woke early and asked an assistant for a bowl of water so that he could perform the daily cleansing ritual he had always practised before his early morning prayers. When he was told that it was too early to wash and that he would be given the chance to bathe when he was being prepared for his operation, he became quite upset because this ritual carried great significance for him. The assistant's attempts to calm him down by suggesting he go back to sleep just made matters worse and she decided that, as he couldn't understand her, there was little point in continuing with the conversation and so she took to ignoring him. The more agitated he became, the more the assistant assumed that he was confused. But to Mr Singh, the reality was very different. It was she who could not understand him, and not the other way round. He *wanted* to go back to sleep, as he did not want to dwell on the procedure to come, but could not do so without observing his religious duties.

- What do you think contributed towards the assistant's assumption that Mr Singh was confused?
- Do you think she was seeing Mr Singh as a unique person? How might she have better understood his perspective?
- Would you have done things differently?

Interdependency and Intergenerationality

Vulnerable older people often express gratitude for the care they receive, but Lustbader (1991) makes the point that being dependent can often make people feel devalued. Having spent much of their lives being busy (as employees, caring for others, being members of communities and so on), they may feel that an important aspect of their identity – the ability to 'give back' – is being denied to them. Promoting *inter*dependency and also intergenerationality – the sharing of expertise and life experience between the generations – can offer a way to counteract dependency, both at a practical level and at the level of an ideology that equates old age with helplessness. Being a citizen of a society involves having rights conferred on you, but also requires you to undertake the responsibilities expected of an adult in that society. Advancing age does not remove those obligations, and many older people would be more than happy to continue to contribute in whatever ways they can, but instead suffer the indignity of being seen as a burden.

Practice study

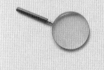

Joe Reid

Joe Reid had always been a busy person before having to move into residential care because of restrictions on his mobility after having a stroke. He hated relying on others but what got to him most was the assumption that he had nothing to contribute any more – after all, he couldn't walk or make speeches, but he was still a skilled man. He hated seeing the kitchen staff rushing about, little repair jobs that needed doing and the greenhouse becoming neglected, but his offers to help were met with comments such as 'you sit there and let us look after you – that's our job.'

- Why do you think that Joe was not allowed to 'give something back'?
- What effect do you think this might have had on how he perceived himself?
- What part do you think ageism might have played here?
- Can you think of any ways in which interdependency, rather than dependency, could have been promoted to everyone's benefit?

Conclusion

Working with older people will always involve care and protection, but the argument here is that care should incorporate promoting autonomy and rights if it is not to be oppressive. As you study and practise, try to put yourself in the shoes of the older person and see the individual, not the stereotype. Individuals can need help at any stage in the life course but they remain a person with problems rather than a problem per se. Every day that you work with older people you will be exposed to ageist assumptions about the type of interventions that are appropriate. The challenge is to try to ensure that older people are treated as adults, with the same range of feelings and aspirations as any other adults, and that they are seen as partners in problem-solving rather than purely recipients of care.

REVIEW QUESTIONS

1 What are the main similarities and differences between the care and empowerment models of work with older people?

2 What do the words 'interdependence' and 'intergenerationality' mean?

FURTHER READING

Arber, S. and Ginn, J. (eds) (1995) *Connecting Gender and Ageing: A Sociological Approach*, Buckingham, Open University Press
   All the chapters in this collection highlight how discrimination on gender grounds continues to be a feature of women's old age, but Chapters 8 and 9 are particularly interesting and relevant.

Thompson, S. (2005) *Age Discrimination*, Lyme Regis, Russell House
   Ageism, and its interaction with other forms of discrimination, are explored here in more detail than has been possible in this short chapter.

As its name suggests, the Open University course Care, Welfare and Community (K202) has a strong focus on issues relevant to those working in social care. While not all the discussions relate exclusively to older people, many of the topics discussed can be applied to work in this field. In particular, Units 3, 18, 19 and 20 are worth a look. The reader associated with this course (Bytheway, B. et al. (eds) (2002) *Understanding Care, Welfare and Community*, London, Routledge) contains some interesting material, especially in Part III, which deals with rights and risk.

WEBSITES: www.cpa.org.uk (Centre for Policy on Ageing)
            www.ageconcern.org.uk (Age Concern)

14 Physical Disability and Sensory Loss

ROBERT ADAMS

By the end of this chapter, you should be able to:

■ IDENTIFY the main features of three major kinds of physical impairment for which society disables people – loss of mobility, loss of sight and loss of hearing

■ DISCUSS the strengths and weaknesses of the main ways of working with disabled people.

This chapter deals with physical impairments in aspects including mobility, communication, and access to social and leisure activities. In order to understand disability, we need to talk to disabled people about their experiences and read what some disabled people, such as Jenny Morris and Michael Oliver, have written. It is possible to make mistaken assumptions about what disabled people want and this can lead us away from responding to their real needs. I attended a service user and carer meeting and said there is a need to ensure that disabled people are more independent, whereupon a disabled person replied that he is more concerned with keeping control over his life. This is an important distinction.

Within the general category of impairments, there are significant differences. A search in the library will show that equal attention is not given to all aspects of physical and sensory impairments. For instance, there is a relative lack of written material on blindness and deafness. We need to ensure that people who have different physical impairments have equal opportunities to make their views and feelings known.

Write the following three headings on three pieces of paper: Loss of mobility, Loss of sight, Loss of hearing. Use personal experience, experience of working with other people or your imagination to write a list under each heading of the problems which arise for the person with the loss.

Keep your notes so you can return to them towards the end of this chapter.

What Disability Means to Disabled People

We should distinguish impairment – the physical condition – from disability – the consequences of living in disabling environments in a disabling society.

Jenny Morris writes about the barriers that exist between disabled and non-disabled people, about the fear and discomfort that accompany non-disabled people turning disabled people into objects of pity, 'comforting themselves by their own kindness and generosity' (Morris, 1991, p. 192). Such attitudes are the basis for the discrimination against disabled people in all the areas non-disabled people take for granted – jobs, housing and so on.

Physical Disability or Physical Impairment

People with impairments often experience discrimination and exclusion, because those around them disable them by their attitudes. Words like deafness, dumbness, blindness, incapacity, immobility, handicap and even disability are regarded by many people with physical impairments as unacceptable general descriptions of their impairment, for three reasons:

- They can be used to apply the impairment to the whole person
- They can reinforce a feeling of being helpless and hopeless
- They can contribute to stereotyping people with more obvious, physical impairments, in contrast with people who have less obvious but no less real impairments.

We use the word 'impairment' deliberately, to emphasise that particular aspects of the person and their life are affected by the physical impairment, rather than the whole person being treated as 'that disabled person'. So we can appreciate that there is a fundamental difference between saying 'John is disabled' and 'John has an impairment'.

Individual and Social Models of Disability

Two models of disability (Oliver, 1983) – the individual and social models – are generally recognised as ways of understanding how practitioners can understand disability and develop more adequate involvement with disabled people. Oliver spelled out what he meant at a workshop on people with locomotor disabilities (Oliver, 1990a).

First, the *individual model* is underpinned by what he calls the 'personal tragedy theory of disability' (Oliver, 1990a, p. 1):

- this includes the psychological and medical aspects of disability
- it describes the disability as a problem within the individual
- it locates the cause of this problem as in the person's assumed psychological losses resulting from their functional limitations, such as inability to walk, see or hear.

The *social model* rejects these three points and states that:

- there is no denying that disability is a problem
- this problem lies in our society that disables rather than in the individual with the impairment (Oliver, 1990b)
- the causes of this problem lie in the failure of society to meet disabled people's needs by providing adequate services through the way society is organised
- this failure falls not only on individuals randomly but systematically on disabled people as a group (Oliver, 1990a, p. 2).

Oliver argues that medicalising disability is inappropriate, because 'disability is a social state and not a medical condition' (Oliver, 1990a, p. 2). 'Disability as a long-term social state is not treatable and is certainly not curable' (Oliver, 1990a, p. 3). This makes the control over disability and medical intervention in it by nurses, doctors and consultants inappropriate. It is inappropriate for them to aim to restore the disabled person to what they assume to be normality (Oliver, 1990a, p. 3).

Oliver is not arguing that medicine has no contribution to make in dealing with disability. He says that while doctors should be working within the medical model to treat illness, it is questionable whether they should be working within the social model of disability (Oliver, 1990a, p. 4). It is inappropriate for the medicalisation of disability to give doctors power over disabled people, leaving them powerless (Oliver, 1990a, p. 5).

Advocacy

The many groups of disabled people adopting an activist stance have acquired the skills of advocacy on their own behalf. Advocacy (see Chapter 40) is a potentially powerful means by which disabled people can assert their views and influence decisions about their services and their lives.

Policy Changes

A major change in government policy towards some disabled people was proposed in 2006 to abolish incapacity benefit and replace it with employment support. This was part of the government's strategy to use measures such as employment advisers to bring approximately one million people off long-term disability benefits, along with a proportion of lone parents, and get them back into employed work. This measure was controversial. Supporters argued that it would be good for disabled people no longer to feel stigmatised as unemployable and 'on the shelf'. Critics argued that it would cause severe financial, emotional and psychological hardship to some disabled people not able to engage in sufficiently rewarding paid work.

Direct Payments

Direct payments are monetary payments by local councils direct to people who use services and to carers, who intend to buy their own services, such as a personal assistant (see Resource File: Charging and Direct Payments, at the end of the chapter).

The benefits of direct payments to people using services have been advocated by campaigners since the early 1990s (Morris, 1993, p. 125). Direct payments are intended to increase their choice in the services they purchase (Leece and Bornat, 2006). Yet with only about 13,000 people using direct payments in 2004, they are still not part of the mainstream of social care services (CSCI, 2005a, p. 3).

Government guidance (DoH, 2003f) points out that while disabled people and adults and carers aged 16 and over as well as people with parental responsibility for a child are eligible to receive direct payments (DoH, 2003f, p. 7), others may not be. These include patients subject to compulsory mental health or guardianship orders and people on probation, licence or after care orders (DoH, 2003f, p. 50). Some people may be put off employing personal assistants by the responsibility of managing their employment, for example tax, national insurance, holiday, maternity, sickness and redundancy pay.

Activity 14.2

Some service users spend direct payments employing carers while others employ personal assistants. Which term do you prefer and why?

Different Impairments

We deal in this part of the chapter with three obvious impairments (partial or total loss of mobility, sight and hearing), but are aware that we are setting to one side the vast range of other impairments from which people suffer.

Loss of Mobility

This is the most visible physical impairment for many people and partly because of this can result in the greatest degree of stigma.

Practice study

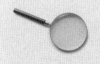

Alan

Alan, 66, is a full-time day user of a wheelchair who lives alone and relies on a part-time personal assistant and his twin sister Sophie, living nearby, for most of his care needs.

Alan is not strong and faces many emotional and physical barriers in his everyday life. He feels labelled as a failure by the people he used to work with. Sophie died last week. Alan needs a community care assessment and Christine, a social work assistant, tried to carry this out in full collaboration with him.

Alan pushed Christine away, maintaining he did not know where Sophie was. He joked that she could be away on a world cruise. Anyway, he stated he did not want any help.

Christine felt that Alan was likely to experience the shock of his bereavement later and put him in touch with an advocate, who would visit him regularly. She was aware from the literature on loss and bereavement that different people react very differently to the death of somebody close to them and not all people move through the so-called stages of bereavement – denial, anger, acceptance – in the same way.

Christine persuaded Alan to have a possum (patient operated selector mechanism) assistive technology system installed, after helping Alan to review different mechanically and electronically operated systems for controlling curtains, hi-fi, phone loudspeaker, room lights, page turner, PC, main plugs and door locks. This would give him independent access to various items of household equipment 'while Sophie was away'.

Some people with multiple physical impairments are enabled to live independently by a combination of assistive technology and resources from a personal assistant or carer. Recently, I met Diana, who has very restricted physical mobility and is blind. With support from her partner and a personal assistant, she is becoming ever more involved in the regional forum that represents the views of people who use services and carers. Not content with airing her views, she plans to campaign on particular issues, to try to change policy and practice. Diana reminds me of the necessity to refer to differing abilities rather than further stigmatising people with physical impairments and perpetuating their exclusion from mainstream society.

Practice study

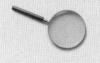

Martha

Martha has multiple sclerosis. She employs two personal assistants from direct payments. They work on shifts during the working week to provide her with care, in conjunction with support on evenings and weekends from a trusted friend with whom she shares her flat. She needs help with feeding and personal hygiene, as well as with writing notes for the service user group she chairs. Having personal assistants enables Martha to take part in many activities in the community and ensures she lives a full and active life.

Loss of Sight (Visual Impairment)

Visual impairment includes the broad range between people who have no sight and those who are affected with a mild impairment which leaves them partially sighted.

Practice study

Henry

Henry has a progressive deterioration in his sight. In his thirties, he lost his job as a taxi driver and decided to make the change from voluntary care work for a disability group to training as a social care worker. He knew about the supported employment scheme in his area. This is used by people with physical impairments to meet their practical needs when at work. He gained confidence through the supported employment scheme and felt confident enough to continue his training. At the end of his training he was successful in his application for a post running a project for people with profound physical impairments.

Hearing Loss (Auditory Impairment)

A whole range of hearing losses are covered by the general word 'deafness'. Hearing loss can be partial or total. Profound deafness usually means severe hearing loss greater than 90 decibels (dB), 25 dB being mild hearing loss or 'hard of hearing'. People unable to hear or understand speech are usually considered 'deaf'. The Royal National Institute for Deaf and Hard of Hearing People (RNID) distinguishes between mild, moderate, severe and profound hearing loss.

Some people lose part of their hearing very slowly, as they grow older. Others, through accident or illness, lose their hearing overnight. Hearing loss can apply to a part of the range of frequencies or the entire range. A person with high or low frequency loss may have good hearing in other parts of the frequency range. This may create several kinds of problems:

- It may be more difficult for other people to accept the real difficulty caused by partial hearing, for instance where much of a conversation is heard perfectly well, but the meaning of some words is misunderstood because the consonants at their ends are inaudible.
- It may be impossible to use a hearing aid because turning up the volume to make the high or low frequencies audible may amplify other sounds to a painful extent.
- Whereas one-to-one conversation in a quiet place may be easy, it may be impossible to hear wherever there are sounds in the background.

Communication problems for the deaf person may create difficulties for them in their relationships, at work, in their social life and in leisure pursuits. They may lose partners and friends or jobs, or be forced to give up pleasurable activities such as sports where hearing sounds is essential for personal safety.

Some people who are deaf 'hear' voices. This includes people diagnosed with schizophrenia. Adam James describes in the Mind magazine *Openmind* several group meetings run by the deaf charity Sign in Balham, south London, where seven people diagnosed with schizophrenia used sign language to discuss their voices (James, 2005, p. 24). The conclusion of the Department of Health (DoH, 2001c, 2002d) is that deaf people, including about 6,000 psychotic deaf patients, are not receiving adequate services. Much useful information on hearing loss is available from the British Deaf Association (BDA), RNID and the National Deaf Children's Society (NDCS).

Ways of Working with Disabled People

General Pointers to Ways of Working

It is generally not a good idea to try to reduce a complex area such as working with people with disabilities to a 'toolkit' of suggestions for practice. However, it is worth creating a checklist that you can check when preparing for, and doing, the practice. Here is the beginnings of such a list:

- Holding to an equality perspective
- Valuing as people first, then 'with impairments', not as 'impaired people'
- Respecting cultural and racial differences
- Not discriminating or stigmatising
- Empowering people, that is, ensuring they participate fully in the process of the work done with them
- Enabling people to choose to claim direct payments if they wish, and employ a personal assistant
- Communicating adequately, that is, accessibly (see Chapter 41)
- Taking account of access, including timing and length of activities and the need for breaks in meetings and support.

Dealing with Problems of Hearing Loss

The assumption that a deaf person suffers less difficulties than a person who is blind is mistaken. Sight and hearing loss present totally different issues and each is potentially as serious for the person concerned, their relatives, friends and other people with whom they interact. A person who loses most or all hearing suddenly may be particularly traumatised. All significant hearing loss involves a serious level of isolation and communication problems.

People with hearing loss may find it daunting to leave their homes and some benefit from a dog trained to guide them, for example in towns where there are busy roads and pavements are crowded with people walking in different directions, pushing prams, with dogs on leads or with young children who stray unpredictably into the path of other pedestrians. It may be difficult for a person with excellent hearing to appreciate the extent to which we rely on our perception of sometimes quite subtle and faint sounds when walking through crowded streets or crossing roads so as to avoid fast-moving vehicles and bicycles.

From an equality perspective, we should regard people with hearing loss as benefiting from a language to enable them to communicate. British Sign Language (BSL) and Makaton are languages used for communication by people with hearing loss. A growing wealth of new technologies are available to support people with hearing impairments, including computer programs recognising speech and converting it to text on the screen, visual telephones with built-in printers and word displays, flashing lights for door bells and environmental alert devices including wake-up alarms with touch stimulation.

Here is a checklist of points to bear in mind when communicating with a person with hearing loss:

- If you are fortunate enough to know enough BSL or Makaton or other sign language, reward yourself for being well prepared
- Work through an advocate with BSL or Makaton
- Otherwise, remember to deal with the situation not as though you are working with a person who has a problem, but as though *you* have the problem, because *you don't know the language*
- Find a place where background activity or noise isn't a distraction
- Keep your face turned towards the person
- Ask if the person needs to lip-read
- Attract the person's attention before speaking
- Speak slowly
- Speak clearly
- Speak expressively by varying the pitch of what you say
- Don't exaggerate in the way you speak
- Don't shout
- Keep your hands away from your face
- Try not to keep moving your hands as you speak
- Remember, a beard or moustache makes lip-reading more difficult
- If you become stuck, try to choose alternative words and use them
- Have a sheet of paper or pad handy so you can jot down words or questions if you become stuck.

Sight Loss

Research bringing together the views of people with visual impairments with a review of the literature has identified seven areas of potential need:

> meeting people and friendship; getting information and advice about other services for people with a visual impairment; finding out about special equipment; having someone to talk to about your personal feelings; building your confidence to go out and do things outside your home; relearning how to carry out everyday tasks in your home; and getting help with practical everyday tasks. (Willis, 2005, p. 32)

Of these, the first was considered the most important by the people with visual impairments. The research made strategic and operational recommendations. The strategic ones included expressing the aims of services in terms of outcomes for people with visual impairments which promoted their inclusion in mainstream provision. The operational ones included individualised programmes supporting people with a visual impairment, empowering them to gain access to mainstream services (Willis, 2005, p. 33).

Loss of Mobility

People with restricted mobility may or may not use wheelchairs. If they do, problems of access are multiplied. Many buildings, especially older ones, do not comply with the Disability Discrimination Act 1995 and provide access for disabled people. Often buildings provide access but toilet facilities are inadequate. Some motorised wheelchairs are too large to fit into the traditional 'disabled' toilet. Many taxis will not accommodate a large, motorised wheelchair. In one northern town, there is only one taxi which will accommodate one resident, a service user whose impairment requires a large, motorised wheelchair and who is an active chair of a local group of service users.

Working with people whose impairments restrict their participation in events requires practitioners to appreciate the degree of frustration and, on occasions, anger this may create. It should also be possible for practitioners to contribute to campaigns to remove some of the barriers that disable people and exclude them from the community and many of its activities.

Activity 14.3

1. Read through the lists you made earlier in Activity 14.1 under the headings: Loss of mobility, Loss of sight, Loss of hearing.
2. Now spend a few more minutes adding further points to your list.

Conclusion

This chapter has surveyed some of the main features of suffering from a physical impairment which disable a person. It has focused on the examples of impairments affecting mobility, sight and hearing, while recognising the wider span of physical disabilities. It has explored some of the main ways of working with people with physical disabilities.

REVIEW QUESTIONS

1 What problems arise for the person experiencing loss of physical mobility, loss of hearing and loss of sight?

2 What points you would bear in mind when working with that person to cope with losses under each of these headings?

FURTHER READING

ADSS, BDA, LGA, NCB, NDCS, RNID (2002) *Deaf Children: Positive Practice Standards in Social Services*, London, RNID

Ballantyne, J. (1993) *Deafness*, London, Whurr

Barnes, C., Oliver, M. and Barton, L. (eds) (2002) *Disability Studies Today*, Cambridge, Polity Press/Blackwell

Lewin-Leigh, Benedict (undated) *Standards for Services for Adults who are Deafblind or have a Dual Sensory Impairment*, London, Sense, enquiries@sense.org.uk

Morris, J. (1991) *Against Prejudice: A Personal Politics of Disability*, London, Women's Press

Morris, J. (1996) *Encounters with Strangers: Feminism and Disability*, London, Women's Press

Oliver, M. (1990) *The Politics of Disablement*, Basingstoke, Macmillan – now Palgrave Macmillan

RNID (1999) *Best Practice Standards: Social Services for Deaf and Hard of Hearing People*, London, RNID

Robinson, C. and Stalker, K. (1998) *Growing Up with Disability*, London, Jessica Kingsley

SCIE (2005) *Transition of Young People with Physical Disabilities or Chronic Illness from Children's to Adults' Services*, Research Briefing 4, London, SCIE

WEBSITES: www.rnib.org.uk (RNIB for blind and partially sighted people)
              www.rnid.org.uk (for people with hearing impairments, including deafness)

Part III

Resource file

Charging and direct payments

Charging for services

Local authorities are guided by section 17 of the Health and Social Services and Social Security Adjudications Act 1983 when they fix what the Act calls 'reasonable' charges. Charges are based on a complicated mixture of flat-rate charges and means-tested rates. Research has found considerable uncertainty about charging policy and practice among people who use services and a lack of knowledge about which charges are mandatory and which are discretionary (McDonald, 2006, p. 124).

Direct payments

Direct cash payments to people who use services are empowered by the Community Care (Direct Payments) Act 1996, later amended to extend the payments beyond the age of retirement (Lloyd, 2003, p. 40). They are consistent with the empowering aims of official policy, for example in relation to people with disabilities (DoH, 2001b). They may be made as a substitute for them receiving services, to enable them to purchase their own services (McDonald, 2006, pp. 125–7). This is usually in the form of a person to do the caring work, usually called a personal assistant. The person using services becomes the employer of the personal assistant and takes on certain responsibilities. Rather than these being seen as a source of barriers and problems, research indicates that people who use services regard them positively (Stainton, 2002).

The government has declared the intention to change

the name of direct payments and to extend their use 'to disabled people aged 16 and over, young people aged 16 to 17 and people who have parental responsibility for who are disabled' (DoH, 2005, p. 86).

FURTHER READING

Brechin, A., Walmsley, J., Katz, J. and Peace, S. (eds) (1998) *Care Matters: Concepts, Practice and Research in Health and Social Care*, London, Sage

Learning Disability **15**

SUE BALDWIN

Learning outcomes

By the end of this chapter, you should:

■ UNDERSTAND the policy context of learning disability

■ IDENTIFY the main features of positive practice with people with a learning disability.

In this chapter we examine some of the main aspects of services for people with learning disabilities. The service provision and quality of life for people with a learning disability has changed dramatically in the past 20–30 years. This has happened as a consequence of a number of important health and social care initiatives. At the heart of these changes, however, has been a fundamental shift in the way people with a learning disability are perceived, and how our attitudes, values and beliefs about this group of people have changed.

Policy Context: From Institutionalisation to Independent Supported Living

It was the second half of the twentieth century before poor standards of care in hospitals for people with learning disabilities were exposed by public inquiries and research. The inquiry into conditions in Ely hospital, Cardiff (DHSS, 1969) followed allegations of ill-treatment of patients which were largely substantiated. In the early 1970s, research into what were called 'subnormality hospitals' found shortcomings in their regimes (Jones et al., 1975). Policy and practice began to change and attitudes towards people with learning disabilities gradually became less punitive and stigmatising. From the 1990s, the growing strength of the disability movement in the UK accompanied policy changes towards enabling disabled people to participate in their own care planning (see Chapters 16 and 39).

Practice study

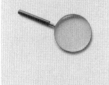

Michael

Michael is in the process of signing his tenancy agreement in preparation for moving into a supported living environment, after spending a lifetime in institutionalised care. Michael has witnessed many of these changes. Institutionalised at the age of five, he was detained in a subnormality hospital under the Mental Deficiencies Act 1913, as an imbecile.

'Imbeciles' was one of four derogatory classifications that reflected the prevailing ideologies towards people with a learning disability in that time period. The other three classifications were idiots, who were people of least ability; feeble-minded persons, who were more able than imbeciles and idiots, but still required protection, or to protect others from them; and lastly, the moral defectives, who were thought to have permanent mental defects, but also had criminal or violent tendencies (Atherton, 2003, p. 50).

The Mental Deficiencies Act was replaced by the Mental Health Act 1959, by which Michael received an informal status, and the new label of 'severely subnormal'. Again the classification under the Mental Health Act reflected society's attitudes towards people with a learning disability. Michael's informal status meant that he was no longer a detained patient, but, as he was only 14 years old, he remained a resident of the subnormality hospital.

Goffman (1961) referred to a variety of residential establishments from monasteries and prisons to hospitals, which shared certain 'institutional' features – including subnormality hospitals – as total institutions. According to Goffman, such total institutions are characterised by the fact that all aspects of life are conducted in the same environment. Inmates are segregated from mainstream society, and are powerless and controlled by rigid routines and block treatment that functions to serve the institution rather than the inmate.

Activity 15.1

Spend a few minutes reflecting on the differences between everyday family life – at its best – and the characteristics of everyday life in one of the total institutions as described by Goffman. Jot down notes under these two headings: 'family life' and 'total institution'. Here are my notes:

Characteristics of *family life*

- living in a house in a street
- part of the local neighbourhood
- all family members 'muck in'
- decisions made by different members

- meals taken when members wish
- hobbies and excursions flexible.

Characteristics of life in a *total institution:*

- living in a large 'warehouse' for storing people
- cut off from surrounding community
- staff in charge of residents/'inmates'
- staff make decisions
- meal times rigid, for residents
- activities programmed by staff.

Michael's memories of the institution are such that he found it difficult to talk about these at first, and a trusting relationship had to be developed, in which Michael felt safe and secure. The relationship also had to be honest and communicated in a manner that was within his level of understanding and communication ability. Michael's childhood through to his early adult life had been marred by a process of dehumanisation. Barton (1976, cited in Birchenall et al., 1997) described this process as one of violence, brutality, bullying, browbeating, harshness, teasing and tormenting.

A number of different outcomes can occur when you live in abusive and extreme conditions in which individuals experience degradation and enforced submission. In Michael's case he freely admits that he 'fought the system', and developed a challenging reputation. Michael's history and experiences are not dissimilar to others who have undergone discharge from the large hospitals. This process began with society becoming alerted to the nature of the institution and the number of inquiries in the 1960s and 70s, including Ely hospital referred to above (DHSS, 1969), which examined the conditions within the hospitals. This culminated in the government White Paper, *Better Services for the Mentally Handicapped* (DHSS, 1971), which led the way for a number of policy reports and service developments that aimed to reduce the number of people within long-stay hospitals. This did not occur in isolation, however, and people with a learning disability experienced the development of new ideologies of care based around the concepts of equality, rights, and the experience of opportunities for conditions of living that equated to those of ordinary community members (Wolfensberger, 2003).

The introduction of the concept of 'normalisation' – meaning the right of people with learning disabilities to have access to resources and support to enable them to fulfil their potential – from Scandinavian and North American philosophies led to a shift in ideology that slowly began to work at revaluing devalued people. This was aimed at society's attitudes towards people with a learning disability and also professionals' working practices.

However, while the 1990s saw a period of hospital closures and the positive effects of the NHS and Community Care Act 1990, Michael remained institutionalised, and when the hospital closed in the mid-1990s, he was transferred to hostel accommodation. The rationale behind this was due to a range of complex needs around his challenging reputation. While living in the institution, Michael developed violent behaviours towards others and property. These behaviours develop for a number of reasons. In some individuals, the behaviour that challenges is because of biological causes, often linked to the cause of their learning disability. However, as no cause of Michael's learning disability had been established, one could assume that he had acquired the behaviours that challenge through learned experiences and his reluctance to conform to the rigidity of his living environment. When individuals see inappropriate behaviours being rewarded in some way, they will imitate them (Wolverson, 2003).

Valuing People: A Person-centred Approach

In 2001 the government published a White Paper entitled *Valuing People* (DoH, 2001b), in which it set out its strategy for service provision for people with a learning disability and their family and friends. *Valuing People* emphasised four key principles underlying service provision, care and support to people with a learning disability. These principles are independence, choice, rights and inclusion.

Valuing People highlighted that even though service provision had shifted to a community-focused service, people with a learning disability still had little control over their lives. Atherton (2003) discusses some of the issues that have led to people with a learning disability still remaining at the fringes of being provided with support to make decisions and take up a valued role within society.

At the centre of *Valuing People* is the adoption of a *person-centred approach*, in which the individual with a learning disability is central to determining the decisions about their lives that ordinary community members take for granted. In essence, person-centred approaches are about establishing, enabling and facilitating a process that will enhance the quality of life for that individual and in which that individual is central. The process is about listening to the individual and the significant people in that individual's life, and enabling that individual to realise their aspirations, dreams and choices in life. For professionals, it means being able to facilitate the process whereby the individual is provided with support, knowledge and skill for them to achieve their goals and make their own decisions. This process is reliant on the professional continually reflecting upon their own attitudes, values and beliefs. Their part in this process is to listen and learn and not to impose their opinion or stamp their own decisions upon the individual's choices.

Michael is at the beginning of this process, which has been an extremely emotional journey for him, given the experiences he has had previously with the learning disability services. In sharing this process with him, we have developed a trusting relationship, which has been extremely important, as person-centred planning is not just asking somebody what they want to do with their life. In Michael's case it has initially been about helping him to deal with his fractured self-concept. Birchenall et al. (1997) talk about the mortification of self, in which it is argued that the institution destroys the vital functions of the self. In essence, Michael has lost his sense of individuality.

We all learn who we are as people from the feedback we receive from other people. This feedback is communicated to us verbally, or non-verbally, when we interact with people. Michael's picture of himself is one in which he is perceived by others as a problem, a troublemaker and a violent person. His past relationships have been based around power, control, violence and aggression. These perceptions have created barriers to him forming relationships with other people. Positive relationships would have enabled Michael to grow as a person and participate in opportunities that would have provided him with the skills to engage in ordinary living.

Sanderson (2003) would argue that person-centred planning is rooted in the principle of *shared power* and *self-determination*. Michael is able to communicate verbally, although he has not developed literacy or numeracy skills. He has been assessed as having a moderate learning disability. If communicated with at a level he understands, he is able to contribute to and participate in meetings set up to determine his appropriate service needs. He has no family contacts and is therefore unable to involve them in the process, but he has identified a number of key people with whom he feels comfortable, and who he wishes to be involved in facilitating the planning process.

Decision-making for people with a learning disability can be a demanding and complex issue. It must be continually borne in mind that people do not develop skills for living, which are required within ordinary living, when they have grown up in impoverished environments. Michael is no different; he developed in an environment that made all life decisions for him, and therefore without his contribution, he never learnt the skills of decision-making. Throughout our discussions, the process of decision-making was addressed, although it is worth pointing out that this occurred over a six-month period. It was a process of trust-building, ensuring that Michael felt valued and enabled, before he felt he was in a position to call his initial person-centred planning meeting.

If person-centred planning is to be meaningful and place the person at the centre of the planning process, then the person has to be equipped with the skills and knowledge in order for them to participate. The person with the learning disability has to feel that they are at the centre of the planning process, and that they are not going to be told what services they can access. In some respects, the individual has to 'bare their soul'. This is how Michael described it, and he went on to infer that all his life he had tried to hide his inner thoughts and feelings because they would have been used against him, or that he would have been laughed at. He likened it to 'us changing our minds', meaning that we now wanted to know what his thoughts and feelings are so that we can help him to achieve them.

Care Planning: Assessment

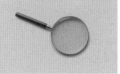

Practice study

Michael (cont'd)

This process was extremely stressful for Michael, but he felt that he was ready to engage in the process, and the initial planning meeting was organised by Michael who

chose who he wanted to attend, and then dictated to his formal carers the invitation letters. Michael then expressed a wish to prepare himself for the meeting. He felt that this was important, particularly as he had no family to help him, and he felt a little nervous about the ways in which he could explain what his aspirations were.

Michael was quite clear about how he wanted to live his life, and as a consequence of our discussions felt that he had some insight as to how he might approach seeking the support he felt he needed. Firstly, he expressed a wish to 'stop being angry'. He recognised that this was important because it was a barrier to achieving his biggest wish, which was for a home of his own. He said to me 'I want to live in a house like you.'

At the planning meeting, Michael outlined his aspirations, and then asked how we could help him work towards living in his own home. Sanderson (2003) writes that 'person-centred planning challenges professionals', and rather than focusing on what skills are required by Michael to achieve this, our practice should be led by what level of support is necessary to achieve this.

Person-centred plans develop a shared understanding in which the individual with a learning disability is enabled to achieve a balance between the issues that are important to them, but secure in the knowledge that they have participated in the decision about how best to support them (Sanderson, 2003). This is not, however, saying that the person-centred planning meeting exists to just give people what they desire. This issue is more complex, and involves discussing realistic aspirations with the person. So, for example, Michael wants to live in his own house, but would require a level of support from carers to enable him to do this while he learns some of the responsibilities he will have in maintaining his role within the community. Michael may not wish to have people invade his home, but may need to accept that it is a level of support that he requires at the present time. The important factor is that Michael has participated, agreed the decision and is also involved in identifying who will give the level of support.

The communication skills of both professionals and the person with the learning disability are essential in this process. Where the person with a learning disability communicates by alternative methods, then the onus is on the professional to acquire the capability to communicate with that person. Likewise, as this is a shared experience and understanding, the professional can facilitate the acquisition of communication skills to assist in the process.

Planning and Implementation

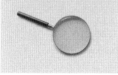

Michael (cont'd)

In Michael's case, he had established his aspirations, and in many respects had identified one of the issues in his life that he had to deal with, that of his anger. He decided

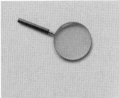

at the planning meeting who he would like to support him, and then engaged in a process of assessment. With the support of a community learning disability nurse, Michael was able to indicate what triggered his anger, and why. More importantly, he was able to work with the community nurse to develop strategies that would support him in best managing situations in which he felt angry. He indicated that instead of somebody trying to tell him how to behave, as had happened in the past, he became more aware that he was choosing to behave in a less angry way. Michael was beginning to realise that he could make life choices that involved making positive relationships with people, based upon friendships.

Activity 15.2

1. Spend a few minutes jotting down notes on how Michael's reflections and attitudes changed during the period described in the Practice study.

Here are my reflections:

- At the outset, Michael was depressed and had a negative view of himself.
- He tended to fight back at the institution containing him.
- He shifted from having low ambition and self-esteem to aspiring to improve his situation.

2. List the main factors that you feel contributed to these changes.

Here are my thoughts:

- Policy and practice changes meant that Michael began to be treated as a person deserving respect.
- Staff listened to Michael's point of view.
- Michael was encouraged to look towards a positive future.
- Michael was empowered by being able to increase his knowledge, skills and available resources.

Person-centred planning is not a one-off event. Simmons (2000) discusses the continual flexibility of the process, in recognition of the changes that will occur when people experience new situations and opportunities. The process is a dynamic engagement with an individual based upon the key characteristics of valuing people, developing a shared understanding and identifying what is important to the person. The support mechanisms needed to achieve their aspirations are then built around the individual. Fundamental to this is the skill of listening and maintaining dialogue.

Professionals require a shift in their skill base, as Sanderson (2003) suggests 'professionals have to move from being experts on the person to being experts on the process of problem solving with others'. In other words, professionals need to start accepting that people generally know how they want to live their lives, but that they don't necessarily have the resources, facilities or support mechanisms with which they can begin to make decisions for themselves.

Greig (2005) believes that the publication and subsequent implementation of *Valuing People* (DoH, 2001b) is a 'government success story', but argues that the work has only just begun. In his report to the secretary of state for community, Greig argues that people are being respected and listened to more, which is a starting point. However, he also stresses that people cannot change overnight. It is worth remembering that the success of any change in the way we approach the development of services for people with a learning disability rests with the attitudes, values and beliefs of that society. Challenging these attitudes will significantly improve the lives of people with a learning disability.

Conclusion

This chapter has outlined theoretical issues from the perspective of one person, Michael. It has explored issues related to the history of learning disability services, making real their impact when examining what it meant in terms of life experiences and opportunities for one individual. Since the publication of *Valuing People* (DoH, 2001b), for the first time in his life Michael is starting to make decisions about how he wants to live his life. The challenge from *Valuing People* for professionals is enabling and facilitating the level of support required for Michael to realise his dreams and aspirations.

REVIEW QUESTIONS

1 What major changes in policy and practice regarding people with learning disabilities have taken place since the 1970s?

2 What is person-centred planning?

FURTHER READING

Atherton, H. (2003) 'A History of Learning Disabilities', in B. Gates (ed.) *Learning Disability: Towards Inclusion*, Edinburgh, Churchill Livingstone
Chapter 4 provides an insightful exploration of the history of learning disability practice.

Goffman, E. (1961) *Asylums: Essays on the Social Situation of Mental Patients and Other Inmates*, Harmondsworth, Penguin
The introduction (pp. 17–22) to this important book describes the key characteristics of total institutions, with direct application to subnormality hospitals, among others.

Jones, K., Brown, J., Cunningham, W.J., Roberts, J. and Williams, P. (1975) *Opening the Door*, London, Routledge & Kegan Paul

Sanderson, H., Kennedy, J., Ritchie, P. and Goodwin, G. (1999) *People, Plans and Possibilities: Developing Person-centred Planning*, Edinburgh, SHS
A short text that provides the reader with an overview of the person-centred planning process and explores different planning frameworks that clearly set the person at the centre of the process.

Stratham, M. and Timblick, D. (2001) 'Self Concept and People who have Learning Disabilities', in J. Thomson and S. Pickering, *Meeting the Health Needs of People who have a Learning Disability*, London, Baillière Tindall

Chapter 10 explores issues of the self-concept and aids our understanding of the importance of positive self-images.

Thomas, D. and Woods, H. (2003) *Working with People with Learning Disabilities: Theory and Practice*, London, Jessica Kingsley

Chapter 4 outlines the principle of normalisation and its impact on the development of person-centred services for people with learning disabilities.

WEBSITE: www.connects.org.uk (Foundation for People with Learning Disabilities portal for mental health and learning disabilities)

Part III

16 Mental Health and Mental Illness

JENNIFER NEWTON

Learning outcomes

By the end of this chapter, you should be able to:

■ EXPLAIN broad categories of mental disorder

■ SUMMARISE a number of different types of support available

■ UNDERSTAND the 'recovery perspective' in mental health.

This chapter introduces some psychiatric terminology, and examines two illustrative examples of people coping with mental health problems. The help available to them is summarised, and the central role of the recovery model to current policy and practice is emphasised.

Words and Labels

While the words 'mental health' and 'mental illness' are commonly used in everyday conversation, and we all believe we know what we mean, defining and explaining these terms is not at all straightforward. The first mistake some people make is to confuse mental illness with learning disability. The latter is a disability caused at conception, during pregnancy or childbirth or shortly afterwards, that is lifelong and cannot be 'cured', although the disability can be greatly reduced by appropriate support and education. It affects the person's ability to learn, is usually associated with impaired intelligence, but can vary in severity from mild to profound (see DoH, 2001b).

By contrast, mental illness is a term used to describe a collection of health conditions that are characterised by alterations in thinking, mood or behaviour, associated with distress and usually with some impaired functioning, problems that have become serious enough to be considered an 'illness'. These can affect any one of us at any time in our lives. Definitions, and use of the term 'illness', are contentious, and lie at the heart of much of the literature promoting differing interpretations of the behaviour of those labelled. This difference of opinion is understandable, given the very negative consequences in Western societies of receiving a psychiatric diagnosis (see Baker and Read, 1996). Mental illness is treatable, and most people recover well, although some experience repeated episodes of ill-health throughout a large part of their lives. People with mental illness are not less intelligent, nor more violent than the average person, nor are they more likely to be old, nor of any particular ethnicity or gender. On the other hand, life difficulties and stresses associated with any personal characteristics or social situation *will* make the person more vulnerable to mental illness (Brown, 1996). Hence, people who are unemployed, those who live in social housing and those recently bereaved or separated have higher rates of depression, for example, than people in work, in owner-occupied housing and married or single.

The next difficulty in definition is determining where the cut-off lies between distress and illness. If, after months of distress and argument following the cot death of their long-awaited first child, Jane Smith has just been told by her partner that he is leaving her, it would not be surprising to find her in depressed mood, hardly eating or sleeping, crying regularly and lacking concentration or motivation. Is this an illness or an understandable response to an upsetting series of life events?

Psychiatrists, psychologists and medical researchers have devised many methods over the years to try to gain some clarity and consistency over such definitions. Distinctions are made not only on the basis of symptoms experienced, but also taking account of the disabling effect of those symptoms, their duration, the person's safety, and their need for formal and informal support (DoH, 1995a). They also categorise mental illness into various diagnoses. This labelling process is central to the *medical model* of psychiatry (Tyrer and Steinberg, 2005). One important distinction is between disorders associated with, and those not associated with, physical damage to or disease in the brain, or brain dysfunction. The former are termed *organic disorders*, and the best known include the dementias, and those psychiatric problems that follow a brain disease or injury. The latter are collectively referred to as *non-organic disorders*.

A second distinction that is frequently made, among the non-organic disorders, is between those mental health problems where there are psychotic features (such as hallucinations or delusions) and those more associated with mood changes (for example anxiety and depression) or behavioural problems (for example eating disorder, addictions, obsessive compulsive disorder).

Practice study

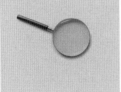

Rik

Rik had become a little distant and increasingly solitary after leaving school with much poorer exam results than his parents had hoped he would achieve. A few months after starting work at an insurance company, he announced he was going away for a few

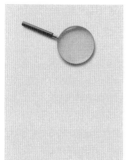

weeks and, without packing a bag, he left for Madrid the next day. A phone call two weeks later from a hospital there led his parents to go to collect him, and this marked the start of recurrent periods of severe difficulty. Rik remains convinced that he was followed during his stay and an attempt was made on his life, and that there are people who wish to kill him who know where he lives in London. From time to time, these beliefs resurface and his psychosis worsens, leading him to keep the curtains closed, hide behind furniture if someone walks up to the house, throw away food cooked by his mother which he believes may have been poisoned, or refuse to leave the house. He is often agitated and upset, and can get very angry at suggestions that he should go out more or move to a home of his own. He has had little work in the 10 years since his ill-fated trip to Spain.

A *psychosis* or a *psychotic disorder* is where the person's difficulties appear to include an inability to distinguish reality from imagination, and he or she may see, hear, feel or believe things that others cannot explain from their own experience of reality. These types of symptoms are termed *hallucinations*, *delusions* and *disorders of thinking*, and one example of a diagnostic label for these types of symptoms is schizophrenia (see Tyrer and Steinberg, 2005, Ch. 6). Problems of this nature are typically present among those labelled as having *severe and enduring mental illness*, who make up the largest group served by community mental health teams (DoH, 1995a). By contrast, those people whose symptoms relate to depression, anxiety, compulsive behaviour, phobias and so on are more likely to be collectively labelled as having a *minor psychiatric condition*, or a *neurotic disorder*, and seen and treated in general practice. Many of their problems are by no means minor or trivial and trying to help them has become a major part of the GP's workload (Armstrong, 1995).

Getting Help

For most people, the GP is the first port of call when feeling ill, distressed or unable to cope, and the GP decides whether or not to refer the person on to psychiatric services, or whether the primary care team can offer the necessary help – the practice nurse, the health visitor, the practice-based counselling service or GP. For this reason the GP is often described as the 'gatekeeper' to psychiatric services. Medication to help sleep, assist relaxation, or to counter depression or anxiety is often part of the help offered. It will initially be the GP who decides whether Jane's problems amount to transient distress or a clinical depression, who writes a probable diagnosis in the notes, and will have first referred Rik to psychiatric services. Jane may be offered a prescription of minor tranquilisers, antidepressant medication and/or a chance to speak to a practice-based counsellor. She would probably benefit from talking to someone who has gone through a similar experience of child bereavement, by contacting SANDS (the Stillbirth and Neonatal Death Trust) or FSID (the Foundation for the Study of Infant Deaths), which provides information and a 24-hour helpline. She may be offered help by one of the 1,000 recently appointed graduate mental health workers, promised in the NHS Plan (DoH, 2000e), who are attached to GP practices and trained in brief therapies.

Practice study

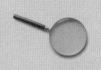

Jane

Jane has experienced a number of major losses: her long-awaited child, her partner, and her job. She had left full-time work and moved away from the city and her friends to a new home and a new role as full-time mother. She is particularly distraught by the belief that she may never be able to have a child, and, in these circumstances, she is a high risk for clinical depression (Brown, 1996). An assessment of her situation should consider whether she has a close confiding relationship to help her through her distress, but also whether she is holding any thoughts about suicide. While suicide is much less common in young women than young men, suicidal behaviour or self-harm that does not lead to death is more common in women than men (see DoH, 1999a, standard 7). If Jane has a strong relationship with a family member or friend, has no history of depression, has good prospects of finding work and was previously a relatively self-confident woman, she will be at much less risk of having prolonged or serious difficulties.

Relationship problems lie at the root of a great number of the reasons for consultation in general practice, with a mixture of depression and anxiety being one of the most common of all health problems seen there. Similar difficulties are also prevalent among the people being helped by social workers in children and family services, and adult services, and they are also widespread among people who do not seek help outside their circle of friends and family. The help any one of us values at this time is similar: someone to talk to, who empathises and helps us to see ourselves as able to cope, as being a worthwhile person, and although we may not be able to see it at the moment, given time, we will see a hope for a better future. Brief therapies, through general practice, local Mind groups or from a psychologist, can be of great benefit, and those who can engage with books and self-help materials can find similar benefits in terms of self-understanding in this way (see Rowe, 1996; Gilbert, 2000).

Working towards Recovery

Psychiatric diagnoses are broadly accepted among a large part of the academic and professional world, and are used by GPs and psychiatrists to label the groups of symptoms that patients present to them when they consult. They are useful in planning, evaluating, researching and treating mental illness. But they are not always welcome labels for a service user. The *social model* is much less fixed about diagnoses, recognising that symptoms and behaviour need to be understood in the context of society as a whole, and that the labels given can create problems of their own. While not necessarily rejecting the usefulness of diagnoses, service users themselves prefer the focus of provision to be guided by the concept of *recovery*.

The National Institute for Mental Health in England (NIMHE, 2005) has issued a guiding statement on the recovery perspective, which it advocates as core to the value base for mental health service provision. It explains that a recovery perspective

> involves a process of changing one's orientation and behaviour from a negative focus on a troubling event, condition or circumstance to the positive restoration, rebuilding, reclaiming or taking control of one's life

and that it reflects a belief in

> both the possibility of improvement in a person's condition and/or experience and the importance of the person assuming an active and responsible life within their cultural and familial context.

As it goes on to explain, the approach is based on successful experiences with self-help and on research into serious mental illnesses.

The view now is that while doctors seek a *complete recovery* in medical terms whereby the symptoms are no longer present, service users feel the most important aspect of recovery is their *social recovery*, that is, their ability to get back to a 'normal' life, to be economically self-sufficient, to have friends, a home and an active, rewarding life. If some symptoms persist but do not interfere too badly with their life, this may not be problematic. Indeed, the Hearing Voices Network, a charity with a helpline, web information and local meetings, has a large membership, who all hear voices but do not all have a diagnosis of mental illness. The groups provide a safe forum in which people can speak freely about their voices, learn to accept them, live with them, and regain control over their lives.

Practice study

Rik (cont'd)

Rik is now helped by the nearby community mental health team (CMHT), and has recently been visited by Lloyd, a support, time, recovery (STR) worker, whose role is to offer *support* and *time*, and thus aid *recovery*. Lloyd is offering friendship, and is working with Rik to rekindle his interest in watching football, introducing him to snooker at the nearby pub, and looking at options at the local FE college with him for courses to help him back to work. Rik has a care plan that he developed with his care coordinator, and although his earlier plans have not worked well, he is now optimistic that with his new STR friend, he will manage to move towards his long-term aim of getting a job again. While it is the community psychiatric nurse (who is also the care coordinator; see Chapter 12) who has drawn up his care programme approach (CPA) plan and also monitors Rik's medication, Lloyd is key to the delivery of the plan.

Rik's CPA plan will be reviewed every six months. The latest plan has been adapted from an earlier one agreed at the end of his last inpatient treatment, which was agreed at a formal, multidisciplinary CPA meeting attended by Rik, a member of the CMHT, a ward nurse, a psychiatrist, and his parents. Future reviews will include feedback from Lloyd, and Rik can involve a friend or someone from an advocacy service if he wishes. The review should check whether specific objectives set in the care plan are being achieved, or whether the plan needs to change.

During a full relapse, Rik is often considered a risk both to himself and others. He will have received a detailed risk assessment, leading to both a crisis and a contingency plan. These notes clarify the warning signs that may indicate a relapse is imminent, and what has been agreed with Rik about what should happen in these circumstances. This is now a required part of practice for all people under the CPA.

Rik's agitation and suspicion over many years have been difficult for his parents, who want to be able to invite friends home, employ a cleaner and have some space to themselves. They have had their own carer's assessment, but have made it clear they want things to change. They have reached a point where they no longer wish to support him in their home, and are hoping the care coordinator will find Rik a place of his own that Rik will be willing and feel safe enough to move to. But plans for moving, which will involve Lloyd taking Rik to see some of the supported housing options available through a local housing association, have been deferred until he has been successfully engaged in some activities outside the home that will help to sustain him after the move.

Rik's local CMHT has several community psychiatric nurses, two social workers, an occupational therapist (OT) shared between their team and one nearby, a psychiatrist and an STR worker. The nurses, social workers and OT are all care coordinators, with a caseload each of people, most of whom have a severe and enduring mental health problem. Their care planning might draw on support and activities available at a mental health day service, and on those provided in the voluntary sector such as local MIND groups. However, using a recovery model and aiming for social inclusion, they will aim to draw on non-specialist activities and existing community and natural support structures too (see Chapter 50).

If Rik experiences a new acute psychotic episode, there is a crisis resolution team to provide intensive support to try to ensure that he does not need to be admitted to hospital again. If, on the other hand, he urgently needs to be admitted, perhaps because he is seen as at real risk of self-harm, or harming others, and has stopped taking his medication, he will be encouraged to come voluntarily into the hospital, but can be compulsorily admitted if it is deemed necessary.

Activity 16.1

Take a look at some voluntary groups, and see what help they can offer. Collect a database of contact numbers and summaries of what they campaign for and what provisions they offer. Start with some of the following: Young Minds, Depression Alliance, Turning Point, Eating Disorders Association, Mental Health Foundation, Manic Depressive Fellowship, MIND, SANE, Rethink, Samaritans.

Legal Basis for Mental Health Intervention

The laws covering compulsory admissions today are the Mental Health Acts 1983 and 2007, assuming the Bill going through Parliament as this book goes to press becomes law. Amendments under the Mental Health Act 2007 will address some issues related to consent to treatment and mental capacity to consent. A person can be detained against their will using a number of different sections of the Mental Health Act 1983, most commonly section 2 (28 days for assessment) or section 3 (six months for treatment). These two can be requested by an approved social worker, or sometimes the nearest relative, and need to be supported by two doctors. The consent of the nearest relative is needed for a section 3. One of the doctors and the social worker will have had additional training to qualify them to take this role. The other doctor should be someone who knows the individual. The proposed changes should enable a wider group of professionals to undertake similar training and take on these roles. People admitted under a section of the Mental Health Act are known as 'formal patients', as compared to the majority (roughly 75 per cent) who are 'informal' or voluntary patients. The law is needed to ensure that people with serious mental health problems that threaten their health or safety or the safety of the public can be treated irrespective of their consent where it is necessary to prevent them from harming themselves or others. The Mental Health Act 2007 clarifies the circumstances in which a person with a mental disorder can be detained for treatment without his or her consent, and sets out the processes that must be followed and the safeguards for patients.

User Involvement

People who have experienced mental health problems are now actively involved in helping to shape mental health policy and practice, and there is a growing literature where they are making clear what their priorities are (see Chapter 39, and Read and Reynolds, 1996). Not surprisingly, they want what any health service patient wants – information (about their diagnosis, the treatment, the services and support available), choices, participation (in decisions about their own care, but also in influencing services), to be able to access help when they need it (including the middle of the night and at weekends), to be treated with dignity and respect, and to have their individual needs taken into account (for example cultural, religious, gender, dietary needs). They have also argued that in the past practitioners have been too pessimistic in their approach, particularly when a person has been labelled as having a severe and enduring mental health problem, and have often failed to consider that the individual may be able and willing to return to work, given adequate support. Policy today is aiming to change these negative views (NIHME, 2005).

Conclusion

Any one of us can develop mental health problems, and very many of us *will* know depression and anxiety at some point in our lives, as it is so prevalent – the common cold of psychiatry. The experience can be devastating, however. Over 4,000 people in England take their own lives each year, including one in ten people with a severe mental health problem (DoH, 1999a).

Most people will be helped in general practice, a small proportion will be referred on to CMHTs or outpatients departments. Many of those who have become 'experts by experience' have written about their experiences and their views on services. As a health and social care practitioner, you will need to familiarise yourself with this literature, and with the preferred recovery model.

REVIEW QUESTIONS

1 How would you describe the following terms: psychosis, learning disability, organic disorder?

2 Why is the recovery model welcomed by service users?

FURTHER READING

Bowers, L. (1998) *The Social Nature of Mental Illness*, London, Routledge

DoH (1999) *National Service Framework for Mental Health: Modern Standards and Service Models*, London, DoH

Golightley, M. (2006) *Social Work and Mental Health* (2nd edn) Exeter, Learning Matters

Heller, T., Reynolds, J., Gomm, R., Muston, R. and Pattison, S. (eds) (1996) *Mental Health Matters: A Reader*, Basingstoke, Macmillan – now Palgrave Macmillan

Read, J. and Reynolds, J. (eds) (1996) *Speaking Our Minds: An Anthology of Personal Experiences of Mental Distress and its Consequences*, Basingstoke, Macmillan – now Palgrave Macmillan

WEBSITES: www.mind.org.uk/Information/ (Mind)
              www.mentalhealth.org.uk/Information/ (Mental Health Foundation)

Part III

17 Children's Services

ROBERT ADAMS

This chapter covers the major area of children's services, a general term used to cover education and social services for children, young people and their families. (Linked material will be found in Chapters 30 and 49.)

Children's Services in Policy Context

Social services departments (SSDs) formerly provided children's social services, under the Children Act 1989. Since 2000, a major policy change in England has resulted in large areas of children's social services being shifted from SSDs and relocated with children's education services in newly created local authority departments. (In Scotland and Wales, generic departments for adult and children's services remain.) So education and social services for children are provided under one department by local authorities. The Children Act 2004 aimed to integrate children's social services and education services in new children's trusts by 2008. Under this later Act, responsibility for children's education and social services lies with the Department for Education and Skills (DfES) and in each local authority is located in one new department for children's services, in recognition of the importance of these services. Two aims of this are to ensure that services are 'joined up' (coherent), their management and delivery being coordinated so that vulnerable children do not 'slip through the net', that is, fail to have their needs recognised and dealt with. A 10-year strategy has been developed (see Resource File: Key Changes in Childcare Policy in the Twenty-first Century, at the end of Chapter 3). Nationally, the government has created a minister for children, young people and families and a children's commissioner. Three factors have highlighted the need for improvement.

First, the children's healthcare, social care and early years sectors have suffered from shortages of training staff for many years. Additionally, the announcement in 2005 of a new single qualification framework, opening up new career pathways, was linked with the specification of a common core of skills across the children's work-force. The Children's Workforce Development Council, the sector skills council for children's work, and Skills for Health, the sector skills council responsible for incor-porating children's work skills into the healthcare area, are working together to implement this, partly through the development of national occupational standards and national vocational qualifications.

Second, increased knowledge and public awareness of the nature and extent of individual and social problems requiring a social services response were beyond the experience and capacity of many local authorities.

Third, the generic SSDs set up after the Seebohm Report (1968) did not respond adequately following the deaths of some 30 children in the years between the inquiry into the death of Maria Colwell in 1973 (Secretary of State for Social Services, 1974), the inquiry into the care of children receiving complex heart surgery at Bristol Royal Infirmary (Kennedy, 2001) and the Climbié report (Laming, 2003).

These three factors contributed to the publication of the Green Paper *Every Child Matters* (DfES, 2004a), the publication of the *National Service Framework for Children, Young People and Maternity Services* (DfES and DoH, 2004; see Resource File: Health Promotion (1) Children, Young People and Maternity Services, at the end of this chapter) and the publication of the action plan for carrying forward policies for children's services (DfES, 2004b). The Childcare Act 2006 sets out the responsibili-ties of local authorities for early childhood services and requires compulsory regis-tration of providers who care for children aged five to seven.

Services for Children

The range of children's services includes:

- working with families of vulnerable children, including those who may be neglected or abused
- health promotion for children
- behaviour support for children in school
- education welfare services aimed at improving school attendance
- education psychology services linked with children's emotional wellbeing
- child and adolescent mental health services

- early years support services to children and families, provided mainly through early education, full daycare, family centres, support for parents with special needs, health services, Sure Start centres and Children's Fund projects
- Connexions services, providing guidance and personal development for young people aged 13–19
- youth services
- services for children with disabilities, including special educational needs, learning difficulties and speech and language difficulties needing speech therapy
- special schools, providing education and support to pupils with statements of special educational needs
- services for children with complex emotional, behavioural and educational needs
- social work services for children and families under the Children Act 1989
- childcare services for looked after children, in children's homes, with foster carers or adopters
- care leavers' services
- family and parenting services
- children and young people who offend (as part of youth offending teams – YOTs).

The 400,000 children receiving social services at any one time in England represent a significant proportion of the total of 11 million children and young people receiving other education and health services (CSCI, 2005b, p. 1). It should be noted that:

1. 'Carer' in this chapter means residential social worker and/or foster carer.
2. Looked after children include those accommodated voluntarily with parental consent, or with their own consent if 16–17; those in care on a care order or interim care order under section 31 of the Children Act 1989; those 'remanded to local authority care', that is, accommodated under section 21(2)(c)(I) of the Children Act 1989; those on an emergency protection order (EPO) under section 44 of the Children Act 1989.
3. There is a variety of secondary services providing information and advice for adults caring for children. For example, in some areas there is a confidential telephone line, the Children's Information Service, offering free information about the range of services for adults caring for children, from registered child-care and free early education places to financial and other support for adults with children.

Children with Disabilities

Parents with disabled children may be able to receive direct payments which may be used – perhaps with other benefits such as disability living allowance – to purchase services, organised and managed by themselves. Direct payments may be spent on personal assistance for the parent or the child, found by the parent or through an agency. They may also be used to provide respite for the parents, by paying for a brief residential or holiday break for the child. Direct payments increase the choice and flexibility of parents and as the child grows older, he or she will have an increased chance to express views about how the payments are spent (see Resource File: Theories and Models of Residential Care, at the end of Chapter 54).

Looked after Children

Children may be taken into care or 'looked after' by the local authority under the Children Act 1989. They may live in a children's home and/or be fostered before returning home, or, if return home is not possible, they may be adopted. Whereas fostering is a temporary arrangement in which the original parental rights are not transferred to the foster carer, adoption is permanent and involves a transfer of parental rights to the adoptive parent. Inspections of children's services indicate that the great majority of looked after children prefer family placements with foster carers or adopters to a stay in a residential childcare establishment (CSCI, 2005b, p. 6).

Residential care

The quality of residential childcare has long been questioned by researchers (Berridge and Brodie, 1998; see Resource File: Theories and Models of Residential Care, at the end of Chapter 54) and highlighted by a succession of scandals and investigations and inquiries (Blom-Cooper, 1985; London Borough of Greenwich, 1987; London Borough of Lambeth, 1987; Butler Sloss, 1988; Levy and Kahan, 1991; Waterhouse, 2000; Laming, 2003).

Efforts are being made to ensure that local authorities respond consistently to the problems of 'runaway' children (LAC, 2002, 17). Each year, an estimated 100,000 children run away from care or from home and research by the Children's Society (2004) shows the additional risks they run, over and above those experienced by other children.

Leaving care

A great deal of attention traditionally was focused on residential care but, until the mid-1980s, the transition from care to the community was badly neglected, to the detriment of children and their families. Stein and Carey (1986) followed up the process of young people leaving care in the early 1980s and found many of them suffered through a lack of preparation and inadequate support in accommodation and job-finding. Although there are still inadequacies (Stein, 2004, 2005; Stein and Dixon, 2006), policy and practice have improved. Under the Children (Leaving Care) Act 2000, every child must have a personal adviser and a pathway plan by the age of 16 and these arrangements must continue until 21 and, if in higher education or training, until 24 years of age.

Activity 17.1

Asher is leaving residential childcare at the age of 17. He was assessed as neglected and was looked after by the local authority for three years.

Spend a few minutes jotting down the kinds of issues that should be incorporated into a checklist for the local authority leaving care team to bear in mind.

In the wake of the Children Act 1989, Bob Broad (1998, p. 254) surveyed the work of 46 leaving care projects working with more than 3,300 young people. He found that a quarter of the 46 local authorities surveyed did not have leaving care policies and the monitoring of leaving care was entirely ad hoc, so it was not possible to ascertain how well the leaving care procedures were working. The Children (Leaving Care) Act 2000 requires local authorities to help children and young people leaving care until they are 21 and provide a leaving care plan with each young person. Research by Roger Morgan, the children's rights director at the CSCI (Morgan, 2006), points to worrying deficiencies in arrangements made by local authorities, including a lack of gradual transition, a lack of adequate information to young people about their leaving care entitlements, and problems obtaining sufficient money and inadequate accommodation and support once they had left. It is clear what works in leaving care arrangements (Stein, 2004), but local authorities still have work to do in bringing leaving care arrangements up to a common standard.

Foster care and adoption

The local authority has responsibility for supervising the welfare of all fostered children. Training and financial support for foster carers may be provided by the local authority, who also may put new foster carers in touch with a network of others. In the past, different local authorities have paid different levels of allowance to foster carers, which potentially leads to geographical inequalities between the services that fostered children receive. The intention of government is to publish national fostering rates (DfES, 2006a). Foster care does not just involve children being looked after by the local authority, but also may be a private arrangement, perhaps made between a parent and someone caring for the child who is not another parent or relative. Once the child has been with this person for more than 28 days, the arrangement becomes private fostering. Under the Children Act 1989, the parents and carers have a duty to inform the local authority of the arrangement. Normally, they should inform the local authority at least six weeks in advance of the beginning of the arrangement. Failure to do so could incur a fine.

Children may go into foster care for many reasons. Often, it is because they have interrupted or unsatisfactory contact with a primary or parental attachment figure, or, as we say, a parent or guardian. While a child is in foster care, every effort should be made to retain the child's contact with the biological parent. If this is not possible, the effort should be directed to building attachment with another adult who can take on the parenting role. Sometimes this will involve preparing for adoption by another person or couple (for further discussion of attachment, see Chapter 7). As well as maintaining contact with biological family members, it is important where possible to maintain the child's sense of continuity and stability while in foster care.

Adoption is the permanent placement of a child with adults who take on full parental responsibility. Since 2000, there have been government initiatives to speed up the process of adoption (DoH Adoption and Permanence Taskforce, 2001), on the grounds that adoption is a benefit which should be made available to as many children as the system can cope with, rather than looking to fit children into what traditionally has been a slow and unwieldy procedure, with losses to the children which were largely hidden (Berridge, 1998; Robinson, 2000). The Adoption and Children Act 2002 represents a major overhaul to the adoption system, aiming to make it less unwieldy and slow.

Asylum-seeking children

A relatively small number of unaccompanied children seeking asylum often present local authorities with complex problems, which, inspections show, they struggle to cope with (CSCI, 2005b, p. 6). Not least of these issues are the tensions between different perspectives on transracial adoptions (Gill, 1983).

Early Years Services

There is a huge quantity of childminding and daycare in England. By 2002, more than 50,000 existing providers had been inspected (Ofsted, 2003, p. 1). Childminding and daycare for children under eight are classified as 'early education' and, since September 2001, responsibility for regulating this provision (that is, registering and inspecting, investigating complaints and enforcing compliance with national standards under the Care Standards Act 2000, amended by the Children Act 2004) has passed from local authorities to Her Majesty's Chief Inspector of Schools (HMCI) at the Office for Standards in Education (Ofsted). Ofsted also regulates government-funded nursery education for children aged three to four.

The regulations governing childcare, including forms of group daycare such as childminding and nurseries, cover the standards of buildings, health and safety, employment of staff, food and hygiene, disability and legislation regarding discrimination (Ofsted, 2005).

Five types of childcare provision are specified and regulated by Ofsted – childminding, full daycare, sessional daycare, crèches and out of school care:

1. A *childminder* is anybody looking after one or more children under eight, not a foster carer and unrelated to them, on domestic premises for more than two hours a day for payment (Ofsted, 2005, p. 4). *Daycare* must be registered if provided for six days or more in any year, for children under eight, for more than two hours at any time of day or night on other than domestic premises (not a children's home, care home, hospital or residential family centre) (Ofsted, 2005, p. 4).
2. *Full daycare* must be registered and involves continuous care for four hours or more in a day, such as is provided by day nurseries, children's centres and some family centres (Ofsted, 2005, p. 7).
3. *Sessional daycare* also must be registered and involves children under eight attending for no more than five sessions of no more than four hours on any single day. Playgroups where morning and afternoon sessions are separated by a lunchtime break, with no children left with the provider, are not regarded as daycare (Ofsted, 2005, p. 8).

4. A *crèche* provides occasional care for children under eight and may be permanent or temporary (for example, the former at a shopping centre, the latter at a conference which the parent attends) (Ofsted, 2005, p. 8).

5. *Out of school care* involves daycare for children aged three to eight before or after school, or during school holidays, for more than two hours in any day and more than five days a year (Ofsted, 2005, p. 8). Older children may use this facility, which includes breakfast and after school clubs, play schemes and summer camps. *Open access schemes* providing supervised play in the absence of parents are included, for children aged five to eight, whether permanent or temporary, although older children may take part (Ofsted, 2005, p. 8). Sometimes children will have support from children's centres or through Sure Start, a government-led initiative to provide additional services for young children and their families.

Face-to-Face Work with Children

Values: The Foundation of Work with Children

The government has put in place a common basis of values, knowledge and skills for all who work with children (DfES, 2004c). Many people – carers, care assistants, nursery assistants, nurses, doctors, dentists, school teachers, careers officers – work with children and young people. Some of these deal with children for just a few minutes at a time, while others, such as parents and foster parents, look after them full time. Residential childcare staff also are in intensive contact with children for long periods of time. Whatever the circumstances, people interacting with children should *treat them with respect* and *with due regard for the diversity of children's own cultures and beliefs*. Parents, of course, do not 'work with' their children. They live with them. Their relationship is personal, while staff, practitioners and workers have a professional relationship with children. There is a tension in that relationship between the friendliness children may expect and associate with 'being normal with me' and inappropriate informality, such as would occur only within a family.

Clearly, agencies have to intervene in some families in order to protect children from harm and ensure that their welfare and best interests are promoted under the Children Act 1989. There is a tension between this and working to empower children, an approach based on assumptions about their right to participate actively in decisions about their health and welfare (see Chapter 40).

Assessment of Needs

Assessment of children's needs has been standardised since 2000 (DoH, 2000a) by the publication of a framework for the assessment of children in need and their families, based on bringing together three overlapping and interrelated 'systems' or 'domains': the developmental needs of the child; the capacities of parents and carers to respond to the child's needs; and the impact on these capacities of wider environmental and family factors. Throughout, the priority is to safeguard the interests and rights of the child, protect him or her from harm and promote his or her welfare.

In completing the assessment, practitioners must note:

- the areas of the child's needs to be tackled
- how progress with the plan will be monitored
- how the child's age and stage of development will be considered
- how the information will be analysed and used in future action (see also Chapters 30 and 51).

Children's Rights

Historically, as reading about the history of child labour in the nineteenth century or a glance at the adult dress of upper-class children in eighteenth-century paintings will show, children have often been treated as miniature adults. Since then, of course, most children have been taken out of the workplace and put into the nursery and the school. Civilised Edwardian parents would have said children should be seen and not heard.

One way of arriving at a view of what good quality work with children should be is to start from a statement of children's rights (see Activity 17.2 below).

So what have children the right to expect? *Childism* involves denying children their rights and is a form of oppression. Children still experience exclusion, lack of power and lack of being taken seriously. Their rights are often neglected or ignored. Advocating that children have rights does not mean treating them as miniature adults. Most children would resent having their opportunities to be childish and play taken away and the responsibilities of adulthood dumped on them. Childhood needs respecting as a stage in the life course.

Activity 17.2

Spend five minutes jotting down a manifesto under the heading 'Ten Rights for All Children Worldwide'.

The following list is in random order. Children have the right to:

- safety
- be cared for
- be loved
- be educated
- be allowed to be children
- not be exploited or abused
- not live in poverty
- not be unnecessarily sick or prematurely die
- be brought up in a loving family
- be well fed.

Effective work with young children rests on the twin foundations of a critical understanding of child development and the careful application of frameworks for assessment (DoH, 2000a) and through the application of messages from research in guidelines and procedures developed by the Department of Health (see DoH, 1995b). When working with children, we demonstrate to them that we are taking them seriously, showing we are listening to them, in the following ways:

- We attend to what they are saying.
- We feed back emotionally (by showing them the effect on our feelings of what they are telling us, without losing control and leaving them feeling unsure or unsafe).
- We repeat what they've said to us, summarising what they've said and reflecting it back to them.
- Where they're using a doll or game, we may use the same medium to reflect back how we're responding to what they're expressing about situations or people.
- We show by our body language, eye contact (sometimes too much eye contact distresses children not used to this), nodding encouragingly, smiling, showing sympathy, demonstrating that we're not being judgemental (adopting a critical view of them), asking questions to invite them to say more, confirming and in places prompting them to clarify and extend what they've said.

Conclusion

This chapter has indicated the range of children's services and highlighted the diversity of provision. It has also indicated some areas of complexity in work with children, especially the tension between using legal powers to intervene in families to safeguard children's interests and, at the other extreme, adopting a children's rights perspective and working with them to empower them.

REVIEW QUESTIONS

1 What range of children's services is delivered by the local authority?

2 What services are covered by the term 'early years'?

3 What rights would you include in a manifesto of children's rights?

FURTHER READING

Clear, H. (2004) *Assessing Children's Needs and Circumstances: The Impact of the Assessment Framework*, London, Jessica Kingsley

Fawcett, B., Featherstone, B. and Goddard, J. (2004) *Contemporary Child Care Policy and Practice*, Basingstoke, Palgrave Macmillan

Milligan, I. and Stevens, I. (2006) *Residential Child Care: Collaborative Practice*, London, Sage

National Children's Homes (NCH) (2003) *Factfile 2002–03: Facts and Figures about Children in the UK*, London, NCH

Richman, N. (2000) *Communicating with Children: Helping Children in Distress*, London, Save the Children

Sinclair, I., Wilson, K. and Gibbs, I. (2004) *Foster Placements: Why they Succeed and Why they Fail*, London, Jessica Kingsley

Vincent, C. (2006) *Child Care Choice and Class Practices: Middle-class Parents and their Children*, London, Routledge

Resource file

Health promotion (1) Children, young people and maternity services

The National Service Framework (DfES and DoH, 2004) establishes national standards to promote children's and young people's health and wellbeing. There are 11 standards:

■ identifying needs and early intervention, through the child health promotion programme led by the NHS in partnership with local authorities (standard 1).

The other 10 standards include:

■ support for parents
■ family-centred services for children and young people
■ growing up to adulthood
■ safeguarding and promoting the welfare of children and young people
■ ill children and young people
■ children and young people in hospital
■ children and young people with disabilities and with complex health needs

■ children's and young people's mental health and psychological wellbeing
■ medicines for children and young people
■ maternity services.

Health improvement for children and young people depends on their active participation and empowerment, by:

■ giving them information about the issues
■ encouraging them to develop opinions
■ offering opportunities to tell decision-makers what they think
■ providing feedback with how their opinions have shaped services
■ ensuring that ways are found of taking account of the views of children and young people from a diversity of ages, abilities, cultures and backgrounds.

FURTHER READING

DfES and DoH (2004) *National Service Framework for Children, Young People and Maternity Services*, London, TSO

DoH (2004) *Disabled Children and Young People and those with Complex Health Needs*, London, DoH

Pike, S. and Forster, D. (1997) *Health Promotion for All*, Edinburgh, Churchill Livingstone, pp. 125–40
A useful chapter covering practice issues regarding children and young people.

Part III

18 Drug Usage: Legislation and Administration MARION GRIEVES

This chapter discusses the general use of drugs in today's society and explores the methods used to protect the public and ensure the best possible effects of administered medicines. The focus of the chapter is to demonstrate the safety mechanisms that the producers and prescribers of drugs and the general public can follow to ensure safe practices when using and disposing of drugs.

What is a Drug?

A drug is a substance that, when taken or applied, may modify one of the body's functions, whereas a medicine is referred to as a drug that is taken in the treatment or prevention of disease. Throughout history drugs have been used for medicinal and social purposes, alcohol being the earliest known substance that caused profound effects on the body, followed by plant derivatives such as leaves, roots and flowers. Tobacco, jasmine tea and camomile lotion provide only a few examples of plant derivatives that are readily available for purchase in the shops.

Drug User or Abuser?

In today's society you hear many comments identifying individuals as drug users or abusers. What does this mean? Considering a drug is a substance that can modify one of the body's functions, you could argue that all individuals in today's society are drug users when they drink alcohol, coffee, tea or fruit juice.

When does a drug user become an abuser? If you define abuse as using something to bad effect, or the improper use of something, then overuse of drugs, taking drugs that are not for the treatment or prevention of disease is considered in this category. This explains why individuals who commonly take drugs such as tea, herbal remedies, paracetamol for headaches, or are on prescribed medication are not considered to be drug abusers, as these activities are not regarded as improper use of a substance.

Activity 18.1

Examine the list below and consider whether the user of each one would be classed as a drug user or a person on medication.

- Alcohol
- Heroin
- Ampicillin
- Senokot
- Paracetamol
- Steroids
- Cannabis

All the list above can be classed as drugs or medication. If you were taking steroids, prescribed by your doctor, for an inflamed knee joint, you would be on medication, whereas if you were taking steroids as a body-building enhancer that were not prescribed, you would be considered to be a drug user/abuser.

All individuals use drugs – it is only why they take them that alters society's classification of the user. Consider what drugs you may have taken yourself in the past and how you would classify your activity.

Legislation

The impact of drugs on society is huge and without safeguards people would be more at risk of receiving drugs that were not fit for human consumption. To overcome this, all countries have their own regulatory boards. In the UK, the Medicines Act 1968, the Misuse of Drugs Act 1971 and the Poisons Act 1972 regulate the use of all medicines and poisons, and these are now discussed.

Medicines Act 1968

The Medicines Act 1968 regulates the manufacture, distribution and importation of all medicines for human use. It identifies three classes of product:

1. *General sales list* (GSL): these are medicines that can be sold to you over the counter without a pharmacist being present. You can often find these medications in your local supermarket, petrol station shop, corner shops and so on.

2. *Pharmacy medicines* (P): these are medicines that can only be sold under the supervision of a pharmacist.
3. *Prescription only medicines* (POM): these are medicines that can only be supplied by retail in accordance with a prescription written by an appropriate practitioner such as doctor, dentist, specialist nurse and so on.

Activity 18.2

Take a few moments and list a few of the GSL, P and POM medicines that you know about or have used.

Often medicines are reclassified, so that you can buy them over the counter instead of going to your doctor to ask for a prescription. Have you recently heard of any medicine that has become available without a prescription?

For centuries, only doctors held the right to prescribe medications, however, recently within healthcare provision there has been a legislative change, whereby nurses and pharmacists can now prescribe from a defined list of medicines after they have carried out a required training programme. This provides the public with further means of accessing medications when they require them.

Misuse of Drugs Act 1971

The Misuse of Drugs Act 1971 is the main government legislation for drugs laws and licensing drugs. Drugs are classified and offences for handling drugs and the penalties are clearly identified.

Table 18.1 Classification of drugs under the Act

Class A drugs	Class B drugs	Class C drugs
Ecstasy	Amphetamines	Cannabis (reclassified in 2004)
LSD	Methylphenidate (Ritalin)	Tranquilisers
Heroin	Pholcodine	Some painkillers
Cocaine		GHB (Gamma hydroxybutyrate)
Crack		
Magic mushrooms (if prepared for use)		
Amphetamines (if prepared for injection)		
Penalties for possession		
Up to seven years in prison or an unlimited fine, or both	Up to five years in prison or an unlimited fine, or both	Up to two years in prison or an unlimited fine, or both

Within the Act drugs are categorised as class A, B and C, with A being the most harmful drug (Table 18.1). Offences under the Act include:

1. Possession of a controlled substance unlawfully.
2. Possession of a controlled substance with intent to supply it.
3. Supplying or offering to supply a controlled drug (even where no charge is made for the drug).
4. Allowing the premises you occupy or manage to be used for the purpose of drug-taking.

Table 18.1 provides examples of the classification of drugs within the Act and the penalties for possession of the drug. More details of the Act can be found at http://www.drugs.gov.uk/drugs-laws/misuse-of-drugs-act/. See also Chapter 19 for discussion of drug abuse.

Poisons Act 1972

The Poisons Act 1972 provides companies and individuals in society with the regulations for the transport, storage and labelling of drugs. All healthcare providers need to adhere to these regulations and you will see the required written details on your prescriptions when you get them from the doctor/nurse/dentist. Not only are there requirements for the prescription but also the labelling. Have a look at any medicine labels you have in your home, what do you see there? The printed information on the medicine container is the legal requirement and is there to safeguard you, your family, service users and carers, and everyone in society.

Why Legislation is Important

When a drug is first developed, there is an immense amount of research done by the drug company, as well as other government-sponsored research agencies such as NICE (National Institute for Clinical Excellence), to ensure that when drugs become available on the market they will be beneficial for people in society and have minimal side effects. Each country has its own strategy and legislation to ensure that drugs are safe and fit for the purpose they have been developed for, so therefore it can take years for a drug to go through the research process before it is licensed and becomes available to the general public.

You may be aware of discussions in the news about drugs that are available in other countries but not in the UK. This is because the strategies utilised by the government to assess the effectiveness of the drug have not been completed by the relevant parties, so a licence has not yet been given for use of the drug in the UK. This process may appear cumbersome at times, however, I am certain you would rather know the drug was safe to use prior to taking it.

How Drugs Work

In general, drugs are in two categories: *systemic*, which are taken into the bloodstream; and *topical*, which are applied to the area where they are needed.

- *Systemic:* When you swallow a tablet or liquid form of medicine, it is absorbed in an area of your gastrointestinal tract – the stomach, the small intestine or the large intestine. The acids in your body need to break down the medicine to enable it to be absorbed into the bloodstream, which is the body's main transport system that carries all the nutrients, fluid and oxygen throughout your body. Once the medicine is in the bloodstream, it is filtered through the liver and kidneys and is excreted in the urine.

- *Topical:* As topical medicines are applied to the area where they are needed, the majority of topical applications are applied to the skin in the form of cream or ointment. However, topical medicines also include sprays, drops, and pessaries and suppositories, for example cream would be used for eczema (skin itching), pessaries for oral thrush, inhalers for asthma, drops for ear, nose and throat and suppositories for constipation (Table 18.2).

Table 18.2 Medication types and routes

Oral	Rectal	Injections	Transdermal	Eye/ear/nose	Vaginal
Solid tablet/ capsule	Enemas	Subcutaneous	Adhesive patches	Cream	Creams
Dispersible tablets	Creams/ ointments	Intramuscular		Ointment	Pessaries
Sustained-release tablets	Aerosol/ foams	Intravenous		Drops	
Enteric-coated tablets	Suppositories	Intra-articular (joints)			
Sublingual		Depot (deep muscles)			
Buccal					
Liquids/syrup					
Lozenge					
Mouthwashes					

How Decisions are Made on the Routes, Dosages and Timing of Drugs

When drug companies develop a new drug, the research they carry out analyses all the processes that would have an impact on the drug – its lifespan, absorption rate, toxic level and side effects.

You will probably have heard of someone who has been on a drug trial. These are continually being carried out throughout the country with volunteers from different age groups, cultures and regions. When drug trials are carried out, there is a vast amount of evidence collected by the researchers, some of which includes data from blood analysis, people's reactions physically and mentally, when maximum effectiveness of the drug is reached, potential effects that the new drug will have on medications already taken, and any adverse reactions throughout the trial. It is from this type of information that dosages, timing and routes of drugs are determined.

Drug Storage

The storage of drugs is very important. You will probably have noticed that some drugs are dispensed in clear bottles, some in coloured bottles and some in sealed plastic cards; this is to ensure that drugs that need to be protected from light and air to stop deterioration are done so through the various packaging methods. The way a drug is stored is extremely important to maintain the maximum effect of the properties within it. The lifespan of the drug can be altered depending on where and how it is stored. Eye drops often need to be stored in the fridge, as warm temperatures reduce their effectiveness and they also expire one month after opening. Some dressings will disintegrate if they are stored in a hot environment.

Therapeutic Levels of Drugs

The routes and dosages of drugs are determined through blood analysis and toxic levels. The most important factor that needs to be considered is the maintenance of the therapeutic levels of the drug within the person's body. Drug regimes are designed to ensure that the dosages and times achieve this level; so if the drug is prescribed as six-hourly, this provides the individual with information to achieve the best possible effect of the drug.

Take a look at Figure 18.1. The drug taken initially takes some time to get to a therapeutic level and then the effectiveness reduces. The timing of the next dosage is purposeful to ensure that the new drug has time to be absorbed into the system so that the therapeutic level is maintained. This is why adhering to the time and dosage of drugs is important.

Figure 18.2 identifies what happens when the timing of the drug is altered. This often occurs with antibiotics. These are often prescribed six-hourly. Can you honestly say that you adhere to the dosage and take the medication on a six-hourly basis?

Many people take a tablet early in the evening about six o'clock and then at bedtime. This might only be four hours after the last tablet. When the second drug

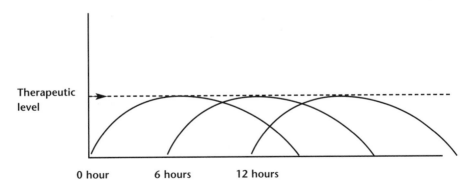

Figure 18.1 A well-maintained and effective drug regime

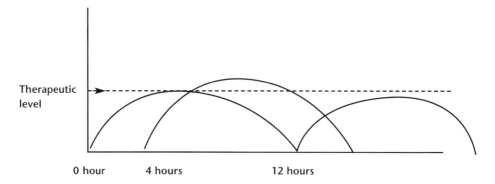

Figure 18.2 A badly maintained and less effective drug regime

is absorbed into the system, the level of drug in the person's system will be higher than the recommended therapeutic level. If the person then takes the next tablet when they get up in the morning – a potential gap of 8–10 hours between the dosages – the effect on the therapeutic level is a reduction.

The Other Determinants of Therapeutic Levels

Not only is it important to take the drug at the prescribed time, it is also important to take the drug in the manner explained in the instructions. If you are directed to take the drug half an hour before food on an empty stomach, this is to ensure that the drug is absorbed into the bloodstream after breakdown by the digestive acids within the stomach. This will gain the most effect from the drug. Some drugs, when absorbed through the stomach, cause acidity for the individual, and in this situation the drug format would be altered so that the person would be given this in an enteric-coated format and be asked to take the drug with food. This will reduce the effect of the acidity and alter the absorption of the drug so that it is absorbed in the small intestine. It is important that an enteric-coated tablet is not crushed in a spoon for someone who cannot swallow drugs easily as the effect of the drug will be reduced.

For people who find tablets difficult to swallow, there are many liquid preparations available as alternatives. Many of these are flavoured, nicer to take and often given to children. When in a liquid preparation, antibiotics, such as penicillin, need refrigeration to maintain their stability and effectiveness.

The absorption of some drugs can be impeded by gastric juices. An example of this is glyceryl trinitrate. This is normally prescribed as a sublingual preparation (under the tongue), which will enhance the absorption and avoid mixing the drug with food and gastric juices.

Hopefully, this brief survey has shown you that there are reasons for prescribing drugs in different formats and the importance of maintaining the prescribed regime.

Administering Drugs and Medication

Practitioners in health and social care cannot take legal responsibility away from the pharmacist and prescribing doctor, who are responsible for 'gatekeeping' and supplying drugs and medication. However, as the practitioner working with the service user, patient or carer taking medicines, you need to ensure that the following points are adhered to:

- Any allergies or reactions the person may have had with previous medication, as well as any other medication the person may be taking at the time, are passed on to the pharmacist, doctor or nurse
- The medicine is the right one
- The expiry date is checked before use, for example ear, nose and eye drops usually have a short lifespan of one month after opening
- The medicine is stored in the recommended way, for example the fridge
- The prescribed timing is kept to, for example six-hourly
- The medicine is taken at the time recommended, for example half an hour before meals
- The right dosage is taken, say, 500mg tablet and the dosage is not doubled if a dose is missed
- If the course of the medication is a specific length of time, the whole course must be taken, for example antibiotics
- The person does not take someone else's medication because they had an illness similar to theirs. They do not know the side effects, whether the drug will be effective for them, or whether the drug will react with other medications they are taking and will make them feel more unwell.

To condense the list and remember the most important aspects, one way is to think about the five Rs:

- Right time
- Right amount
- Right person
- Right drug
- Right route.

Safe Disposal of Drugs

The final aspect of using drugs is the disposal of out-of-date drugs, drugs you have discontinued or those you have found in the cupboard and do not know what they are for.

The process for returning unwanted drugs is to take them to a local pharmacist for destruction. A written response to a question posed to the secretary of state for health in the House of Commons in June 2006 identifies that the Department of

Health estimates that unused medicines returned to pharmacies are probably worth £100 million per year (Hansard, HC, vol. 74529, col. 385W, 5 June 2006). Although returned drugs cannot be reused as the pharmacist does not know if they had been stored correctly, if the drugs are stable or if there has been any cross-contamination, the pharmacists are able to have the drugs destroyed appropriately to maintain environmental safety. It is *never* recommended to throw drugs down the drain as the substances can transfer into local drainage systems and streams and may cause harm to the general public and the environment.

Individuals who have been prescribed injections and need to use needles and syringes must always consider the safe disposal of these. They are provided with sturdy sharps bins for the safe disposal of used needles and syringes to ensure that there is no danger of needlestick injuries to anyone handling the disposed of items.

Conclusion

This chapter has considered the legal context for the regulation of drugs and drug-taking. It has also examined briefly the implications for the administration and handling of drugs by professionals including practitioners in health and social care.

REVIEW QUESTIONS

1   What would you do if you found out one of your parents, or the person with whom you are working, was taking another relative's painkillers?

2   What would you do if you found needles and syringes in the park?

3   When might an enteric-coated tablet be prescribed for a person?

FURTHER READING

Dewing, J. (2002) 'Older People with Confusion: Capacity to Consent and the Administration of Medicines', *Nursing Older People*, **14**(8): 23–8

Griffith, R. (2003) 'Administration of Medicines, Part 1: The Law and Nursing', *Nursing Standard*, **8**(2): 47–53

Hopkins, S.T. (2005) *Drugs and Pharmacology for Nurses* (13th edn) Edinburgh, Churchill Livingstone

Jordan, S. (2003) 'Administration of Medicines, Part 2: Pharmacology', *Nursing Standard*, **18**(3): 45–6

Mallik, M., Hall, C. and Howard, D. (2004) *Nursing Knowledge and Practice: Foundations for Decision Making*, Edinburgh, Baillière Tindall

Resource file

Policies to tackle drug and alcohol abuse

National Alcohol Harm Reduction Strategy (2004)

The Prime Minister's Strategy Unit (2004) published this interim report, which contributes to the development of an alcohol harm reduction strategy for England to reduce binge-drinking, with its consequences of health problems, premature deaths and alcohol-related crimes, disorder and injuries.

Other points from the report are:

- Taxes on alcohol raise £7 billion per year. Alcohol contributes £30 billion a year to the economy and half a million people are employed in the industry
- Moderate drinking can reduce the likelihood of coronary heart disease for older people
- Regular heavy drinkers suffer greater health problems and die younger
- 150,000 hospital admissions per year are alcohol-related accidents and illnesses
- About 40 per cent of admissions to A&E are alcohol-related
- 15,000–22,000 deaths per year are alcohol-related
- Parental alcohol problems affect up to 1.3 million children in the UK
- Young people are drinking twice as much now as 10 years ago
- In 2001–2, there were 1.2 million alcohol-related violent incidents.

UK-wide Drug Strategy (updated 2004)

The government produced the Drug Strategy in 1998 and updated it in 2002 and in a document from the Home Office Drug Strategy Directorate (2004), with similar publications in Wales, Scotland and Northern Ireland. The strategy aims to reduce the harm caused by illegal drugs.

By 2008, the strategy aims to:

- Reduce availability of drugs and put drug dealers out of business
- Prevent people, especially young people, using drugs
- Treat and rehabilitate existing drug users, especially the most serious users
- Use the criminal justice system to tackle drug-related crime and treat and rehabilitate those committing crime to finance their drug-taking
- Extend drug intervention programmes to 30 more areas
- Introduce legislation to steer more drug-related criminals away from crime and into treatment
- Introduce tougher legislation for the police and courts to tackle drug dealers
- Improve treatment and prevention schemes.

FURTHER READING

Home Office Drug Strategy Directorate (2004) *Tackling Drugs. Changing Lives – Keeping Communities Safe from Drugs*, Drug Strategy Progress Report, London, Home Office

Prime Minister's Strategy Unit (2004) *National Alcohol Harm Reduction Strategy*, London, Cabinet Office

RESOURCE FILE: Health Promotion (2) Stopping Smoking, at the end of Chapter 19

19 Problems of Alcohol, Drugs, Tobacco and Food ROBERT ADAMS

Learning outcomes

By the end of this chapter, you should be able to:

■ IDENTIFY the main social and medical problems associated with alcohol, drug, smoking and food abuse

■ DISCUSS some of the main approaches to working with people who abuse different substances.

The abuse of alcohol, drugs, tobacco and food has huge medical, psychological and social costs in common, although the problems and issues raised by each differ widely. It is common to discuss problems of dependence as though they only apply when a person's daily functioning is seriously affected. However, as this chapter indicates, many people's difficulties with drugs, alcohol and food are hidden by themselves, their partners and other family members. Tobacco is in a different category, since although tobacco is now banned in public places in several European countries including Britain, in many private situations people continue to smoke.

Problems of Alcohol, Drug, Smoking and Food Abuse

Alcohol and drug abuse pose formidable problems for the health and social services. To take drug abuse first, illegal drug-taking is the source of criminal activity that has knock-on effects for those who are its victims. Large-scale thefts and burglaries in some localities are overwhelmingly due to addicts stealing in order to sell the proceeds of crime to fund their habit. The consequences of addiction are no less serious for addicts themselves, for their nearest relatives and others with whom they share their households and their lives. Jobs, friendships and relationships all can be wrecked by substance abuse.

There is controversy about which substances are more addictive and which drugs are more harmful and whether alcohol or drugs are more harmful to the individual. Addiction is the concept which links the problems of all these substances, including food, an addict being *a person with a physiological need to continue to take the substance.* The concept of addiction is not sufficiently broad to enable the individual and social implications of substance use and abuse to be examined. Smoking addiction may not lead to criminal activity and social problems, in constrast with excessive heroin use and alchohol consumption. Addicts to class A drugs such as heroin may need to steal in order to find more than £100 a day to feed their addiction. The social costs of alcohol consumption in terms of criminal violence – particularly by men against women – and the costs to the health services of smoking and alcohol abuse are very great (Hammersley, 1999, pp. 408–33).

Alcohol Abuse

In 2004, the government published the National Alcohol Harm Reduction Strategy for England, concentrating on harm to people's physical and mental health rather than people's behaviour when abusing alcohol (Prime Minister's Strategy Unit, 2004). Government policies, particularly social and taxation policies, express markedly conflicting attitudes to people's alcohol problems. The availability of cheap, alcohol-based drinks has increased since the 1960s and there is much emphasis in the mass media on advertising alcohol as a lifestyle choice, linked with pleasure, fun and having a life. The downside of this is the increase in *social problems* related to alcohol consumption. On the one hand, governments benefit more from increasing revenues by taxing people's increasing drinking. On the other hand, statutory and voluntary agencies devote huge resources to dealing with – treating and trying to prevent – excessive drinking. Drunkeness is correlated with committing crimes, particularly crimes of violence and sex crimes. In 2002–3, 1.2 million alcohol-related crimes were committed and 44 per cent of all violent crime was alcohol-related (Hunter, 2005, p. 55) Research indicates that many perpetrators of sexual violence against women have drunk alcohol immediately previously (Grubin and Gunn, 1990) and many victims of sexual attacks develop alcohol problems as a consequence (Darves-Bornoz et al., 1998).

Medical problems arising from alcohol abuse include:

- *the consequences of intoxication:* acute alcohol poisoning, gastritis and pancreatitis (inflammation of the stomach and pancreas)
- *excessive consumption:* brain damage, degenerative conditions of the liver, particularly cirrhosis and chronic hepatitis leading to jaundice and liver failure, problems of weight gain, with increased risks of diabetes, circulatory and heart disorders
- *alcohol dependence:* alcoholic hallucinations and dementia (Institute of Alcohol Studies, 2002, p. 1).

A great variety of causes of problem drinking have been proposed over the years, none of which has solid scientific research evidence to support it: 'alcoholism', the so-called illness of excessive drinking; the 'alcoholic personality' with the tendency towards alcoholism; and an allergy to alcohol. A number of more plausible theories have more research evidence to support them: genetic factors, involving an inherited proneness to alcohol in a small proportion of cases; instability at home; modelling on parents' behaviour; and cultural and social factors that make it acceptable for people to turn to alcohol (Velleman, 1992, pp. 8–15). The fact that most social work with families focuses, in effect, on women with children has led perhaps to a concentration on men's problem drinking, rather than recognising that alcohol abuse affects men and women from the teenage years upwards, throughout the life course. Since the mid-twentieth century, women have taken on more demanding roles in society; more single mothers have become family breadwinners; and more women have competed successfully for careers that formerly were male preserves. The pressures on women to succeed in and out of the household have increased and alcohol is readily available as a form of relaxation. However, the reality is that for people of similar weight, young and adult women are physically more vulnerable than men to damage their liver by alcohol (Kent, 1990, p. 99). Thus, women need help and support with problem drinking just as much as men (Kent, 1990, p. 96).

Drug Abuse

There are circumstances in which most drugs are legally available. However, whereas some substances such as amphetamines and barbiturates are more often legally available on prescription, the availability of heroin, crack cocaine and other so-called 'hard' drugs is largely outside the drug treatment system (see Table 18.1 for classification of these drugs).

Drug abuse has consequences for the health of the individual, through new cases of HIV, hepatitis B and C following injecting with dirty needles, drug-related mental health problems, overdoses and deaths. It has consequences also in increased crimes such as burglaries, thefts and robberies (MacDonald et al., 2005, p. 4).

Drugs are classified (see Chapter 18) under the Misuse of Drugs Act 1971 and regulated under the Medicines Act 1968, and penalties arise for misuse under more recent legislation. Supply or intent to supply class A drugs can result in life imprisonment and a heavy fine. Supply or intent to supply class B or class C drugs can result in a maximum of 14 years' imprisonment plus a fine. A strong argument is advanced by some experts to have drugs reclassified according to their potential for harm, in which case ecstasy and LSD would be lower risk and alcohol and cannabis would move markedly up to higher risk.

One of the main problems of illegality is that access to supplies of heroin is controlled by illicit gangs and networks. Those who become addicted may be drawn into crime simply through being driven by their craving to pay the dealers who supply them. Another problem is that users may become diseased (for example infected with HIV/AIDS or hepatitis) and pass on infections by sharing dirty needles.

Women are particularly vulnerable to abuse by men and may be drawn into coercive relationships, or even resort to prostitution in order to finance their habit.

Cannabis was downgraded from class B to C in January 2004. Following further research into links between cannabis use and mental health problems, the Advisory Council on the Misuse of Drugs (ACMD, 2005) stated that cannabis had 'real and significant' effects on mental health. At the same time, the government left cannabis in the lowest category of risk (C), following the ACMD's view that it was still less harmful than the class B drugs, amphetamines and barbiturates, and following indications that cannabis usage by young people had not increased since the late 1990s (Leason, 2006, pp. 28–9). This view may still be reconsidered.

Tranquillisers

If tranquillisers – especially minor tranquillisers such as benzodiazepines – are used for a short while, they can provide relief, but uncontrolled use of 'bottled happiness' can grow into dependence or addiction. Medicines can become a commodity in the health service where market principles exist alongside professional values and the government's commitment to prioritise the interests of the patient, service user and consumer. There are dangers of the pharmaceutical industry, driven by the profit motive, undermining the interests of patients by offering prescribing doctors inducements to promote their products. Against this, prescribers are bound by their professional values to prescribe in the best interests of patients. Whereas doctors may prescribe initially at a consultation, dangers arise where repeat prescriptions are made available without further consultations. The tension is uneasy, in a setting where the resource of time may be too scarce to enable each patient to be interviewed at length to establish the root cause of the problem.

Solvent abuse

Sniffing substances is not new. People sniffed ether in the nineteenth century and the better off would hold ether-sniffing parties (Ives, 1986, p. 5). Nitrous oxide, or laughing gas, was also used. From the 1950s onwards, the harmful habit grew of sniffing a range of modern glues and chemical solvents such as cleansing agents and paint thinners containing trichloroethylene and toluene (Ives, 1986, pp. 6–7).

Smoking

Despite efforts by health campaigners to reduce tobacco companies' influence over people's smoking habits, the tobacco industry continues to exploit those sectors of the market that are still vulnerable. In Britain, this includes young women, whose smoking habits are still increasing. Outside Britain, many developing countries are targeted as new and expanding markets by the tobacco companies. The World Health Organization (WHO) set up the Tobacco Free Initiative in 1998 and noted in 2004 that tobacco consumption was spreading, particularly affecting poorer families and causing suffering and grief through illness and premature deaths (Esson and Leeder, 2004, p. viii).

This context indicates that smoking continues to be a market created and sustained by large corporations driven by the profit motive. We should bear in mind also that the government benefits enormously from the tax revenue from tobacco sales and, were it to disappear, would need to replace it from elsewhere. It follows that in Britain individual people should not be blamed for smoking, as though the ill-health it causes is purely a sign of their moral weakness. Traditionally, smoking has been identified alongside drinking alcohol as a refuge for hard-pressed people, a way of relaxing from the cares of life. However, increasingly, the dangers to health of excessive smoking and exposure to smoke (passive smoking) have been recognised. In recognition of this, by 2007, smoking in many public places was illegal in Britain.

Food Abuse

The turn of the twentieth and twenty-first centuries has witnessed an increasingly high priority given by government to problems of obesity, which, among children and young people as well as adults, is increasing (BMA, 1999, 2003) and has now reached epidemic proportions (BMA, 2005, p. v). The relationship between many men and women and food is increasingly problematic. The mass media, and particularly advertisements for clothes, dieting, plastic surgery, makeovers and makeup, are often blamed for promoting a link between quality of life and a particular body shape, which, even if desirable on health grounds, many people find difficult to attain. The problems of eating and not eating often revolve around control and it is as common to encounter difficulties of undereating (anorexia) as it is to find that some people overeat and also repeatedly induce vomiting (bulimia). These eating disorders are becoming more common among males. However, feminists argue that dependence on various substances, and food particularly, as it is linked with their weight, body shape and how they look to others, is one aspect of women's dependence on men, in a world where predominantly male consultants and others in power in the health services are making the healthcare decisions about how women should be treated (Ettore, 1992, p. 109). The feminist argument is that it is women more than men who are pressured into their obsession with how they look, measured against the so-called 'ideal' female body, a form which, ironically, varies markedly from culture to culture. Despite many theories about the causes and nature of eating disorders, the fact remains that, in general, their origins are not adequately understood (Abraham and Llewellyn-Jones, 2001, pp. 45–60).

Working with People Dependent on Alcohol, Drugs or Food

Problem Drinking

Traditionally, approaches to problem drinking were based on the view that 'alcoholism' was a physical addiction, an illness or a disease, with biological and physiological effects on the body that could not be controlled by the person. We saw in

Chapter 7 how the development of learning theory and cognitive theories in psychology have been applied in helping people to control their own behaviour. Such self-management approaches have contributed greatly to the curbing of problem drinking (Baldwin, 1990, p. 67). The self-help group approach of Alcoholics Anonymous is the most well-known example of this approach.

One of the commonest problems associated with alcohol abuse is secrecy. Problem drinkers often go to great lengths to conceal the extent of their drinking and people whose partners drink to excess often conceal the consequences – which may include physical abuse and money problems. Families also will tend to try to absorb such problems (Fanti, 1990, p. 125). In work with women, Kent (1990, p. 120) has identified the need for the worker to clarify whether the main focus of help with problem drinking personally, in a relationship or in a household, should be upon managing any crisis which has arisen, reducing long-term harm to the drinker and other family members, or focusing on techniques that enable the drinker to self-manage.

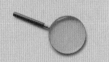

Practice study

Shelley

Siobhan is a volunteer worker with a women's community organisation, working with Shelley, a young, single parent, living in a women's refuge. She has a serious drink problem going back to her mid-teens. She has experimented with many different drugs, but at present claims not to be taking any non-prescription drugs.

Shelley states that her drinking began when her stepfather began to physically abuse her. It fell to what she describes as a normal level when she applied for a job and left home to work in another town. She married and after a year her drinking became a problem again when her husband started to beat her up when he returned home from the pub late on some evenings. Seven months pregnant, she left him and lived with a girlfriend for several months before meeting another man, taking her baby daughter with her and moving in with him shortly afterwards. Within a few weeks they began to argue and he became violent towards her. Six months passed and the violence became worse, so she took her baby and went to live in the women's refuge.

Activity 19.1

How should Siobhan focus her discussions with Shelley?

Siobhan decides to enable Shelley to examine the links between her past and her present. She suggests to Shelley that she focuses on how her previous experiences of abuse are affecting her life now – her relationships, her self-esteem, her aspirations, her self-confidence and her drinking patterns. Siobhan discusses with Shelley how the refuge can provide physical and emotional support to enable her to break the pattern of abusive relationships and turning to alcohol when abused.

Over a period of months, Shelley is able to persuade her retired mother to provide childcare support for the baby. Siobhan takes the role of advocate for a short period to encourage Shelley to apply for jobs. After several failed attempts, she obtains a part-time job and feels emotionally strong enough to leave the refuge and return home to live with her mother. Her aim in the medium term is to rent a flat, but for the present she has stability and independence in her life and with support from her mother and continued regular meetings with Siobhan is managing without resorting to alcohol. However, realistically, the possibility of relapses is high (Marlatt and Gordon, 1985).

The *Healthy Care Programme Handbook* (Chambers, 2005, p. 34) contains examples of how Healthy Care Partnerships can contribute to services for children and young people. These include alcohol and drug education, drug and alcohol teams, and a substance misuse policy involving training in alcohol and drug education of all staff across all services, including foster carers, residential care staff and looked after children's nurses. Children themselves have taken part in drama workshops, writing and performing a play about the problems associated with substance abuse and a music recording and training project leading to a CD on the theme of educating people about alcohol and drug abuse.

Illegal Drugs

Young people leaving care are especially vulnerable to being drawn into drug misuse, through four particular factors: negative childhood experiences; feelings of loss and disconnection associated with living in care; interaction with other young people normal at that age; and the challenges associated with leaving care (Ward et al., 2003, p. 49). Ways of countering these problems include educating young people and giving them more support when encountering difficulties, adopting specialist approaches to particular problems as well as a holistic approach with young people in general (Ward et al., 2003, pp. 50–2). This strategy could easily be adapted and applied usefully to other vulnerable groups.

Sniffing solvents

Ives (1986, p. 11) makes the useful distinction between recreational, experimental and dependent drug use, pointing out that the last, smallest group presents the greatest challenge in terms of prevention, treatment and control. Two workers in the Sunderland Solvent Abuse Clinic found that the most effective method of working with young solvent abusers was a groupwork programme, using a wide variety of techniques (Biddle and Gardiner, 1986, p. 48). They concluded that since most of the young people experimented with sniffing, if they could be supported through the crucial adolescent years, the abuse of solvents tended naturally to disappear (Biddle and Gardiner, 1986, p. 49). Those who dropped out tended to be the young people from social services whose social worker stopped being involved, leading to the young person dropping out (Biddle and Gardiner, 1986, p. 50).

Empowering Women Substance Abusers

Traditional self-help groups such as Alcoholics Anonymous focus on equipping the individual to overcome his or her weakness. More radical women's therapy groups challenge the clinical model of dependence as akin to illness and emphasise that women need to educate themselves and raise each other's consciousness in order to challenge society's tendency to put them into the role of victim. The aim of women's liberation, it is argued, is to enable women to use their solidarity to take political action to overcome their oppression. Thus, women deal with their substance abuse as an aspect of taking control of their lives (Ettore, 1992, pp. 134–8).

Conclusion

This chapter has dealt with some of the most difficult aspects of people's problems to work with, namely dependence-forming and addictive substances and behaviour. The approaches to treatment are as many as the problems are various, so it is inevitable that this has been a brief survey. The list below contains further reading for following up particular areas.

REVIEW QUESTIONS

1 What are the main social and medical consequences of alcohol abuse?

2 How are benzodiazepines, cocaine, speed and ecstasy classified under the Misuse of Drugs Act 1971?

3 What are the main differences between bulimia and anorexia?

FURTHER READING

Alcohol

Collins, S. (ed.) (1990) *Alcohol, Social Work and Helping*, London, Tavistock/Routledge

Davidson, R., Rollnick, S. and MacEwan, I. (1991) *Counselling Problem Drinkers*, London, Routledge

Velleman, R. (1992) *Counselling for Alcohol Problems*, London, Sage

Drugs

DoH (1997) *Substance Misuse and Young People*, London, DoH

DoH, Scottish Office, Welsh Office and Department of Health and Social Services Northern Ireland (1999) *Drug Misuse and Dependence: Guidelines on Clinical Management*, Clinical Guidelines on Drug Misuse and Dependence Working Group, London, TSO

Eating disorders

Able, J. (1997) *Counselling Skills for Dieticians*, Oxford, Blackwell Science

Abraham, S. and Llewellyn-Jones, D. (2001) *Eating Disorders: The Facts* (5th edn) Oxford, Oxford University Press

Duker, M. and Slade, R. (2003) *Anorexia Nervosa and Bulimia: How to Help* (2nd edn) Buckingham, Open University Press
Provides detailed accounts of theories and practice.

Hepworth, J. (1999) *The Social Construction of Anorexia Nervosa*, London, Sage

Schmidt, U. and Treasure, J. (1993) *Getting Better Bit(e) by Bit(e): A Survival Kit for Sufferers of Bulemia Nervosa and Binge Eating Disorders*, Hove, Psychology Press

Waskett, C. (1993) *Counselling People in Eating Distress*, Rugby, British Association for Counselling

RESOURCE FILES: Policies to Tackle Drug and Alcohol Abuse, at the end of Chapter 18
Health Promotion (2) Stopping Smoking, below

Resource file

Health promotion (2) Stopping smoking

Tobacco has been taken by people since prehistoric times, although its use in Europe is limited to the past 500 years. About a quarter of adults in the UK smoke more than 15 cigarettes per day and 15 per cent of children aged 11–15 smoke at least once a week (Munafò et al., 2003, p. 1). The nicotine content of tobacco is highly addictive and chewing tobacco, sniffing it as snuff and smoking cigarettes, cigars and pipes all increase the risk of disease and premature death. Smoking increases the proportion of poisonous carbon monoxide in the blood and is the largest single cause of preventable illness and premature death in Britain (Munafò et al., 2003, p. 19).

The most common diseases caused by smoking are cancers of the lung, cervix, pancreas, kidney and bladder, mouth and throat, breast and anus. Smoking also increases the risk of death from coronary heart disease and thrombosis and increases the incidence of breathing conditions such as bronchitis and emphysema. Smoking during pregnancy adversely affects the health of unborn children, and children and other adults can be harmed by so-called 'passive smoking', that is, inhaling smoke from other smokers.

A range of pharmacological, behavioural counselling and psychological techniques may be used to try to eliminate smoking.

Pharmacological methods include behavioural methods such as aversive therapy involving requiring the person to smoke too much to the point where unpleasant symptoms of nicotine overdose are experienced. The aim is to associate smoking with unpleasant effects in the hope that the habit may be discouraged. Another drug approach is the more supportive and gradual nicotine replacement therapy (NRT) using nicotine-based chewing gum or nicotine patches on the arm, which may be reduced in strength over a period of time.

Counselling may take the form of behavioural treatment (see Chapter 45), linked with a range of other measures aiming to reduce the temptation to restart smoking during the 'withdrawal' period.

Anti-smoking initiatives by governments in different European countries are driven in part by the high cost to health services of the treatment of smoking-related diseases. Smoking in enclosed public places is now banned in the UK and the Irish Republic.

FURTHER READING

British Heart Foundation (2001) *Stopping Smoking*, London, British Heart Foundation

Butler, C., Rollnick, S., Cohen, D., Russell, I., Bachmann, M. and Stott, N. (1999) 'Motivational Counselling versus Brief Advice for Smokers in General Practice: A Randomised Trial', *British Journal of General Practice*, **49**: 611–16

DoH (1998) *Report of the Scientific Committee on Tobacco and Health*, London, TSO

DoH (1998) *Smoking Kills: A White Paper on Tobacco*, Cm 4177, London, TSO

DoH (2000) *National Service Framework for Coronary Heart Disease*, London, TSO

McEwen, A. and West, R. (2000) 'Smoking Cessation Activities by General Practitioners and Practice Nurses', *Tobacco Control*, **10**: 27–32

Munafò, M., Drury, M., Wakley, G. and Chambers, R. (2003) *Smoking Cessation Matters in Primary Care*, Abingdon, Radcliffe Medical Press

WEBSITES: www.ash.org.uk
                   www.gasp.org.uk
                   www.quit.org.uk

Part III

Working with Young Offenders

TERRY THOMAS

Learning outcomes

By the end of this chapter, you should be able to:

■ UNDERSTAND welfare and justice approaches to work with young offenders

■ WORK THROUGH the process of work with a young offender

■ APPRECIATE tensions in practice over such aspects as confidentiality.

The problem of young people engaging in antisocial behaviour and criminality is a long-standing one. Shakespeare summed it up some 400 years ago:

> I would there were no age between ten and three-and-twenty, or that youth would sleep out the rest; for there is nothing in the between but getting wenches with child, wronging the ancientry, stealing, fighting. (Shakespeare, *The Winter's Tale*, 3.3.65–9)

Each generation seems to produce young people who duly threaten the adult population and then, in turn, grow into that same adult population who will be equally threatened by the new youth coming through. In contemporary Britain over the past 50 years, we have identified subcultures of young people as teddy boys, mods, rockers, punks and 'hoodies', who have come to represent both a moral decline and 'all that is wrong with young people'. It is almost a normal pattern repeated endlessly as youth grows out of youth, and achieves adult status.

Such an overview might provide us with some comfort but is, of course, no relief to the direct victims of youth crime, whether as individuals or communities blighted by graffiti, vandalism or worse. The overview also avoids the idea of youths growing into a permanent adult criminal career. In these circumstances, a simple standing-off in order to 'leave the kids alone' is not an option and we ask our workers with young offenders to intervene to reduce youth crime and change the behaviour patterns of young people.

In this chapter we outline the traditional approaches to working with young offenders in terms of having to balance a welfare and justice perspective to the work. We look at the organisational contexts of work with young offenders and the various components of that work, which includes assessing and planning work before actually intervening. The significance of evaluation, and whether or not the work has been effective is considered, as is the question of the confidentiality within which the work takes place.

Let us begin with an example from practice.

Practice study

Rosie

Rosie is aged 14 and currently lives in a local authority secure children's home. Until the age of 11 she had never been in any trouble. At that point in her life her mother left home to start a new life in Scotland with a new partner. Rosie's younger sister went with her mother. Rosie stayed with her father and older brothers.

Rosie was upset at her mother's departure. She started missing school and taking to alcohol and drugs. In turn this led to Rosie being aggressive in a random manner to, sometimes, complete strangers. Violent incidents followed in the form of fights involving head-butting, punching, stamping and kicking. In school a chair was thrown at a teacher following a comment about her mother.

Rosie showed little remorse for her violence and a youth court appearance for assault led to her present placement.

Rosie sees her future beyond the secure children's home as being foster care, where she can experience a new family and where she is 'the only child' – a children's home would not be suitable (in Rosie's view). She claims not to trust her mother or her father. She hopes for a long-term career in social services or childcare to help others on the basis of her experience (see Chapter 17 for material on children's services).

Given this information:

■ Is there sufficient information to complete an assessment (see Chapter 30)?
■ Would you wish to question Rosie in any more areas, or contact any other possible sources of information?
■ Are you yet in a position to devise a plan?
■ What are your initial thoughts on suitable interventions for Rosie?

Traditional Approaches

The conventional approach to working with young offenders holds that workers are caught between two stools. As offenders, they have to face law enforcement and the consequences of their actions. As young people, however, they are said to be entitled to more understanding and help in growing up because they are not yet fully fledged adults. These are usually described as the *justice* or *welfare* approach respectively, and the two approaches can be seen as opposite ends of a continuum.

The police, the courts and prosecuting agencies are examples of agencies and practitioners that tend towards the 'justice' end of the continuum. Social workers, education welfare officers, residential care workers and probation officers would tend towards the 'welfare' end. Working together, these practitioners would work out a customised intervention based on a mix of justice and welfare for the individual young person before them.

Children and young people are also recognised as moving from positions of dependency on parents or carers to positions of independence as young adults. This movement takes place across the physical and emotional changes that all children experience through adolescence, and involves the almost normal testing of boundaries to find the edges of acceptable behaviours.

The activities of children and young people may legally start to be designated 'criminal' after the age of 10 (in England and Wales). From the age of 10–18 we recognise a developing sense of maturity – and responsibility – in young people, leading to an acceptance of full responsibility as an adult when the eighteenth birthday is passed. This is mirrored by a gradually diminishing level of parental responsibility for the parents or carers.

The age of criminal responsibility was fixed at 10 years (in England and Wales) in 1963; before that it was 8. Other countries have fixed their age higher (for example Germany 14, Denmark 15). Ireland moved the age from 8 to 12 in 2002, while Scotland has set the age at 8, but 'offenders' appear before a Children's Panel rather than a court.

The age of 10 as the age of criminal responsibility in the UK is recognised as being the lowest in Europe. Other countries still have children acting in a way we would call *criminal*, but they have to deal with them in ways that do not involve a criminal justice process. In terms of the welfare–justice continuum, these countries have *only* the welfare perspective at their disposal in working with these children. From the child's perspective, it means a welfare approach that tries to understand and help, without the 'interference' of the justice approach.

Organisational Contexts

Social care work with young offenders takes place within a variety of organisational contexts to which we have already alluded. Some workers are located in residential care facilities including 'secure' facilities, some in multidisciplinary teams such as youth offending teams and others in specialist 'children and family' social work teams or education welfare departments. Whatever the setting or context, social care workers should try to retain some basic underlying standards – professional standards – in their work with young people and in turn ensure that these standards and principles are taken on and reproduced in the various policies of their employing agencies.

The organisational settings for work with young offenders may also have standards imposed upon them by those overseeing their work. The most conspicuous of these are the 'national standards' produced by the Youth Justice Board (2004) for all youth justice services (see Resource File: Key Childcare Policy Changes in the Twenty-first Century, at the end of Chapter 3).

The youth courts may also impose certain constraints or standards on workers with young offenders, when the child or young person in question has been formally placed 'in care' or made subject to forms of 'supervision'. If we break the word 'supervision' down into its component parts, it simply means a form of overlooking (super and vision) of the young person's behaviour on behalf of the court. That behaviour may have also had certain conditions placed on it by the courts, which the worker may be obliged to enforce and report back to the court if there are any breaches of those conditions.

The organisational context of the agency and the courts will both influence the environment within which the worker with young offenders has to operate.

The Working Relationship

To return to our practice study, no effective work can be done with Rosie in the absence of an effective working relationship. All workers with young people need to form a working relationship with those young people. Sometimes this is referred to as 'striking up a rapport' with them. It is the worker's opportunity to use their sense of 'self' to make an individual connection to the young person within the organisational context (see above) and as a platform for more formalised approaches (see below).

The working relationship is the basis for all other work. Workers proceed at the pace of the young person, and use language that the young person can understand. It is the basis on which trust can be established. The working relationship is *not* the same as a friendship and is *not* an end in itself.

Effective Practice

Working with young people such as Rosie is difficult and demanding and working with young people who are engaged in offending behaviour can be even more difficult and demanding. The work cannot be simply left to individuals to carry out in their own individual way and on an ad hoc basis, in the vague hope that some 'good' will come of it. A framework for this work usually follows the same sequence, whereby an assessment is made of the young person and their circumstances, a plan of action formed and then carried through, using various interventions, and finally an evaluation is made of the effectiveness of the intervention.

Assessment

Rosie and her offending behaviour need to be assessed before any meaningful work can take place. As the worker starts to build their working relationship, the process of assessment also starts, and ultimately a formalised assessment is arrived at.

Assessment means putting together a picture of Rosie and her circumstances, in the form of family, friends and neighbourhood, on well-established lines (DoH, 2000a). It tries to answer the question 'why' she is offending, and what are the blocks or difficulties that need to be removed if behaviour is to change and offending patterns reduced. This is also sometimes referred to as *assessing the risk of future offending*.

Assessment requires an understanding of the difficulties confronting all young people in terms of adolescence, maturing and finding out about the adult world. It involves understanding the racial or cultural characteristics of the young person.

It may be appropriate to ask other professionals or agencies with knowledge of Rosie to contribute any relevant information they may have that will help with your assessment. This information may confirm what you already know, or take you into new areas that improve the picture you are putting together.

In direct work with the young person, assessment needs to proceed at their pace. As workers, we may see the picture emerging quickly, but it may still be necessary to allow the young person to construct that picture in their own words and at their own timing. A good assessment is a partnership between worker and young person.

As workers, we may have various aids to assist us in our assessment, such as our knowledge and understanding of young people and how they function. This knowledge and understanding might come from our experience of working with other young people, or it might come from books we've read or classes we have attended.

Some agencies provide their workers with other aids to assessment, such as prescribed formats to guide them through the questions they should be asking and the leads they should be following up. These aids are sometimes referred to as 'instruments' or 'tools' and include, for example, ASSET, the common assessment tool now used by all workers in youth offending teams (Baker, 2005).

If the assessments start throwing up questions that are particularly specialist, we may have to look elsewhere for help and guidance in making an assessment. Child psychologists or psychiatrists might make an input to an assessment. Educational specialists might also make an input. Workers need to know when they are getting 'out of their depth' and need to involve these other practitioners to help complete the assessment picture.

Planning

Only when the assessment of Rosie has been completed can we start to think of planning what needs to be done. Committing ourselves to a plan of action without an assessment is an example of trying to work in the dark.

The plan might be short or long term or have components of both short- and long-term planning. An immediate situation or crisis may have to be dealt with in such a way that it hardly deserves the title of 'a plan'. But thereafter we have to consider the long-term plan, which will include the work – the interventions – that will need to be done over the forthcoming months or years.

Planning – like assessment – is carried out in the context of the working relationship that has been established, and should always take into account how the young person sees their future, as well as other significant people in their immediate family or household.

Interventions

With an assessment completed and a plan outlined, the worker with Rosie can proceed to the interventions – or work – considered necessary to help to resolve her problems, alleviate difficulties confronting her and ultimately reduce her offending. Just as a plan cannot be completed without an assessment, so too interventions should not proceed without a plan.

Planned intervention means that the worker knows what they are doing each time they meet the young person in question because it has all been thought through in advance. It avoids ad hoc meetings that are aimless and not thought through and are ultimately just 'chats' about nothing in particular. When the young person has been involved in the initial assessment and plan, they too will have an expectation that the interventions are going to be meaningful and ultimately fruitful.

The working relationship that has underpinned the process of assessment and planning now forms the bedrock for the interventions or 'real work' that is to be carried out. These interventions may be individualised or 'one to one' between the worker and Rosie, or they can constitute group activities. Either way they are discrete programmes, which may take weeks or months to complete and need to be monitored to ensure that they run according to the original plan.

It may happen that during the interventions, new information comes to light about the young person and their circumstances that is so significant we have to go back to the assessment and rethink that assessment and its attendant plan. Such reassessments should only take place when the new information is judged so important and significant that it cannot be ignored.

Individualised interventions

Individualised interventions include:

- *Pro-social modelling:* where the worker demonstrates to Rosie an example of measured and desired behaviour. This can be done informally or spontaneously as part of other programmes or as part of a naturally occurring one in, say, a residential care setting. It also involves the worker in reinforcing and rewarding Rosie's own pro-social expressions and actions, while showing an interest in her and offering reflective listening.
- *Mentoring:* a form of pro-social modelling that is usually held to involve an older, more experienced person guiding a younger one.

- *Motivational interviewing:* a form of engagement seeking to draw out Rosie's own desires and motivation to become involved in changing her behaviour – as opposed to having that change imposed on her.
- *Counselling and psychotherapy:* more in-depth forms of individualised work that require an element of added expertise on the part of the worker. These interventions may help Rosie to reflect and understand her past and present 'difficulties', with a view to moving past the 'obstacles' they present to her personal growth and development. In doing this, counselling and psychotherapy also seek to change behaviour and reduce patterns of offending.

We turn now to consider the potential of working with Rosie through groups.

Groupwork interventions

Groupwork interventions include:

- Working with 'natural' groups Rosie relates to that might have arisen in the community, that is, detached or outreach youth work, or groups within residential care settings.
- Working with more formalised groups including Rosie, brought together by the worker for the purpose of changing attitudes or behaviour. This may be done through, for example, discussing attitudes to crime and issues of being a victim of crime (sometimes using techniques such as cognitive-behavioural techniques), practising new social skills to replace offending behaviour patterns or offering mutual support to members in moving towards more acceptable behaviour.

The worker clearly has a central role in these more formalised groups and will need a degree of expertise in 'conducting' groups in order to ensure their continuity and success.

Evaluation

There is an increasing emphasis on questioning the effectiveness of all interventions in all forms of social care. This is often referred to as the *evidence base* of the work and tries to ensure that the interventions actually work and do make a difference.

The practitioner working with Rosie is also required to look back on their work to ask how effective it was and to learn from evaluation, whether the lessons be positive or negative. The evaluation looks back at the assessment, plan and interventions to see if they were justified and as accurate or effective as they could have been.

Confidentiality

One problematic aspect of all social care work with young offenders is the degree of confidentiality that can be accorded to young people when they are talking to practitioners, in that there is a tension between protecting their right to confidentiality and sharing with others, including professionals, information about their criminality. Guidance may be given on this question by the law (for example Crime and Disorder Act 1998, s. 115), 'national standards' or employing agencies, but the bottom line is usually that an unqualified 100 per cent total confidentiality policy is not permissible.

If confidentiality is, therefore, to be qualified, at what point might we have to breach it when working with young people? Presumably, this would be if information was forthcoming about a serious crime, and that information had to be brought to the attention of the police or other law enforcement agencies.

Some agencies talk of the 'confidential space' they allow their workers and young people to communicate and interact within. The greater the space, the more open and trusting the working relationship can be. The smaller the space, the less trusting and more closed it may be.

Questions about confidentiality are not easily answered. What, exactly, for example, is a 'serious' crime compared to a 'non-serious' crime? At present, a degree of discretion is allowed to workers (within various guidelines from employers and national standards) but each situation needs to be carefully weighed.

Conclusions

Work with young offenders such as Rosie is difficult and demanding, but a structured and organised approach that gets below the immediate offending behaviour to see what is really going on, and how best we might approach this work, is inevitably going to produce better results for everyone.

REVIEW QUESTIONS

1   What does 'the age of criminal responsibility' mean and what is it in the four countries of the UK?

2   What are pro-social modelling and motivational interviewing?

FURTHER READING

Baker, K. (2005) 'Assessment in Youth Justice: Professional Discretion and the Use of ASSET', *Youth Justice*, **5**(2): 106–22

Burnett, R. and Roberts, C. (eds) (2004) *What Works in Probation and Youth Justice: Developing Evidence-based Practice*, Cullompton, Willan Publishing, especially Chapters 3, 9, 10 and 12

Eadie, T. and Canton, R. (2002) 'Practising in a Context of Ambivalence: The Challenge for Youth Justice Workers', *Youth Justice*, **2**(1): 14–26
Discusses balancing 'justice' and 'welfare' within a context that minimises the latter.

Pitts, J. (1990) *Working with Young Offenders*, Basingstoke, BASW/Macmillan
This text is a bit old but still useful.

Youth Justice Board (2004) *National Standards for Youth Justice Services*, London, YJB

21 Nutrition

LYN JACKSON and JO SMITH

Learning outcomes

By the end of this chapter, you should:

- UNDERSTAND the contribution of nutrition to a person's health
- KNOW what good nutrition entails
- APPRECIATE the importance of nutrition in health and social care work.

The importance of nutrition cannot be overestimated; in a nutshell, it is essential for life. Nutrition is required by the body for energy, growth, maintenance and repair. An individual's nutritional intake should be appropriate to their particular needs if health is to be maintained; for example a teenager will have different requirements to an older person and likewise someone with diabetes will have different needs to someone who hasn't a pre-existing condition. An important part of a health and social care practitioner's role is helping a person to meet their nutritional needs, which may be as simple as removing clingfilm from preprepared food to more complex issues such as feeding someone who, for whatever reason, cannot do it for themselves, or who is unable to take food orally. This chapter will explore these issues in more detail.

Nutrition and Health

A good starting point is to look at the relationship between nutrition and health and why in recent years it has gained such prominence.

In the past, dietary intake was largely governed by the availability of food, income of the family and cultural influences. Dietary deficiencies were commonly seen as a result of a lack of one of the five major food groups, for example vitamins. However, in the early 1990s, a body of research highlighted the importance of nutrition in the maintenance of health and recovery following illness (King's Fund Centre, 1992). It was also apparent that it was not uncommon for people in care environments, for example hospitals, to be malnourished (McWhirter and Pennington, 1994). It is important to remember that when we talk about being malnourished, we mean not only an inadequate intake of food, but also obesity or an imbalanced diet. All these factors have a detrimental effect on the health and wellbeing of the individual, and therefore we need to identify those people who are, or are at risk of becoming, malnourished. Nutritional assessment is the process of gathering detailed information about the nutritional status of the person and factors that actually and/or potentially influence their dietary intake, for example preferences, weight, history of weight loss or gain, pre-existing conditions, medications, age and holistic factors, to name a few. This information is then used to plan and deliver appropriate care, in collaboration with other healthcare professionals, for example dieticians, to meet their individual needs and prevent the complications associated with being malnourished.

Activity 21.1

Pick one factor, either inadequate intake of food, obesity or an imbalanced diet, and identify the potential detrimental effects on the health and wellbeing of the individual. Remember to think about not only the physical effects, but also the psychological and social effects.

Here is our list that could apply to one or more of the factors identified above:

- delayed wound healing
- reduced ability to rehabilitate
- increasing susceptibility to infections
- prolonging hospital stay
- increased susceptibility to skin damage, for example pressure sores
- changes in mood and behavioural problems, for example hyperactive children
- loss of self-esteem and changes in body image
- reduced energy levels and fatigue, for example a father not being able to play football with his children due to being overweight
- cessation of menstruation in underweight females
- poor dental health
- dietary-linked health problems, for example cardiovascular disease, non-insulin-dependent diabetes and anaemia. Diet is now being implicated in a range of other disease processes and conditions, from cancer to asthma.

Holistic Aspects of Eating

Eating and drinking are not just about the physical wellbeing of a person. They are closely linked with the social and psychological aspects of our lives. We have all heard the term 'comfort food' and you will be able to think of something you would eat if feeling a bit low, fed up or ill. This is the psychological aspect of food at its most simple. More complex examples can be seen when you explore the relationship a person has with food when they have an eating disorder. However, we also use food and drink in a social way. Most people enjoy going out for a meal with friends and the eating is part of the pleasure, but the other element is the socialisation, which is also important in maintaining a balanced healthy life. One of the main pleasures of eating and drinking is the taste, however, in reality, we only taste salt, sour, bitter and sweet. The more diverse tastes we experience come from our sense of smell. Appetite is also stimulated by the visual appearance of food, the more attractively it is presented, the more appealing it seems.

Different cultures use this aspect of food and socialising in different ways. Food is an integral part of many religious festivals (for example restricting food intake during Ramadan) and is used to express personal beliefs and values. While sitting down together as a family for a meal is becoming rarer in the UK, it is still an important part of healthy family life in many parts of the world. The thought of a TV dinner on a tray, or eating alone, would be considered very strange and unattractive in many countries.

Another factor closely linked with culture is religion. Many religions have specific restrictions on some foods. Also, it may dictate other requirements such as which hand is used to eat the food. Unless you are part of a religion, the reasons for these restrictions may not be readily apparent, however, they must be respected by carers to avoid causing distress and affront to the client.

Activity 21.2

Think of a religion or set of particular values or beliefs, different from your own, then identify and list its particular dietary restrictions and conventions around eating.

Here are some examples drawn from Andrews and Hanson (2003):

- A Jewish person has strict dietary laws and:
  - does not eat pork or pork products
  - does not mix milk with meat products
  - is not allowed shellfish, whereas fish with fins and scales are acceptable
  - eats meat killed humanely, using ritualistic practices passed down through the generations; such meat is considered 'kosher'.
- A Muslim person has strict dietary laws and:
  - does not eat pork or pork products
  - eats meat killed according to the 'halal' practice
  - does not drink alcohol
  - fasts during the festival of Ramadan; however, if individuals are unwell or frail, for example an older person, they can be excluded from fasting.
- A Hindu person does not eat meat and generally adopts a vegetarian diet.
- A vegetarian person excludes or reduces animal products and derivatives from the diet.

However, there are degrees of adherence; some people are devout while others are more liberal and may deviate from traditional practices.

Part III

Another aspect of why people eat what they do is income. The whole concept of food has become a multibillion pound business, with large companies exerting pressure on food producers in terms of cost and quality. In years gone by, food would have been grown and sold locally and the price dictated by availability. Now large companies control the supply and the cost. For families on low incomes this may be a significant problem. It may be easy to shop in a large supermarket where everything is under one roof, but it may be cheaper to buy your fruit and vegetables in a local greengrocers or market. Yet a lot of these have difficulty competing on price. The food industry has responded to this need for cheap food by producing a huge range of processed foods; however, to keep the cost low, the quality of the ingredients may well be very poor. Mechanically extracted 'meat' is used, even if it bears no likeness to meat as we would recognise it. To give it texture, flavour and colour a range of artificial additives are then often added. It is the long-term effects of these additives which are now being questioned, particularly for children, for example the effect of certain additives on children's behaviour. The other problem with processing food is that its nutritional value may be reduced.

The knock-on effect of processed, preprepared food is that people are now losing the skills to cook and a fast-food culture is developing in its place. If you think about it, being able to feed yourself a healthy, balanced diet is a basic life skill. Many people used to learn how to cook from their parents, now we have some parents who have never really cooked, feeding their children convenience foods and equally unable to teach their children how to cook. It is easy to see how this could soon become a skill lost to significant sections of society, unless cooking is highlighted as a key skill, for example in schools and health education campaigns.

In reality you can cook nutritious food on a limited budget, but it does need the skills and knowledge to do so. Many would argue that it is a misconception that if you have a limited budget, you can't afford to eat a nutritious diet, and, conversely, that relying heavily on processed, convenience foods is not especially cheap and may not provide a healthy diet.

We also need to remember that for many people who live alone, the social element of eating and drinking may have been lost to them. Whether they are single, divorced or widowed, there is not much motivation to cook a nutritious meal just for one. If the person is also elderly, they may not be able to cook themselves a meal anymore, a factor that may be made worse by medical conditions or ill-health. All these factors will impact on the quality of their diet and thus their health.

What is Nutrition?

Nutrition consists of the different elements our bodies extract from the food we eat. There are five major food groups:

- fats
- proteins
- carbohydrates

- vitamins
- minerals.

To maintain health, foods containing the above need to be included in the diet, the amount depending on a number of factors:

- physical activity
- age
- health status, presence or absence of disease
- cognitive/developmental/psychological issues
- personal choice
- cultural and religious preferences
- income.

Activity 21.3

Identify and list specific foods in the five major food groups and describe their particular function in maintaining health and wellbeing.

Here are some examples (Rosdahl and Kowalski, 2003; Harkreader and Hogan, 2004; Green and Jackson, 2006):

- *Fats:* provide energy and fatty tissues for insulation, improve taste and texture of food, and are necessary for the transportation and absorption of the fat-soluble vitamins A, D, E and K. For example: butter, cream, cheese, margarine, cooking oil, lard, olive oil.
- *Protein:* ensures the growth and repair of tissue, from the smallest cell to a large wound. It is important in the production of red blood cells. The body cannot store protein, so it should be eaten on a daily basis. For example: meat, fish, poultry, cheese, nuts, pulses, eggs, soya.
- *Carbohydrates:* the primary energy source for the body. For example: cereals, flour, cakes, bread, potatoes.
- *Vitamins:* essential in small amounts for healthy body functioning at all levels:
  - Vitamin A – found in green leafy vegetables, red, orange and yellow fruit, dairy products and liver; deficiency leads to dry skin, fatigue; essential for healthy skin, hair, bones, teeth and night sight.
  - Vitamin B_1 (thiamine) – found in meat, rice, pasta, whole grains; deficiency leads to nervous disorders, confusion, fatigue.
  - Vitamin B_2 (riboflavin) – found in dairy produce, eggs, green leafy vegetables, whole grains; deficiency leads to skin rashes, anaemia.
  - Vitamin B_6 (pyridoxine) – found in beans, whole grains, fish, poultry, lean meat, avocado; deficiency leads to muscular weakness, anaemia, dermatitis.
  - Vitamin B_{12} (cyanocobalamin) – found in seafood, meat, dairy produce; deficiency leads to tiredness, anaemia.
- *Minerals:* include calcium, potassium, magnesium, sodium chloride and phosphorus, needed in minute quantities.

Also very important are trace elements, for example iron, zinc, selenium. Vitamins, minerals and trace elements are mostly found in protein, fruit, vegetables and cereals.

You will see from the list you have compiled that some foods fall into more than one food group, for example cheese contains both protein and fat.

Activity 21.4

Spend a few minutes considering the patients or service users with whom you work. What types of condition are they likely to have that have required them to adapt their diet?

Responses you could have given include diabetes, coronary heart disease, renal failure, coeliac disease, eczema, children with attention deficit hyperactive disorder (ADHD), and clients taking monoamine-oxidase inhibitors (MAOIs) used in the treatment of mental health problems.

How Dietary Requirements Change Through a Person's Lifespan

The dietary requirements of children will change considerably as they grow and develop, however, for the purpose of this chapter the focus is on adults' needs. There are several factors during our lives that directly influence our nutritional requirements. Changes in employment or lifestyle may necessitate an increase or decrease in calorific intake. Health-related issues may result in someone having to adapt their diet; for example someone diagnosed with high blood pressure is likely to be advised to reduce their salt and saturated fat intake. Women go through several developmental stages in adult life that may also require dietary modification, for example pregnancy and the menopause.

Age is a subjective state. Some people remain very active into their seventies and eighties, however, in general, as you age your metabolism slows down and your level of activity often decreases, and consequently your nutritional requirements change. Protein, fruit, vegetables, vitamin and mineral intake should remain unchanged, but Marieb (2004) supports the general principle that carbohydrates should be reduced because of the decreased level of activity. The advent of dementia can present particular problems for service users and challenges for family and carers, and patience and understanding are often needed in abundance.

Assisting People to Eat and Drink

When we feel unwell, our appetite and interest in food often decrease; however, whether you are young or old, this is the time when health and social care workers can play a key role.

There are a number of key aspects you need to consider when helping people to eat and drink, be it in the home or healthcare environment:

■ Actively involve the person in decisions about choice and amount of food.
■ Ensure the person is not rushed and, where appropriate, fed at a pace comfortable to them.
■ Small amounts often are much more appetising and more manageable than large meals.
■ Ensure food is attractively presented – remember what we said earlier about eating involving senses other just than taste.
■ Wrapping should be removed. Clingfilm placed over food can protect the contents, but may cause problems for people who have reduced dexterity, for example rheumatoid arthritis or injuries such as fractures. Some may have upper limb weakness due to strokes or other neurological conditions or have venflons inserted in their hand or arm.
■ Food should be placed within easy reach and cut into small manageable portions, if appropriate.
■ Food and fluids should be presented at the optimum temperature, not too hot or cold.
■ Provide hand washing facilities before and after eating, for both the person and anyone else involved in the process. There is nothing more off-putting than unclean hands; it also reduces the risk of cross-infection that may further compromise the health of the person.
■ People who have swallowing difficulties may prefer some privacy when eating. Drawing curtains round the bed, if in hospital, can reduce self-consciousness, particularly if they are prone to dribbling. However, remember this should be done in consultation with the person as it can also increase their sense of isolation.
■ Eating surfaces should be clean and clutter-free. Remove unnecessary articles from tables, for example ashtrays, dirty tissues and male urinals.
■ Provide gentle supportive encouragement, as getting irritable will not help the person to regain their appetite and enjoy the eating experience.
■ Sit the person as upright as their condition allows, as this helps the swallowing process and reduces the risk of food going into the lungs, which can be life-threatening, particularly for people with swallowing difficulties.
■ When assisting with feeding, sit at the person's level, engaging them through eye contact and appropriate conversation. Remember, the purpose is to encourage the person to eat, therefore avoid using demeaning, childlike language that people may find offensive and off-putting.
■ Use utensils appropriate to the person's needs and preferences. Using a spoon for everything may seem convenient, but, remember, people may already feel embarrassed about being fed. Using a spoon is reminiscent of being a child, which can further increase feelings of inadequacy and loss of dignity; a fork can be used just as easily for most consistencies of main courses.

■ People with swallowing difficulties may be prescribed what we call a 'modified textured diet'. This is where food consistency is changed, for example pureed or minced. You will need to make sure that you have the right consistency for the person.

Activity 21.5

In the previous sections, we have discussed various issues relating to nutrition. Think of a particular person and identify how you could help them to meet their nutritional needs.

Issues you could have thought of include the holistic aspects considered in this chapter, also identification of problems or issues service users may have, which need to be passed on to a more senior practitioner.

While food in our diet is usually taken orally, there are a number of conditions, not necessarily age-related, which require an alternative route. For example, people who have suffered a stroke may be fed initially through a nasogastric tube and, if swallowing difficulties persist, this is usually replaced by a medium- to long-term feeding tube, for example a percutaneous endoscopic gastrostomy (PEG). This is inserted through the stomach wall and is positioned on the external abdominal wall above the waistline. If these routes are used, normal food is not given; instead, it is administered in the form of a specially prepared liquid with a balanced nutritional value. Carers involved with people who have these special needs should receive appropriate training and be able to demonstrate competence in this area.

If you would like to learn more about these routes and the required care, refer to CREST (2004) in Further Reading below.

Conclusion

We have discussed the holistic nature of eating and drinking. Although the physical implications of a healthy diet are important, these cannot be considered in isolation. It is essential that practitioners recognise the social, cultural, religious and economic needs of individual service users in relation to their nutrition. A healthy diet includes foods from the five main food groups and it is important that these are consumed in balanced quantities, appropriate to the individual needs of the person. We have also identified key factors in assisting people to eat and drink. Many of these factors could be considered common sense; however, that does not diminish their importance from the service user's perspective.

REVIEW
QUESTIONS

1 Why has the relationship between nutrition and health become more highlighted over the past generation?

2 What are the main contents of a healthy diet?

3 What main hints would you give to a person caring for someone at home, who was helping them to eat?

FURTHER
READING

Chapter 19 Further Reading for material on eating disorders

WEBSITES: http://www.bda.uk.com/latest-food-facts.php (British Dietetic Association
http://www.nutrition.org.uk/home.asp?siteId=43&sectionId=s (British Nutrition Foundation)
http://www.nice.org.uk/page.aspx?o=cg032niceguideline (NICE CG 32 (2006) Nutrition Support in Adults: NICE Guidelines)
http://www.crestni.org.uk/tube-feeding-guidelines.pdf (Northern Ireland Clinical Resource Efficiency Support Team – CREST)

Hand Hygiene in Infection Prevention and Control RACHEL MORRIS

By the end of this chapter, you should:

- ■ UNDERSTAND why hand hygiene is essential to health and social care work
- ■ KNOW the elements of hand hygiene.

In a variety of hospital, residential and home-based settings, health and social care workers will encounter a number of patients, carers and service users who will have an infection. Simple precautions are necessary to prevent the spread of these infections to others (Horton and Parker, 2002; Lawrence and May, 2003; Wilson, 2006). There are also risks of bringing infection to a person from an external source. The worker may be visiting a succession of people, travelling in the car, carrying a diary and papers, shaking hands, touching door handles, work surfaces, clothing and bedding. These are necessary in a day's work, but from the point of view of infection prevention and control, they require particular attention to hygiene. One of the main areas identified is the importance of correct hand hygiene. This chapter will discuss the crucial importance of when and how to wash hands, and why hand washing is essential.

Activity 22.1

You are helping your friend Ann to plant seeds in her garden. Ann offers to make you a drink. On returning with your coffee, you notice that her hands are still covered in soil from the seed planting. Ann has obviously not washed her hands before making your drink.

- ■ List the reasons why you think Ann should wash her hands before preparing a drink.

- Consider why it is important to wash your hands either before or after the following activities:
  - before food preparation
  - after going to the toilet
  - before every meal
  - when your hands are visibly dirty after a particular activity
  - after touching animals.

Check your answers in the following section, which details the importance of hand washing.

Why it is Important to Wash Hands

Hand hygiene is crucially important, as it is the most basic measure to help prevent cross-infection. This simple procedure, however, is often forgotten and poor hand hygiene has been acknowledged repeatedly. Infectious diseases such as the common cold, flu and infectious diarrhoea are commonly spread by hand-to-hand contact. It is therefore important that hands are washed regularly. *Microorganisms* (germs) such as viruses or bacteria can be transferred onto hands from a variety of sources such as dirt, water, food, contaminated surfaces and ill people. These microorganisms are invisible to the naked eye and if you have them on your hands, you can unwittingly pass them through touch to your mouth, eyes, nose or even to another person. It may then be possible to develop an infection or pass an infection on to other people. These microorganisms are known as *transient organisms*. They are loosely attached to the surface layer of the skin, but are easily removed by routine hand washing. Hand washing frequency will, however, vary depending on your surroundings and what activity you are undertaking. Special attention needs to be considered, for example, in healthcare and food preparation settings. Healthcare workers often acquire transient organisms by direct contact with patients or contact with contaminated surfaces near to the patient. Transient organisms are most frequently associated with healthcare-associated infections (HCAI – an infection that develops as a result of healthcare treatment, which was not present or incubating on admission to hospital), such as methicillin-resistant Staphylococcus aureus (MRSA). It is critically important, therefore, that hands are washed regularly and effectively to reduce the risk of cross-infection.

Hand Hygiene

Activity 22.2 | Washing Hands

Go to a sink and wash your hands in the normal manner. Consider whether you have cleaned all areas of your hands. Which parts do you think you missed? How did you dry them?

Did you remember to wash all the areas of your hands including your thumbs and fingertips? The following gives a description of how to wash and dry your hands correctly:

- Using running water, wet your hands before you apply the soap. Applying soap to dry hands is like putting shampoo on dry hair. Wetting the hands first allows the soap to create lather.
- Move the lather over all areas of your hands by rubbing them together for about 10–30 seconds. This friction helps to remove the transient germs (remember, these are germs that are loosely attached to the skin's surface and can pass onto other people during touch if they are not removed).
- Make sure you wash following the six-stage hand washing technique (Ayliffe et al., 1978; ICNA, 2002):
  1. rub palm to palm
  2. rub palms over back of opposite hands
  3. rub palm to palm fingers interlaced
  4. rub interlocked fingers together
  5. rub thumbs and wrists
  6. rub finger tips onto palms of opposite hands.
- Rinse your hands under running water to remove the remaining soap.
- Make sure you dry your hands carefully on a clean towel (leaving soap residue on the skin or incomplete drying can contribute to dermatitis).

Drying Hands

Microorganisms transfer more easily on wet surfaces than dry ones, therefore drying methods have to be effective. Paper towels are the best option in healthcare settings as they are disposable and therefore limit the risk of cross-infection. Care should be taken, however, with the disposal of paper towels. Foot-operated bins are the preferred option, as hands are not contaminated when opening the bin lid.

Hand Hygiene Facilities

When caring for people in a care home or hospital environment, hand hygiene facilities are likely to differ from those in your own home. The taps are usually elbow- or wrist-operated. This makes it easier to operate the taps without having to touch them with your hands. There are usually cleansing products in liquid dispensers next to the sink area. This enables you to apply a measured amount of soap onto your hands.

What Product Should you Use to Clean your Hands?

There are many cleansing products available for hand hygiene use, including plain soap available in bar or liquid form, antibacterial soaps, or alcohol-based hand sanitisers. The necessity and availability of these will vary depending on your surroundings. Plain soap and water is extremely effective and will eliminate most microorganisms. This method is essential if soil or dirt is visible on your hands.

Alcohol-based hand sanitisers or antibacterial wipes are useful alternatives if soap and water are not available (for example, when travelling in the car, before eating outside or when camping). In addition, the use of alcohol-based hand sanitisers by healthcare personnel is an excellent method for hand hygiene. This is particularly helpful when there are no sinks available and where many more hand hygiene episodes are required, for example when caring for a group of people, hands need to be cleansed between each person. Alcohol-based sanitisers will destroy most common microorganisms, they work within seconds and water is not needed. They can, however, dry out your hands. It is essential therefore to check that the product you are using includes a moisturiser. It should be borne in mind, however, that hands must be visibly clean for the alcohol gel to be effective. The hand hygiene technique is slightly different when using alcohol gel:

■ Apply the recommended amount of alcohol gel onto the palm of one hand and rub both hands together, covering all the surfaces of hands and fingers, until the hands are dry.

Activity 22.3

Look at the following table and suggest which cleansing product could be used for the chosen activity. Check your responses in the previous section.

	Soap	Alcohol gel
Before preparing a meal		
Between patients in a hospital setting		
Following removal of surgical gloves		
After a walk with the dog		
Before assisting in surgery		
After using a public lavatory		
After digging in the garden		

Other Considerations

For hand hygiene to be effective, nails need to be kept clean and short. Long or false nails can harbour bacteria, and may scratch a client/patient. Jewellery such as bracelets or rings should also be kept to a minimum as they discourage energetic hand washing. It is easy for hands to become dry, especially when working in an environment that necessitates regular washing. Using a moisturiser regularly should protect hands.

Conclusion

This chapter has discussed simple but essential precautions that are necessary to prevent and reduce the level of cross-infection. The main preventive measure relates to correct and effective hand hygiene. Other simple methods of prevention, including waste management, use of protective clothing and cleanliness, are described in the next chapter. You should now be able to list when, how and why you need to wash your hands. Correct hand washing is the single most important way of preventing the spread of infection.

REVIEW
QUESTIONS

1   Why is hand hygiene by staff essential in an environment where people are cared for?

2   When caring for a person in a care home with a wound infection, how would you carry out hand washing so as to avoid cross-infection?

FURTHER
READING

DoH (2002) 'Getting Ahead of the Curve: A Strategy for Combating Infectious Diseases', http//:www.doh.gov.uk
   This is the government's strategy for combating infectious disease.

Horton, R. and Parker, L. (2002) *Informed Infection Control Practice* (2nd edn) Edinburgh, Churchill Livingstone
   Explores the changing nature of infection and essential infection control knowledge.

Infection Control Nurses Association (2002) *Hand Hygiene Guidelines*, http://www.icna.co.uk
   Provides guidelines relating to the importance of hand hygiene.

Lawrence, J. and May, D. (2003) *Infection Control in the Community*, Edinburgh, Churchill Livingstone
   Explores the diversity of settings in the community and the infection control implications.

Wilson, J. (2000) *Clinical Microbiology: An Introduction for Healthcare Professionals* (8th edn) London, Ballière Tindall
   Provides clear and concise information about microorganisms, how they cause infection and how they can be treated.

Wilson, J. (2006) *Infection Control in Clinical Practice* (3rd edn) London, Ballière Tindall
   Gives a comprehensive guide to the principles and practice of infection control.

23 General Infection Prevention and Control

ELIZABETH STUART-COLE

Hygiene is of central importance in all aspects of health and social care because, from care provided in the home to primary care, nursing home care and acute hospital care, infection is ever present. This chapter underlines the principle that good awareness of how infection is transmitted and prevented is pivotal in the provision of effective health and social care.

All health and social care workers should be educated about occupational risks and should understand the need to use universal precautions with all patients and service users at all times, regardless of diagnosis.

Threats from Infections

A healthcare-associated infection (HCAI) is one acquired as a result of contact with the healthcare system. Despite the recent media hype regarding 'killer superbugs' and so on, HCAIs are not a new phenomenon. According to a report published by the Department of Health, between 5 and 10 per cent of patients admitted to hospitals in the UK, Europe, America and Australia contract some form of HCAI (DoH, 2004e).

To some extent, the healthcare system is a victim of its own success. Greater awareness, advances in medical therapy and technology, more emphasis on primary and community care, longer life expectancy, increases in invasive procedures and immunosuppressant therapy are but a few of the factors contributing to the recent upsurge in HCAIs. But the main preventable cause of infections is poor hygiene. Carrying out simple preventive procedures, such as hand washing and good personal hygiene, can notably reduce the incidence of HCAIs.

Not all hospital infection is avoidable but a lot can be prevented with increased awareness of infection risks and good hygiene techniques. The Department of Health has produced guidelines, *The Management and Control of Hospital Infection* (DoH, 2000d), which outline the following standard principles:

- strengthen prevention and control of infection in hospital
- secure appropriate healthcare services for patients with infection
- improve surveillance of hospital infection
- monitor and optimise antimicrobial prescribing.

The Health Protection Agency (HPA) is an independent body set up in 2005 to protect the health and welfare of the population, play a crucial role in curbing infectious diseases and prevent harm from incidents involving hazardous chemicals and radiation. At a more mundane, but no less important, level in the workplace, healthcare professionals are duty-bound to adhere to workplace policies regarding personal hygiene (for examples see DoH, 2003e, 2006b; NHS, 2004). These are but a few examples of how the government and the NHS are working together to try to ensure that patients are treated in a clean environment and that the risk of contracting a healthcare associated infection is kept to a minimum (for internet access to regular Department of Health updates, type in 'Department of Health towards cleaner hospitals and lower rates of infection').

Types of Infection

Hospital-acquired infections (also known as nosocomial infections) can be caused by various bacteria, viruses, fungi, or parasites. These microorganisms may already be present in the patient's body or may come from the environment, contaminated hospital equipment, healthcare workers, or other patients. Nosocomial infections are the leading cause of death among long-term care residents (Albrecht et al., 2002).

Some groups of people are more likely to develop infections than others. This is often because of their general state of health and because the longer people remain in hospital, the more likely they are to develop an infection. Those more likely to develop infections include:

- those with frequent admissions to hospital
- those with underlying medical conditions
- surgical and intensive care patients

■ those with catheters and other medical equipment such as a tube or line inserted into the body

■ sick, frail elderly people

■ those with immunosuppressed conditions.

Spread of Infection

Pathogenic microorganisms need to gain access to the inner body in order to cause disease. Routes into the body may be natural (for example mouth, nose, eye, ear, anus, vagina) or unnatural (for example accidental or surgical wounds, catheters, drains, invasive procedures and so on). Individuals may harbour potentially pathogenic microorganisms without suffering from any symptoms. They are known as *carriers*. Microorganisms can be spread by direct or indirect methods. The former may be from physical contact with an infected person or carrier and the latter via contaminated objects, food or animals/insects. Bacteria living harmlessly on or in one part of the body may cause infection if transferred to a different area, for example anal microorganisms transferred to the urethra/vagina.

MRSA

MRSA stands for methicillin-resistant Staphylococcus aureus. *Staphylococcus aureus (S. aureus)* is a common type of bacterium which, in most cases, lives innocuously on the skin. In the right circumstances, it causes a number of common problems such as boils, impetigo and wound infections. Methicillin is an antibiotic drug related to penicillin. MRSA includes several types of the *S. aureus* bacteria that are not sensitive to the antibiotics usually effective against them. For people who become infected with MRSA, symptoms can include:

■ Boils and abscesses in any part of the body
■ Impetigo
■ Septic wounds
■ Heart valve infections
■ Food poisoning
■ Toxic shock syndrome
■ Pneumonia.

Long term, the worry is that *S. aureus* will become resistant to all antibiotic drugs. For this reason, it is important that everybody is aware of the problem, practises good hygiene, antibiotics are only used when necessary, and the full course of a drug is taken when it has been prescribed.

Universal Precautions

Universal precautions are basic infection control measures that aim to reduce the risk of transmission of blood-borne pathogens through exposure to blood or body fluids among patients and healthcare workers. The basic principle of universal precautions dictates that blood and bodily fluids from *all* persons should be treated as if infected, regardless of the alleged HIV/hepatitis status of the individual. Infection cannot be seen. By assuming everybody is potentially infected, healthcare workers protect themselves as well as their patients, and ensure anti-discriminatory practice in all cases. Simple ways of encouraging universal precautions include:

- washing hands with soap and water before and after all procedures with all patients
- vigilant use of protective barriers, such as gloves, gowns, aprons, masks, goggles, when in direct contact with blood and other body fluids
- immediate disposal of contaminated sharps without recapping
- use of new, single-use disposable injection equipment for all injections
- appropriate disinfection of instruments and other contaminated equipment
- as little contact as possible with soiled linen. Gloves and leak-proof bags should be used where necessary. Cleaning should occur outside patient areas, using the appropriate detergent and hot water. This should apply to all cleaning procedures.

Hand Washing

Health and social care practitioners maintain that hand washing is the easiest and most effective way (both practically and financially) of preventing the transmission of infective agents and thus reducing the incidence of HCAIs. (See WHO Hospital Infection Control Guidance at www.who.int/esr/surveillance/infectioncontrol/en/; Why is handwashing important? at www.unicef.com/handwashing.) Evidence abounds that healthcare professionals' hands become contaminated with microorganisms from close contact with service users (NAO, 2000; Plowman et al., 2001; Pratt et al., 2001). All healthcare personnel, patients, family members and both formal and informal carers must be encouraged to practise effective hand washing. The single most important thing we can do to prevent infection and the spreading of illness to others is to clean our hands. Thorough hand *antisepsis* removes or destroys the transient microorganisms that can cause disease. Hands may be washed under running water using soap for 10–30 seconds or decontaminated with a waterless, alcohol-based hand gel or hand rub for 15–30 seconds, which is only recommended for hands that are not visibly soiled.

Many healthcare professionals assume that wearing gloves eliminates the need for hand washing. Gloves may even offer a false sense of security, because contamination can occur even when they are used properly. It is recommended that gloves be used as an adjunct rather than a substitute for hand washing (Larson, 1988, 1997).

Barrier Nursing

Patients who are suffering from contagious infections are often treated and cared for in isolation using a procedure known as *barrier nursing*. This is a technique developed to protect the hospital environment (and patients) from contagion with dangerous pathogens. Infected individuals are segregated. Anything that comes into direct contact with them is treated as infective and is either sterilised before being reused or, if this is not possible, incinerated before disposal. Healthcare professionals in contact with barrier-nursed individuals are required to wear personal protective equipment.

Reverse Barrier Nursing

Vulnerable service users, that is, those most at risk of acquiring infections while in hospital, such as elderly people, those with immunosuppressed conditions and organ transplant recipients, may benefit from a form of reverse barrier nursing. Attending staff and visitors are required to wear personal protective clothing before entering the area and any equipment entering must be sterilised beforehand. These precautions help to protect the patient against infectious agents within the health-care environment.

Personal Protective Equipment

Personal protective equipment (PPE) includes any specialised clothing, barrier products, or breathing devices and equipment used to protect individuals from serious injuries or illnesses while in contact with patients. When caring for individuals, PPE helps:

- protect against infection or contamination from blood, body fluids, or respiratory secretions
- reduce the chance that healthcare professionals will infect or contaminate other patients or colleagues
- reduce the chance of transmitting infections from one person to another
- protect against harmful chemicals or other hazards in the healthcare environment.

Examples of personal protective equipment include hair cover, eye wear, mask, gown, apron, gloves and shoe covers.

Cleaning

One of the most fundamentally important aspects of healthcare hygiene is cleaning. The job of a cleaner is an important one. It is not just about making things look nice and tidy. It is about ensuring a *safe, infection-free environment*. The principle aim of cleaning is to remove visible dirt. The mechanism behind it is purely mechanical. The dirt is dislodged, dissolves in the water and is removed with rinsing. Soaps act by promoting mechanical removal and, unless specifically formulated, they have no anti-microbial properties. Thorough cleaning will remove approximately 90 per cent of microorganisms. If not carried out properly, in some cases a poor attempt at cleaning can spread microorganisms over a wider area, increasing the chance of transmission.

Cleaning alone is for low-risk items, such as floors, furniture and mobility aids and so on. Cleaning must take place before either disinfection or sterilisation if these techniques are to prove effective.

Disinfection

This is carried out after initial cleaning with soap and hot water. The aim of disinfection is to reduce microorganisms to a level that will not harm health. It can be achieved by both physical (heat) and chemical means. The choice of the disinfectant to be used depends on the particular situation. Some disinfectants have a wide spectrum, killing nearly all microorganisms. Others kill a smaller range of disease-causing organisms but are preferred because they are less corrosive or relatively non-toxic to humans.

Sterilisation

Sterilisation is the elimination of all transmissible microorganisms and can be performed by both physical and chemical means. Physical methods include auto-claving, dry thermal or wet thermal sterilisation, irradiation and titration. Chemical means include gas sterilisation, and immersion in a disinfectant solution with steril-ising properties. The principle of sterilisation counts more than these technical terms.

Needlestick Injuries

A needlestick injury can be defined as a penetrating stab wound from a needle or other sharp object that may result in exposure to potentially infected blood or other body fluids. The pathogens of primary concern are the human immunodeficiency virus and the hepatitis B and C viruses. Several measures can help to reduce the risk of needlestick injuries (NHS Plus – Health at Work, http://www.nhsplus.nhs.uk):

■ Avoid sharps usage where possible, and where it is essential, exercise particular care in handling and disposal.
■ Avoid wearing open footwear in situations where sharps are being handled.
■ Wear gloves; consider double-gloving.
■ If possible, no more than one person should work in an open wound/cavity.
■ Use a 'hands-free' technique, where the needle is not touched by more than one person and hand-to-hand passing of sharps during operations is avoided.
■ Clearly tell all colleagues where the needle has been placed. Ensure that it is in a safe area.

■ Ensure that all needles and sharps are not left exposed.
■ Always use instruments rather than fingers for retracting and suturing.
■ Direct needles and instruments away from own, or assistant's, hand.

Figure 23.1 details what to do if you or a colleague suffer a needlestick injury.

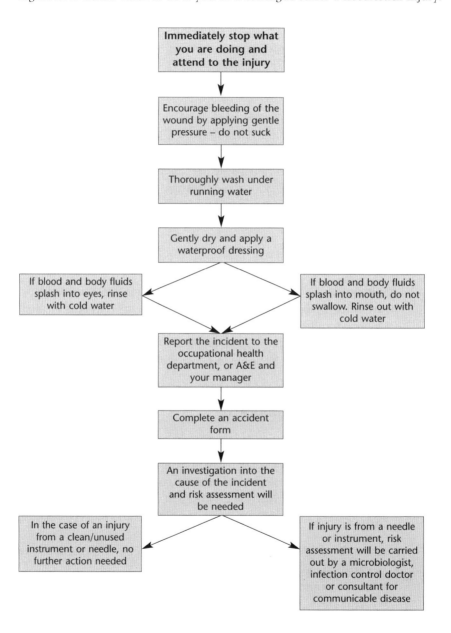

Figure 23.1 Management of a needlestick injury

HIV/AIDS

HIV stands for human immunodeficiency virus. It is a type of virus known as a *retro-virus*. HIV destroys white blood cells known as CD4 T-cells, which are an important part of the immune system. These cells are vital to protect the body against various bacteria, viruses and other 'germs'. AIDS stands for acquired immunodeficiency syndrome. This term covers the range of infections and illnesses that can result from a 'weakened' immune system caused by HIV. When an individual first becomes infected with HIV, they do not have AIDS. Generally, there is an interval of several years between first being infected with HIV, and then developing infections and other AIDS-related problems. People with HIV can pass the virus on to others whether or not they have any symptoms (Table 23.1).

Table 23.1 Transmission of HIV

Causes of transmission	Details of transmission
Sexual transmission	This is the most common way the virus is passed on. It is transmitted during sex with an infected individual (vaginal, anal or oral sex). Semen, vaginal secretions and blood from an infected person contain HIV
Needle-sharing	HIV and other viruses such as hepatitis B and C can be transmitted by drug users who share needles
Accidental needlestick injuries	There have been cases where healthcare workers contract HIV, having been injured accidentally by contaminated needles
Infected blood	Although now rare in this country, HIV may be transmitted by infected blood transfusions and other blood products
From mother to child	About 1 in 3 untreated pregnant women with HIV pass the infection on to their babies during pregnancy or childbirth
Other causes	Some cases have been reported where HIV has been transmitted through organ or tissue transplants, and by contaminated medical or dental equipment which has not been sterilised properly

You cannot catch HIV from ordinary contact with someone with HIV such as hugging, shaking hands, touching and so on, or from sharing food, cups, plates, towels, swimming pools, toilet seats and so on. Worldwide, 42 million people are living with HIV. Of these, 38.6 million are adults (19.2 million are women) and 3.2 million are children under 15. Since 2002, 5 million new cases have been diagnosed and 3.1 million deaths have occurred as a consequence of HIV and AIDS-related illnesses (WHO Aids Epidemic Update, December 2002, www.who.int/hiv/pub/epidemiology/epi2002/2n/). The number of people diagnosed with HIV in the UK has increased dramatically in the past few years. In 1998, it was estimated that 30,000 people were living with HIV, of whom one-third were undiagnosed (DoH, 2001h, p. 7).

The main way to prevent infection by HIV is to increase general awareness, practise good hygiene and universal precautions and avoid risky activities such as sharing needles and having unprotected sex.

Hepatitis B

Hepatitis B is a virus that in most cases causes an acute infection, which may or may not show symptoms. Following infection, a small proportion of infected individuals go on to develop a persistent infection called chronic hepatitis B. These people may not suffer any symptoms but can still pass the virus on to others. Some people develop more serious chronic liver problems. The virus is mainly transmitted by the same routes as HIV, sexual contact, sharing needles to inject drugs, or from mother to baby and so on. A vaccine against hepatitis B is widely available. Three doses of the vaccine are needed for full protection. The second dose is usually given one month after the first dose, and the third dose five months after the second dose. One month after the third dose a blood test is performed to check immunity.

Anyone who is at increased risk of being infected with the hepatitis B virus should consider being immunised. These include:

- workers who come into contact with blood products, or are at increased risk of needlestick injuries, assault and so on. Examples include nurses, doctors, dentists, medical laboratory workers, prison officers and staff at daycare or residential centres for people with learning disabilities where there is a risk of scratching or biting by residents
- individuals who inject illegal drugs (their sexual partners and children are also at risk)
- individuals who are sexually promiscuous
- individuals who live in close contact with someone infected with hepatitis B, for example prison inmates
- individuals with specific kidney or liver diseases
- individuals who live in shared residential accommodation, particularly those for people with learning disabilities
- individuals who regularly receive blood transfusions
- travellers to countries where hepatitis B is common.

Legislation

The most important legislation relating to hygiene is the Health and Safety at Work Act 1974, and the Management of Health and Safety at Work Regulations 1999. As well as a whole range of health and safety issues, these detail how all organisations are legally obliged to produce and enforce a personal hygiene policy. This policy will instruct individuals on expected standards regarding appearance, health and personal hygiene. Another important area in the legislation is risk assessment. Guidelines clearly stating when, where, how and on whom risk assessment should be performed should be clearly available in all workplaces. It is the employer's responsibility to ensure that all employees are aware of the policy and procedures surrounding hygiene. Besides the Health and Safety at Work Act itself, there are other pieces of guidance and legislation that contain important information. These include:

- Management of Health and Safety at Work Regulations 1999: require employers to carry out risk assessments, make arrangements to implement necessary measures, appoint competent people and arrange for appropriate information and training.
- Workplace (Health, Safety and Welfare) Regulations 1992: cover a wide range of basic health, safety and welfare issues such as ventilation, heating, lighting, workstations, seating and welfare facilities.
- Personal Protective Equipment (PPE) Regulations 1992: require employers to provide appropriate protective clothing and equipment for their employees.
- Provision and Use of Work Equipment Regulations (PUWER) 1999: require that equipment provided for use at work, including machinery, is safe.
- Manual Handling Operations Regulations 1992: cover the moving of objects by hand or bodily force.
- Health and Safety (First Aid) Regulations 1981: cover requirements for first aid.
- The Health and Safety Information for Employees Regulations 1989: require employers to display a poster telling employees what they need to know about health and safety.
- Employers' Liability (Compulsory Insurance) Regulations 1969: require employers to take out insurance against accidents and ill-health to their employees.
- Reporting of Injuries, Diseases and Dangerous Occurrences Regulations (RIDDOR) 1985: require employers to report certain occupational injuries, diseases and dangerous events.
- Control of Substances Hazardous to Health Regulations (COSHH) 1999: require employers to assess the risks from hazardous substances and take appropriate precautions.

Conclusion

This chapter has dealt with the major threats to hygiene and ways of tackling them. It is not possible to regulate infection out of the workplaces of health and social care. We need to maintain constant vigilance, a self-critical approach and a willingness to remind our colleagues of the need to maintain high standards in order to protect health and, in some cases, avoid life-threatening risks.

REVIEW
QUESTIONS

1 What are the main threats to good hygiene?

2 What are the main ways of maintaining good hygiene?

3 What are the main laws governing hygiene?

FURTHER READING

Babb, J.R., Davies, J.G. and Ayliffe, G.A. (1983) 'Contamination of Protective Clothing and Nurses Uniforms in an Isolation Ward', *Journal of Hospital Infection*, **4**: 149–57

Bryan, J.L., Cohran, J. and Larson, E.L. (1995) 'Hand Washing: A Ritual Revisited', *Critical Care Nursing Clinics of North America*, **7**: 617–26

DoH (2004) 'Standards for Better Health', www.dh.gov.uk

Hambraeus, A. (1973) 'Transfer of Staphylococcus Aureus via Nurses' Uniforms', *Journal of Hygiene*, **71**: 799–814

Hambraeus, A. and Ransjo, U. (1977) 'Attempts to Control Clothes-borne Infection in a Burns Unit', *Journal of Hygiene*, **79**: 193–02

Larson, E.L. (1995) 'APIC Guidelines for Hand Washing and Hand Antisepsis in Health Care Settings', *American Journal of Infection Control*, **23**: 251–69

Loh, W., Ng, W. and Olton, J. (2000) 'Bacterial Flora on the White Coats of Medical Students', *Journal of Hospital Infection*, **45**: 65–8

Madeo, M. (2004) Commentary on Bennett, G. and Mansell, I. (2004) 'Universal Precautions: A Survey of Community Nurses' Experience and Practice', *Journal of Clinical Nursing* **13**: 413–21, in *Journal of Clinical Nursing*, **13**(8): 1017–19

NHS Executive (1995) 'Hospital Laundry Arrangements for Used and Infected Linen', HSG(95)18

NICE (2003) 'Infection Control: Prevention of Healthcare-associated Infection in Primary and Community Care', Clinical Guidance 2, www.nice.org.uk

NMC (2004) *The NMC Code of Professional Conduct: Standards for Conduct, Performance and Ethics*, www.nmc-uk.org

Parker, M.T. (1978) *Hospital-acquired Infections: Guidelines to Laboratory Methods*, Copenhagen, WHO Regional Office for Europe, European Series, No. 4

Perry, C., Marshall, R. and Jones, E. (2001) 'Bacterial Contamination of Uniforms', *Journal of Hospital Infection*, **48**: 238–41

RCN (2005) *Uniform Approach: Key Points for Nursing*, London, RCN

Salisbury, D.M., Hutfilz, P., Treen, L.M., Solin, G.E. and Gautam, S. (1997) 'The Effects of Rings on Microbial Load of Health Care Workers' Hands, *American Journal of Infection Control*, **25**: 24–7

Scottish Executive (2002) The Watt Group Report, 'A Review of the Outbreak of Salmonella at the Victoria Infirmary', www.scottishexecutive.gov.uk

Speers, R., Shooter, R.A., Gaya, H. and Patel, N. (1969) 'Contamination of Nurses' Uniforms with Staphylococcus Aureus', *Lancet*, **2**(7614): 233–5

Wong, D., Nye, K. and Hollis, P. (1991) 'Microbial Flora on Doctors' White Coats', *British Medical Journal*, **303**: 1602–4

Promoting a Healthy Bladder and Bowel

RUTH MCDONALD

By the end of this chapter, you should be able to:

■ UNDERSTAND the contribution of bladder and bowel function to health

■ KNOW some of the main causes of urinary incontinence and constipation

■ ENABLE the management of urinary incontinence and constipation.

This chapter discusses how health and social care practitioners can promote and maintain the health of a patient's or service user's bladder and bowel. First we examine the psychosocial effects that individuals with bladder and bowel problems may experience. Then we explore the incidence and prevalence of two often hidden and taboo bladder and bowel problems: urinary incontinence and constipation. We also examine first-line interventions to relieve and treat them.

The Psychosocial Effects of Bladder and Bowel Problems

Activity 24.1

Imagine you are working with a person with little or no control over their bladder or bowel. Consider how they may feel and how they may manage their problem in the following situations:

■ Going shopping at the local supermarket
■ Spending a night at a friend's house
■ Going on holiday
■ Going on a date.

A bladder or bowel problem creates considerable social, psychological and hygienic problems for sufferers (DoH, 2000f). People with little or no control over the emptying of their bladder or bowel worry constantly that they will have an 'accident'. They often feel dirty and worry that they smell of urine or faeces, resulting in distress, embarrassment and inconvenience and a perceived lack of personal control. These feelings can leave individuals reluctant to go out of the house, to the detriment of their work and leisure activities. They may withdraw from friends and family and dramatically reduce sexual intimacy with a partner. This enforced social isolation at a time when individuals often need a lot of support and reassurance can lead to low self-esteem, anxiety-related conditions and sometimes more serious illnesses, such as clinical depression.

People with poor control over their bladder or bowel may be unable to be spontaneous. Even going to the shops or visiting a friend require careful, time-consuming planning. Prior to leaving the house, many reduce their intake of fluid and food and consider wearing dark, loose fitting clothes, so that marks or stains are not evident and they can be removed quickly if the person has to use the toilet in a hurry.

These problems are compounded by the fact that bladder and bowel problems are a taboo subject presenting hidden problems. Two common misconceptions are shared both by those suffering in secret from the problem, for fear of stigma or unfair judgement by others, and by those providing professional care:

- It is a problem only experienced by very young children or older people.
- Nothing can be done to resolve the problem, except to hide it using appliances and aids, such as absorbent products or sheaths.

People with bladder or bowel problems may be unable to discuss them and may not know with whom to raise the subject. Practitioners need to develop skills, encouraging people to talk about their problems (see also Chapter 41). Once a practitioner has developed a good relationship with the patient or service user, when they broach the subject they will often find that the person is relieved to share their problem with someone who understands. Inoffensive questions can be used to initiate discussion: Do you know how common bladder and bowel problems are? Do you have any problems getting to the toilet in time? Have you ever had an accident or a leakage prior to getting to the toilet?

The Department of Health (2000f), in *Good Practice for Continence Services*, states that everyone with a bladder or bowel problem has the right to a thorough, individualised assessment of their condition and appropriate treatment by a person knowledgeable in this aspect of care. However, if practitioners reinforce common misconceptions about bladder and bowel health, are unaware of available services and lack the knowledge and skills to promote a healthy bladder or bowel, then people in their care will continue to suffer in secret. We now examine urinary incontinence and constipation and interventions to tackle them.

Urinary Incontinence

The bladder acts as a storage vessel. Urine collects in it following excretion by the kidneys, is stored until the bladder reaches its capacity (approximately 500 ml) and is expelled through the urethra. Bladder emptying is controlled by a combination of muscles and nerves, working together. As the bladder reaches its capacity, sensory nerve impulses initiate the urge to void (empty the bladder), the detrusor muscle contracts and the urethral sphincter relaxes, allowing the urethra to relax so that urine is expelled from the bladder. These nerve impulses and muscular contractions must coordinate so the bladder empties at an appropriate time and place.

Urinary incontinence has been described by members of the International Continence Society as a 'Condition where there is involuntary loss of urine, and is a social or hygienic problem' (Abrams et al., 1988, p. 403). Urinary incontinence is a common problem affecting men and women of all ages. Research shows a wide variation in the incidence of urinary incontinence, but there is general agreement that it is a large problem affecting 1 in every 3 women and 1 in every 11 men (DoH, 2000f). At certain times in their lives, women and men are more likely to develop the problem. In women, urinary incontinence peaks at around child-bearing age, then in mid-life around the time of the menopause, and then further peaks in old age. The pattern is slightly different in men. They are unlikely to suffer from urinary incontinence until their mid-life, unless suffering from illness or an accident which directly affects their bladder function. Men, like women, are likely to suffer urinary incontinence as they reach old age. However, old age alone is not a cause of urinary incontinence; old age does not make it inevitable, but the presence of other conditions can make it more likely.

The four types of urinary incontinence are caused by different parts of the bladder (or other parts of the body) not functioning correctly:

1. *Stress incontinence* predominantly occurs in women due to constipation, or a weakness in their pelvic floor muscle, following childbirth and after the menopause. Symptoms of stress incontinence include small amounts of leakage following exertion, such as coughing, sneezing, standing and walking.
2. *Urge incontinence* is also known as 'overactive' or 'unstable bladder'. It is caused by a number of factors such as medical conditions, urinary tract infections (UTIs), drinking fluids that irritate the bladder, concentrated urine and constipation. Symptoms include a strong urge to pass urine with increased frequency both day and night, passing only small amounts of urine and often being unable to reach the toilet in time.
3. *Overflow incontinence* is often caused by an obstruction, such as an enlarged prostate in men, a urethral stricture or constipation. Often the bladder retains large amounts of urine due to an obstruction, which makes UTIs more likely to occur. Other symptoms include frequently passing small amounts of urine and dribbling constantly or after passing urine.

4. *Functional incontinence* refers to urinary incontinence that occurs as a result of another health condition or disability. The individual's bladder may be healthy, but problems such as reduced mobility, poor dexterity and environmental factors may create incontinence. People are unable to get to the toilet in time to empty their bladder and often will lose large amounts of urine at once.

Several factors (Table 24.1) affect normal bladder function. Normally, a person diagnosed with a urinary problem will suffer from several of these.

Table 24.1 Factors affecting normal bladder function

Medical history
■ Certain medical conditions such as multiple sclerosis, Parkinson's disease and stroke
■ Previous surgery, such as gynaecological, prostate and pelvic surgery
■ Taking certain medications
■ Childbirth
■ Menopause
■ Urinary tract infections
■ Low fluid intake
■ Obesity
■ Constipation
■ Chronic cough
Inability to cope with demands on bladder
■ Cognitive or memory problems, such as dementia
■ Sensory conditions, such as poor eyesight
■ Environment, inadequate or unsuitable toileting facilities
■ Reduced mobility, not able to get to the toilet quickly enough, if at all
■ Poor manual dexterity – unable to unfasten clothes
■ Lack of help and support

Activity 24.2

Lily Smith is an 81-year-old woman, living alone in a three-bedroom house, with one toilet, upstairs. Lily has found that recently she has had episodes of urinary incontinence and when she gets the urge to pass urine, she is often unable to get upstairs to use the toilet in time. She has been buying small sanitary pads from her local chemist, but has been using several per day to contain her urinary incontinence, and is reluctant to leave the house for long periods of time in case she has an accident. Although Lily has good mobility, she is worried that she may fall on the stairs in her hurry to reach the toilet. She says her urine is dark in colour and smells strong. She confesses to drinking three to four small cups of milky coffee a day.

■ What advice would you give Lily and what practical steps could you take as a practitioner to relieve her bladder problems?

Strategies to Promote a Healthy Bladder

Whatever the cause of urinary incontinence, there are a number of first-line interventions that can be used to greatly enhance bladder function, and these are now discussed.

Increasing appropriate fluid intake

It is essential to drink around two litres of fluid per day to maintain bladder health. This prevents urine from becoming concentrated, which can irritate the bladder wall, increasing the sensation of needing to pass urine even if the bladder has not reached its full capacity. Normal urine should be straw-coloured; dark urine can indicate that fluid intake is insufficient. People with urinary incontinence and those caring for them should observe the colour of the urine. Practitioners need to ensure that the person understands the importance of sufficient fluid intake as a reduction can worsen urinary symptoms. Drinking two litres can often seem an impossible task for some people, especially if they have managed their continence problem by reducing their fluid intake. It may help to suggest that they drink little and often during the day, rather than large amounts at one time.

The right type of fluid should be consumed. Drinks containing caffeine, such as coffee and tea, cola and hot chocolate, can irritate the bladder and increase the urge to void. Advising people to reduce or avoid caffeine-based drinks and to drink water and juices is often difficult, but it can help to offer decaffeinated tea and coffee.

Avoid constipation

Constipation can adversely affect the functioning of the bladder. The fibre in fruit and vegetables, cereal and wholemeal bread and drinking fluid can help to prevent constipation (see below).

Facilitate and encourage increased mobility

People with reduced mobility often experience urinary incontinence, when unable to reach the toilet in time, if at all. These individuals can have a perfectly functioning bladder, but their restricted mobility means they leak urine before arriving. Preventive strategies include:

- encouraging the person to leave sufficient time to reach the toilet
- ensuring that they can call someone easily to help them reach the toilet
- observation by practitioners who can learn to detect signs that the person needs to pass urine and intervene in a timely manner.

Everyone should be encouraged to use the toilet, but for chair- or bed-bound people many different aids and appliances exist to promote continence. Commodes or urinals – more accessible than toilets – are available from local NHS resources and social services agencies or adult care services, or a health or social care practitioner.

Toileting techniques

Toileting techniques can promote and maintain a healthy bladder. Using these, practitioners can ensure that when people go to the toilet, they empty their bladder effectively. Without this, more frequent visits to the toilet or increased episodes of urinary incontinence can result. The following can be helpful:

- The person should sit properly on the toilet. The pelvic floor muscle needs to be relaxed in order for the bladder to empty fully. The person should be encouraged to sit comfortably on the toilet with both feet flat on the floor and never to hover over the toilet.
- The person should have sufficient time and not be interrupted when passing urine. Being hurried or a lack of privacy can lead to the bladder being only partially emptied.
- A final check to ensure that the bladder is as empty as possible involves encouraging the person when they have finished voiding to lean forward or stand up and then sit down again. This movement changes the position of the bladder and allows any remaining urine to be expelled.
- A common reason why women in particular suddenly become incontinent of urine can be a UTI. UTIs can occur when bacteria transfer from the anus to the urethra. Practitioners should encourage women, after they have passed urine, to wipe themselves from front to back, which reduces the chance of transferring bacteria that can cause a UTI.
- Many people, particularly those with urinary incontinence, have a tendency to empty their bladder before setting out, 'just in case', rather than when it is full. Emptying the bladder when it is not full can be harmful, especially if habitual, as it reduces the bladder's capacity, resulting in more frequent visits to the toilet. If someone already has a small bladder capacity, practitioners can work alongside health professionals and the patient or service user to design individual toileting plans and retrain the bladder to increase its capacity.

Constipation

In order for the body to function effectively, people need to eat and digest a healthy diet (see Chapter 21). The essential nutrients present in food are required to give the body energy and for the growth and repair of cells (Chapter 6). Once eaten, food is digested and waste products are removed from the body. The transit time for food, from entering the body to the bowel emptying, is 24–36 hours. The bowel comprises the small and large intestine and the rectum. The waste products following digestion are propelled along the bowel by peristalsis. *Peristalsis* is the contraction of the muscles in the bowel, pushing the waste product (faeces) through the bowel. Peristalsis occurs naturally after a meal and is further stimulated by the bulk (size and weight) of the faeces. The faeces reach the rectum, where they are stored until the appropriate time and place to defaecate.

A normal bowel movement should be a semi-solid form, of a soft consistency and a good brown colour. When emptying the bowel, individuals should not feel a great urgency or have to strain. The longer the faeces remain in the bowel (that is, the slower the transit time), the more water is reabsorbed back into the body, making the stool harder, lighter and more difficult to pass. Constipation has been defined as 'the passage of hard stools less frequently than the patient's own normal pattern' (Medicines Resource Centre, 1999).

Constipation is present if a person:

- strains on defaecation for a least 25 per cent of the time
- has lumpy or hard stools for a least 25 per cent of the time
- has a sense of incomplete evacuation for a least 25 per cent of the time
- has two or less bowel movements a week.

Constipation is a very prevalent condition, with an estimated 1 in every 2 people suffering from constipation at some time during their lives and over three million people in the UK on a frequent basis (Potter et al., 2002). Pregnant women and those in long-term residential care are more likely to experience constipation (see Table 24.2), as are older people, being likely to possess more risk factors causing constipation. As people live longer, the incidence of constipation is likely to increase, causing yet more people to suffer and increasing the staggering cost the NHS has to meet each year in prescriptions for laxatives.

Table 24.2 People at a greater 'risk' of constipation

■ Those taking more than five medications
■ Those with no or limited mobility
■ Residential and nursing home residents
■ Those with certain medical conditions, such as Parkinson's disease, diabetes, multiple sclerosis, stroke
■ Those with a low fluid intake
■ Those with a poor fibre intake

Simple constipation is not necessarily harmful, but can have a great impact on a person's quality of life, often leading to a loss of wellbeing, feelings of discomfort and anxiety, loss of appetite and reduced mobility. The symptoms of constipation are wide-ranging (see Table 24.3).

Activity 24.3

Norman Wade is 76 and has suffered from constipation since his stroke six months ago, when he moved into a nursing home, being unable to manage at home. Norman has a pronounced weakness in his right side and finds it difficult to mobilise unaided and to use a knife and fork at meal times. He requires help with walking and eats only small amounts. Norman only has a commode in his room, where he often stays, not wanting to bother staff.

- What practical steps could you take to help Norman relieve his constipation?

Table 24.3 Symptoms of constipation

■ Altered bowel habit
■ Frequent hard pellet-like stools
■ Feelings of incomplete evacuation
■ Abdominal pain
■ Bloating/flatulence
■ Nausea and vomiting
■ Urinary dysfunction – urinary incontinence or retention of urine
■ Poor appetite
■ Tiredness
■ Faecal incontinence due to obstruction and overflow

Strategies to Prevent and Manage Constipation

Preventing and relieving constipation is straightforward, but it needs to be tackled sensitively. Most interventions involve giving advice and encouraging changes to lifestyle and diet.

Increasing dietary fibre and fluid intake

One of the main causes of constipation is an inadequate intake of fibre and fluid. Fibre is generally undigested by the body and as it travels through the bowel, it helps to retain water and increase the bulk of the stool, thereby increasing peristalsis, transit time is faster, and the stools are soft and easier to pass. In our busy modern world, there has been a trend towards processed and convenience foods, low in dietary fibre, which can promote constipation. Good sources of fibre include fruit, vegetables, nuts, cereals and pulses. An adult should consume an average of 18–30 g of fibre a day. In the UK, the average daily consumption is only 12–13 g. Recent studies (Medicines Resource Centre, 1999) show that a daily intake of 25 g can increase the frequency of bowel movements in those with simple constipation. Practitioners can help to manage or prevent constipation by educating and encouraging the person to consume more dietary fibre. Simple advice includes:

■ Making wise food choices by eating five portions of fruit and vegetables a day and changing from eating white or processed products to wholemeal and natural options.
■ Checking the labelling of food for fibre content; even small changes can help to increase fibre intake, for example eating an apple provides 1.8 g of fibre, whereas choosing a pear is better as it contains more fibre, 3.7 g.
■ It may be useful to encourage the service user or patient to keep a food diary, so that they can monitor their intake of fibre and become aware of what types of foods help their bowels to work more effectively.

As well as eating sufficient fibre, it is also essential to maintain an adequate fluid intake. Like dietary fibre, water increases the bulk of the stool, keeps the stool soft and increases bowel efficiency. A dehydrated body means less water in the bowel, the stool is solid and hard and the transit time slower. Practitioners can encourage people to drink one and a half to two litres of fluid per day, preferably water, sipping little and often, ensuring it is within easy reach when the practitioner is absent.

Exercise

Increasing physical activity and exercise helps the bowel to function effectively. Regular activity stimulates the contraction of the abdominal muscles, which in turn stimulate the bowel muscles. Many people with a healthy bowel find that following exercise they feel the sensation of needing to empty the bowel. Service users or patients with very limited mobility can be encouraged to exercise, even if it is minimal and for short periods of time. For example, helping a chair-bound person to stand for a couple of minutes each hour or ordering equipment such as Zimmer frames and walking sticks can encourage people to become more independent and active.

Promoting a routine

Bowels benefit from routine, and those people with a healthy bowel often empty their bowels at the same time each day – it is most common for people to want to defaecate in the morning, or after a meal. For many reasons, including lazy lifestyles, fear of using unfamiliar toilets, lack of privacy, missing meals and stress, people often delay or avoid emptying their bowels, even when they get the sensation to go to the toilet. This is referred to as 'ignoring the call to stool'. If people continually ignore this call, the bowel contents remain in situ for longer periods of time, drying them out, as water is reabsorbed into the body, resulting in constipation. This in turn creates a vicious circle, as often defaecation is painful and time-consuming so the call to stool is ignored further. Over time this causes the urge to open the bowels to weaken and disappear, further exacerbating the constipation. This can result in the impaction of faeces, which requires more intensive treatment to relieve.

Three strategies can promote a healthy bowel and develop a bowel routine:

- Encourage the person to listen to their bowel and use the toilet on the urge to go.
- Ensure the person has privacy (closed door) and time (no interruptions) to empty their bowels fully.
- Ensure toileting facilities are appropriate – the person should be able to sit on the toilet correctly and safely. It is important to sit comfortably with both feet firmly on the floor, allowing the pelvic floor muscle to relax and complete emptying of the rectum.

Taking medication

Simple lifestyle and dietary changes can improve the motility of the bowel; however, medication may be needed to relieve constipation. Laxatives should be used correctly in order to have maximum effect. They can be prescribed or bought over the counter in chemists. There is a wide variety, each working on different parts of the bowel with different side effects. Although laxatives can be useful in treating constipation, if taken unnecessarily over a long period of time, they can harm the bowel. People using laxatives to relieve their constipation should understand how the medication works, its dosage and frequency. Practitioners can help the service user or patient with the necessary information enabling them to take their laxatives wisely. However, practitioners should refer the person with persistent problems for specialist advice from a suitably qualified health professional.

Conclusion

This chapter has surveyed some common problems people may experience with their bladders and bowels, highlighting a number of interventions that practitioners can use to help alleviate urinary incontinence and constipation. The key message from this chapter is that something invariably can be done for people with bladder and bowel problems, which should be identified and treated and not kept secret. Often simple and straightforward interventions can improve a bladder or bowel condition and greatly enhance a person's quality of life. The interventions discussed in this chapter are first-line treatments only and people with complex problems who do not respond to them may benefit from more specialised interventions delivered in partnership between the patient or service user, the practitioner and a qualified specialist.

REVIEW QUESTIONS

1 Is urinary incontinence inevitable in old age?

2 What can be done for people suffering from urinary incontinence?

3 What are the main causes of constipation?

4 What dietary changes can be made to prevent or treat constipation?

FURTHER READING

Abrams, P., Blavis, J.G. and Stanton, S.L. (1988) 'Standardisation of Terminology of Lower Urinary Tract', *Neurological Urodynamics*, **7**: 403–27

Ashbury, N. and White, H. (2001) *Don't Make Me Laugh: How to Feel Better about Living with a Weak Bladder*, Newcastle Upon Tyne, Northumbria Health Care Trust

Button, D., Roe, B., Webb, C., Frith, T., Colin-Thorne, D. and Gardner, L. (1998) *Continence: Promotion and Management by the Primary Health Care Team – Consensus Guidelines*, London, Whurr

Doughty, D.B. (ed.) (2006) *Urinary and Faecal Incontinence: Current Management Concepts*, St Louis, Mosby Elsevier

Royal College of Physicians (1995) *Incontinence: Causes, Management and Provision of Services*, London, Royal College of Physicians

WEBSITES: http://www.aca.uk.com/ (Association for Continence Advice – ACA)
http://www.continence-foundation.org/ (Continence Foundation)
http://www.incontact.org/ (In Contact)

Illnesses and Conditions: Signs and Symptoms ROBERT ADAMS

Learning outcomes

By the end of this chapter, you should be able to:

■ UNDERSTAND the basic signs of disease and ill-health in a person

■ BE AWARE OF the range of conditions and diseases which could be responsible

■ APPRECIATE the dangers of ill-informed attempts to diagnose.

The shift towards closer collaboration in the health and social services makes it more important that all practitioners should have acquaintance with each other's knowledge base. This chapter introduces those vital signs and symptoms with which you should be familiar as health and social care workers. It is impossible to give a comprehensive picture of this topic, but there is space to provide an indication of the major areas of relevance. One main purpose is to familiarise social care workers in particular, who may not come into regular contact with medical practitioners, with the main conditions and illnesses responsible for ill-health and some basic terms and their meanings. It is probably useful to read this chapter in conjunction with Chapter 6, which provides a summary of the functions of the main organs of the body.

The Main Conditions and Illnesses

It is necessary to emphasise at the start that no health and social care practitioner is professionally qualified to make diagnostic statements on the basis of signs and symptoms as described in this chapter. People should always be referred to a qualified medical professional. The purpose of this chapter is to provide a map to guide the non-expert, not to substitute for extensive medical training.

Diseases of the Blood

These can affect the formation of blood cells. For instance, anaemia is the condition resulting from a decrease in the level of haemoglobin in the blood. There may be no symptoms, or there may be fatigue, headaches, faintness, angina, breathlessness or palpitations. The most common cause of anaemia is iron deficiency, which through reasons of poverty and inadequate diet affects about 500 million people in the world – between a quarter and a third of the population. Older people may suffer from pernicious anaemia, which is associated with faulty vitamin B_{12} absorption. Anaemia can also be associated with leukaemia or various cancers, in which case there will be other serious symptoms.

Diseases of the Nervous System

A wide range of conditions occur, with a huge variety of signs and symptoms. Some may have very minor and unimportant causes while others are progressive and life-threatening. They include, for example, headaches, shingles, epilepsy, Parkinson's disease, meningitis, multiple sclerosis, brain injury, tumours of the brain, dementia, cerebral palsy and motor neurone disease. Many of these diseases, such as shingles, create pain, others such as Parkinson's bring about nervous tremors and loss of control over basic movements and functions.

Liver, Bile and Pancreatic Diseases

In Western countries, the main cause of liver disease (of which cirrhosis is perhaps the best known) is alcohol consumption, whereas in developing countries it is the hepatitis B and C viruses. Anaemia may be a symptom of liver problems and various blood tests are also used in diagnosis. The typical yellowish skin colour symptomatic of jaundice sometimes results from faulty functioning of the liver, as well as from other causes such as blockages of the bile duct. Symptoms and causes are likely to vary according to the age and lifestyle of the person. For instance, in a younger person, jaundice is more likely to indicate hepatitis and questions may be asked about alcohol use and sexual activity. In an older person, jaundice accompanying loss of weight may result from cancer.

Hepatitis A is the most common form of viral hepatitis worldwide and is spread by poor and dirty living conditions. Anorexia – characterised by drastic loss of weight – and nausea are common symptoms, along with jaundice. Hepatitis B affects a large proportion of the world's population, more obviously in developing countries. The virus is commonly transmitted in semen and saliva, and drug addicts often pass it on in infected needles. Hepatitis C is less common and can be transmitted in blood transfusions and about four-fifths of patients develop chronic liver disease, with a proportion developing liver cirrhosis or cancer. Hepatitis D is particularly passed on by drug users. Cirrhosis of the liver is usually irreversible and progressive, with about 50 per cent of patients dying within five years. Transplants can be used for this and other liver diseases, but may not work where the infection, or cancer, has spread outside the liver.

Rheumatological and Musculoskeletal Disorders

A huge variety of conditions affect mobility, through affecting the bones and joints of the body, and upwards of a quarter of a GP's patients may be afflicted with them. Often, especially in healthy, younger people, injuries or other problems are temporary and correct themselves without help, or with simple painkillers or physical treatment such as physiotherapy or osteopathy. Some conditions such as arthritis or osteoporosis ('brittle bone disease') are progressive and no simple 'cure' may be possible. Inflammatory arthritis may be worse in the morning and after rest. Rheumatoid arthritis may flare up in an unexplained way, when the linings of the joints and tendon sheaths become inflamed and cause acute pain. Often these are conditions that affect older people and restrict their mobility, so new arrangements – walking frames, electric carriages, adaptations in the home – have to be made to support their day-to-day living and maintain the maximum degree of independence. Problems of back pain are widespread and can result from a specific vehicle accident – as in whiplash injury – or may result from spondylosis, a condition which affects the vertebral joints, as in the trapped nerve of an older person. Although children rarely suffer from arthritis, rheumatic conditions can occur at any age.

Bone diseases can restrict mobility unless treated successfully. Perhaps the most widely known is osteoporosis, in which the bone mass decreases and the risk of fractures increases. Often a sudden fracture is the first symptom of the disease.

Digestive and Gastrointestinal Conditions

Many diseases and conditions affect the different parts of the digestive system, including cancers, gallstones, gastritis or inflammation of the stomach lining, irritable bowel syndrome (IBS), peptic or duodenal ulcers and colitis or inflammation of the bowel, of which Crohn's disease – with its pains in the joints, weight loss, loss of appetite, fever and bleeding from the rectum – can be an extreme form.

About 1 in 5 of all cancers occurs between the oesophagus (the 'eating tube' below your throat) and 'gut', that is, stomach, colon and rectum ('bottom'). Often there are no symptoms for colon cancer until it is very advanced. However, in general, symptoms of gastrointestinal cancers include weight loss, anorexia and passing blood. Some people suffer quite regularly with more minor conditions, such as indigestion, nausea, vomiting, flatulence, diarrhoea and constipation. Many of these are treatable by giving attention to the lifestyle – particularly exercise and diet – of the person.

A great number of infections of the gut can occur through lack of personal cleanliness and through flaws in institutional cleanliness routines. Often food that is imperfectly cooked or reheated using microwave ovens is susceptible to infections such as *E. coli* or *Salmonella*. Symptoms can include fever, severe stomach pains, sickness and diarrhoea. The consequences can be fatal for children, older people and other people whose health is fragile. Gastritis – inflammation of the gastric region – can be painful and other conditions such as peptic and duodenal ulcers can lead to extreme pain, sweating, faintness and palpitations. People can lose weight, as they can when suffering from gastric cancer.

Urinary and Renal Diseases and Conditions

Ageing, illness and injury can cause urinary problems. The kidneys can lose efficiency at removing wastes and can slowly develop chronic kidney disease (CKD) and the muscles of the two ureters and bladder can weaken, creating incontinence. Kidney stones are more likely in men, can form in the kidney and move through the urinary system and may create painful obstructions, which these days can be removed by non-surgical means. Men tend to suffer also from prostatitis – inflammation of the prostate gland which sits under the bladder – sometimes causing frequent and painful urination. Cancer of the prostate affects about a third of older men. Women get urinary tract infections (UTIs) more than men and drinking plenty of fluids helps to flush out the bacteria causing them. Gynaecologists specialise in the female reproductive system and urologists specialise in the urinary system and male reproductive system. Constipation – the retention of waste in the bowel – is dealt with further in Chapter 24.

The urine is the main indicator of renal (kidney) health or disease. Unfortunately, the appearance of the urine – apart from when it is obviously 'bloody' – is not an indicator of kidney health. Having said that, jaundice or various drugs can create very dark urine. A low salt and protein, high fat and carbohydrate diet creates a lower excretion of urine ('passing water'), whereas a high salt diet creates a greater thirst and a higher rate of excretion. Some illnesses cause the kidney's function of concentrating the urine to fail and more has to be excreted. A total lack of urine indicates a blockage in the urinary tract. Tests of the urine for the presence of blood, protein and sugar establish whether renal disease is present.

Respiratory Conditions

The most widespread and well-known diseases and conditions of the respiratory system affect the lungs and impair breathing, including asthma, bronchitis, tuberculosis (TB) and cancer, although cancer also affects other parts. Asthma is brought about by allergies and involves mucus clogging the airways and thus restricting the flow of air. Bronchitis is an inflammation of the bronchial tubes, made worse by smoking or air pollution.

A wide range of symptoms are extremely common and, in the case of a runny nose for instance, it may be extremely difficult to distinguish a cold from a different condition such as an allergy. A cough, similarly, may be a sign of heavy smoking, lower respiratory (breathing) tract (passageway) infection or a symptom of asthma. Sputum (mucus) is produced and coughed up normally, but if stained with large quantities of yellow or green may indicate a bronchial condition. Blood-stained mucus may indicate chest infections such as TB or cancer. Breathlessness needs to be assessed with reference to the person's lifestyle. It may be normal for an older person to become out of breath after climbing two flights of stairs, whereas chest pains with breathlessness may indicate other conditions that need investigating by a medical practitioner.

Cardiovascular Conditions

Heart disease may not have any symptoms, but can also be evident from dyspnoea (abnormal awareness of breathing), 'Cheyne-Stokes respiration' (irregular but rhythmic breathing with temporary cessations – apnoea), chest pains – the most common symptom, palpitations (irregular heartbeats), oedema (swelling) of ankle or calf, particularly later in the day, and fatigue (tiredness).

Sexually Transmitted Diseases

Sexually transmitted infections (STIs) bring about a group of the most common illnesses in the world, sexually transmitted diseases (STDs), which occur in all societies. STIs include thrush, genital herpes, chlamydia infection, non-specific urethritis, syphilis and gonorrhoea. Symptoms vary, with conditions such as gonorrhoea causing urethritis (inflammation of the urethra), vaginal discharge in women, pelvic pain as the infection ascends and intermenstrual bleeding. Syphilis is a chronic systemic disease which can be caught through sexual contact or passed on 'congenitally' (from parent to child). In the early stages, the disease shows as a small ulcer which heals within a few weeks and at this stage the disease can be treated. Between a month and three months later, the secondary symptoms appear and can include a sore throat, fever and general malaise. Other illnesses can develop, with general skin rashes, including hepatitis, arthritis and meningitis. At a later stage, possibly years later, tertiary symptoms of lesions occur on the skin and in the bones.

HIV/AIDS is the fourth biggest killer in the world, with more than 2.5 million deaths annually (see also Chapter 23). Two-thirds of the new infections annually occur in the African continent. Infections occur through sexual intercourse, sharing contaminated needles, receiving contaminated blood transfusions and organ transplants and transmission from mother to baby including through breast-feeding. Diagnosis is by a test to establish the presence of HIV antibodies, plus the development of an opportunistic infection or a low CD4 T-cell count (the immune system's white blood cells, which protect against such infections). Symptoms are diverse, because the disease suppresses the immune system (creating 'immunodeficiency') and patients are susceptible to cardiac, respiratory, eye, blood and gastrointestinal infections and complications.

Diabetes

Diabetes is a disease of the metabolism (speed at which the body 'lives') and is associated with a relative deficiency of insulin and consequent inability of the body to deal with excess glucose (sugar). The body needs glucose in order to remain healthy. Diabetes appears to be associated with being overweight, although some forms of the illness can result in depletion of liquids and actual weight loss. The symptoms of diabetes can vary, but at an extreme an insulin deficiency can result in drowsiness, akin to a drunken state, leading to coma and even death.

Type 1 diabetes mellitus results from the loss of the ability of the pancreas to produce insulin, which therefore has to be injected or taken orally. About four-fifths of patients with type 2 diabetes are obese (overweight). If type 2 diabetes is diagnosed between the ages of 40 and 60, this may mean a reduction in life expectancy of 5–10 years. If diagnosed after 70 years, it has little significant effect on life expectancy. Keeping slim, eating what would be regarded as a normal healthy diet and taking plenty of exercise are likely to delay the onset of type 2 diabetes or even prevent it altogether.

Conclusion

This chapter has surveyed a great many of the most obvious illnesses and conditions, but it would require many complete books of this size to do justice to signs and symptoms for the huge variety which occur. Sufficient information has been provided, hopefully, to give the basis for further reading in any particular area where you come into contact with a person suffering from a specific condition. It can be very reassuring for a service user or carer if you know enough to be able to empathise with the problems caused by a condition, even though, clearly, the purpose of this chapter is not to encourage you to trespass into the territory of medical professionals responsible for diagnosis and treatment.

REVIEW QUESTIONS

1 How may hepatitis A and hepatitis B be passed on?

2 What are dyspnoea and apnoea?

3 What are the changing symptoms of syphilis as the disease develops?

4 What deficiency in the body's function creates diabetes?

FURTHER READING

Champney, B. and Smiddy, F.G. (1979) *Symptoms, Signs and Syndromes: A Medical Glossary*, London, Ballière Tindall
    A clear, alphabetical reference book of signs and symptoms.
Kumar, P. and Clark, M. (eds) (2002) *Clinical Medicine* (5th edn) Edinburgh, WB Saunders/Elsevier

Pain Management **26**

CAROL HAIGH

Learning outcomes

By the end of this chapter, you should be able to:

- UNDERSTAND the nature of acute and chronic pain
- KNOW how to assess pain
- APPRECIATE how to manage pain.

This chapter gives an introduction to pain and its management. Good pain management is one of the most important and most difficult parts of health and social care practice. This chapter introduces two different types of pain, acute and chronic (there are others but these are the ones you are most likely to come across), and will explore how practitioners can help patients and service users to cope.

What is Pain?

Although most of us will have experienced pain to a greater or lesser degree at some time or other in our lives, defining pain is extremely difficult. This is because, apart from the physical elements of pain, there are psychological, behavioural, emotional and social components that vary from person to person. So, pain means different things to different people and it is difficult to define it clearly. We know that it is often associated with some form of tissue damage and most of the definitions of pain tend to concentrate on that. For example:

> An unpleasant sensory or emotional experience associated with actual or potential tissue damage, or described in terms of such damage. (International Association for the Study of Pain, 1986)

Other definitions prefer to take a simpler viewpoint: 'Pain is whatever the experiencing person says it is and exists whenever they say it does' (McCaffery and Beebe, 1994). Unfortunately, the first definition is often seen as too simplistic, since it disregards other factors that may contribute to pain in an individual, and the second one is rarely translated into understanding or dealing with an individual's self-reported pain. This is because very few nurses are willing to believe patients when they say they are in pain, preferring to put professional experience over patient reality (Carr and Mann, 2000). However, the important things to remember about any type of pain are:

- It is different things to different people
- It is something that cannot ever be ignored
- One of the key elements of good pain management is accurate, holistic assessment by healthcare practitioners.

Although it is possible to argue that managing pain is more important than defining it, there are some things that we do need to know about a person's pain before we can manage it appropriately. Understanding the cause and mechanisms of someone's pain not only affects the sort of treatment used but also the type of pain assessment carried out. Health and social care practitioners need to be aware that the origins of a person's pain may lie some distance, physically and emotionally, from the symptoms.

Acute Pain

Acute pain is usually recognised to be pain from injury (including surgery) or pain due to conditions like toothache or heart attack. It is generally intense, localised to a specific area and time-limited, in that as the injury heals or the disease abates, the pain lessens.

The Causes of Acute Pain

Acute pain is sometimes referred to as *nociceptive pain*. *Nociception* refers to the central processing of information (that is, by the brain) of a stimulus that damages tissue or has the potential to do so. The pain can arise from bone, joints, muscle, skin or connective tissue. It can also occur in visceral organs such as the gut or the pancreas. It can be sharp, stabbing, aching or throbbing in quality and is well localised.

There are pain receptors throughout the body. They respond to heat and/or cold, twisting or crushing and chemical stimulus. Acute pain is felt when the damaged cells at the site of injury or disease release chemicals that sensitise the pain receptors. The pain receptors communicate the pain stimulus to the brain via nerves and the spinal cord. Two main types of nerve fibres are involved in this communication. A-delta (sometimes written as Aδ) fibres conduct the pain impulses very quickly, at

35–75 metres/second. They are responsible for the first sharp pain that accompanies the injury as it happens. The second type of nerve fibres, the C fibres, are much slower (1–2 metres/second) and are responsible for the dull aching pain that follows the initial pain. So, if you put your hand on a hot kettle, it is the Aδ fibres that make you snatch your hand away quickly and the C fibres that give you the dull pain that tells you that your hand is burnt.

When the pain impulses reach the brain, they are recognised and interpreted and the conscious experience of pain begins.

How Acute Pain is Managed

Acute pain responds well to drug therapy, which is the treatment of choice when dealing with nociceptive pain. These drugs, called *analgesics*, can be separated into three groups with increasing pain-relieving properties – non-opioid drugs, weak opioids and strong opioids. These drugs may be administered alone or supplemented with other medication. A three-step approach was devised by the World Health Organization in the early 1980s. Although directed primarily at those with cancer pain, the general principles behind the analgesic ladder apply to most patients requiring potent pain relief:

- Step 1: *Non-opioid drugs* are the first line of analgesia. They usually control mild pain and where necessary may be supplemented with other drugs. Non-opioids are often underestimated as analgesics and there is a tendency to forget how useful they can be.
- Step 2: If the regimen employed in step 1 fails to control the pain, or the patient reports increasing pain, then the second line of analgesic therapy is to move to a *weak opioid*. This weak opioid may be given with the non-opioid or used to completely replace the non-opioid drug. Again, other drugs may be used if necessary. Bear in mind that the other medications may include laxatives to overcome opioid-induced constipation as well as other analgesic drugs.
- Step 3: Continuing pain demands the use of a *strong opioid*. The drug of choice in the UK is generally morphine.

So, it can be seen that there are a number of options available to health practitioners when managing pain. These drugs can be given in a variety of ways (Table 26.1).

Some patients and a considerable number of nurses are afraid of the opiate class of drugs, fearing that they will cause addiction. While the opiate drugs do have the capacity to cause addiction if used recreationally, the risk of becoming dependent on them, particularly when being used in acute pain management, is so small it is insignificant (Ferrall et al., 1992). In addition to the appropriate and efficient use of drug therapy, the most important part of satisfactory pain management is regular and accurate assessment.

Table 26.1 Common methods of administration of pain medication

Method of administration	How it works
Sublingually	Medication is placed under the tongue and allowed to melt
Intravenously	Medication is injected directly into the veins. Used in episodes of severe pain. The principle behind patient-controlled analgesia (PCA)
Orally	Medication is swallowed. The commonest form of administration but does not work if people are vomiting
Intramuscularly	Medication is injected into muscle, typically in the thigh. Good if patient is vomiting but the drug is absorbed slowly by the body so it can take a while before the effects are felt
Spinally	Medication is given directly into the epidural space of the spine, either as a one-off injection or via a continuous pump. It is commonly used after surgery but these patients require extra monitoring as side effects can be severe
Subcutaneously	Medication is given via superficial injection into the patient's skin. Can be used as a one-off administration or as long-term pain relief via a pump (common in palliative care settings)
Rectally	If a patient is vomiting, or if a drug is known to cause stomach problems, it can be given via the rectum. A lot of migraine medication can be given this way. This very efficient method of administering drugs is not particularly popular in the UK
Nasally	Medication is held in solution and sprayed into the nose. It is quickly absorbed into the body in this format, but this method is not widely practised in the UK at present

How Acute Pain is Assessed

If pain is to be managed appropriately and to the satisfaction of the patient, it should be assessed on a regular basis. A good pain assessment is more than just asking 'have you any pain?', it should include the use of a recognised measurement tool and formal and accurate documentation.

Commonly used acute pain assessment tools include visual analogue scales (VASs). Sometimes referred to as a 'pain thermometer', a VAS consists of a 100 mm line, vertical or horizontal with either verbal descriptions or numbers from 1 to 10 (see Figure 26.1). Patients are asked to describe, mark or 'score' their pain at two- to four-hourly intervals or within 20 minutes of being given analgesia.

Other sort of assessments use a 0–3 scale where 0 is no pain, 1 is mild pain, 2 is moderate pain and 3 is severe pain. The difficulty with this approach is that it is sometimes difficult for patients to decide whether their pain is mild or moderate. Also, with both types of pain assessment tool, patients will often hesitate to describe their pain as 'severe' or rate it as '10', preferring to keep something in reserve in case the pain gets worse. It needs to be made clear to patients that they should make full use of all the choices that the assessment tool provides them if their pain is to be managed appropriately.

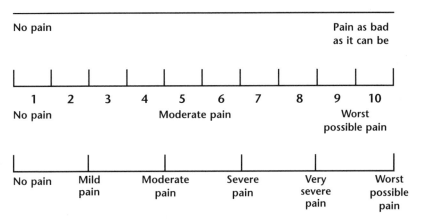

Figure 26.1 Examples of visual analogue scales

Sometimes, healthcare practitioners are reluctant to believe a hospital patient's report of pain, especially if the patient concerned has been sleeping, leaving the ward area to smoke or even sitting quietly watching television. The feeling is that if they can do those things, they cannot possibly be in the amount of pain they say. This is a dangerous and unprofessional assumption, as any one of those activities may help to act as a distraction for the patient, helping them to cope with their pain, but cannot be taken as proof that the patient is overestimating the amount of discomfort they are in.

There are three important things to remember, whatever methods of pain assessment are being used:

1. Pain should be assessed regularly
2. The results of pain assessments should be recorded and acted upon
3. The patient should always be believed.

The social care aspects of acute pain

When patients are in acute pain, their main focus of concern is having it controlled and the underlying problem corrected. However, issues such as where to recuperate, the maintenance of benefits and supply of any aids to independent living do take precedence as the patient progresses towards regaining their health and normal patterns of living.

Chronic Pain

Chronic pain is generally accepted to be pain that lasts for a long period of time. It lasts beyond the time of healing of an injury and often there is no identifiable cause or explanation for it (International Association for the Study of Pain, 1986). It is associated with the abnormal processing of sensory input by the peripheral or central nervous system. It is not usually responsive to opioids; treatment usually includes different analgesics.

The Causes of Chronic Pain

Unlike acute pain that is initiated by trauma or chemical stimulus, chronic pain is allied to the abnormal processing of information. Chronic pain can be described as centrally generated or peripherally generated pain. *Centrally generated pain* is associated with injury to either the peripheral or central nervous system. For example, phantom limb pain may reflect injury to the peripheral nervous system. *Peripherally generated pain* relates to painful neuropathies. In patients who suffer from these, pain is felt along the distribution of many peripheral nerves. It is often bilateral and always diffuse. It can be caused by metabolic disturbances or toxic agents, for example diabetic neuropathy. Unlike acute pain that is initiated by chemical release, chronic pain is reliant upon 'abnormal' nerve excitation.

How Chronic Pain is Managed

Many of the drugs used to manage acute pain are also used to manage the early stages or the occasional 'flare up' of chronic pain. However, current medical practice is to try to avoid long-term or strong opiate use for these patients for obvious reasons. In addition to the methods of administration outlined in Table 26.1, Table 26.2 shows other methods used in the management of chronic pain.

Table 26.2 Additional methods of administration of pain medication, common in chronic pain management

Method of administration	How it works
Spinally	Medication is given directly into the epidural space of the spine, sometimes as a one-off injection. This is used to manage chronic back pain
Transdermally	Medication is given via a patch placed on the body, in the same way a nicotine patch is used. The drug is absorbed through the skin and takes a few days to build up in the patient's system. Much used in chronic and palliative care
Subcutaneously	Medication is given via superficial injection into the patient's skin. Can be used as a one-off administration or as long-term pain relief via a pump (common in palliative care settings)

Although non-pharmaceutical methods such as distraction can be used in acute pain management as a supplement to drug therapy, in chronic pain such measures play a more central role. So, treatments such as relaxation, imagery, exercise, hypnosis, complementary therapies and disciplines such as physiotherapy, clinical psychology and counselling are used either on their own or in conjunction with analgesia and other drug therapies to control or reduce the patient's pain. A further distinction between acute pain and chronic pain is that whereas acute pain is for the most part completely or significantly reduced by treatment, chronic pain may prove more intractable and difficult to cope with. Sometimes the best that can be achieved is a slight reduction in the chronic pain that a patient suffers and when this is the case, the treatment focus moves to coping strategies instead.

How Chronic Pain is Assessed

It has already been emphasised that pain is more than simply a physical reaction to stimuli. In acute pain, the patient's fear or anxiety may contribute to how they perceive their pain severity and such factors play an integral part in the life of the chronic pain sufferer. It is sometimes difficult for such patients to be taken seriously by the medical, nursing and social care professionals who, if there is no clear organic cause for the pain, may imply that the patient is faking their symptoms for reasons of their own, to obtain benefits for example, or assume that the root cause of the patient's behaviour is psychological in origin. Therefore chronic pain sufferers tend to become depressed, anxious, demanding and angry, which can make them a challenge to look after.

Given the extremely complex nature of the chronic pain experience, the assessment of pain that is appropriate for such patients must be in more depth than the assessments used for acute pain sufferers. Figure 26.2 shows an example of a chronic pain assessment sheet, which is far more complex that those outlined in Figure 26.1.

NAME _____   DATE_____

Please tick any of the words that describe your pain under the column that describes its intensity

	None	Mild	Moderate	Severe
Throbbing				
Shooting				
Stabbing				
Cramping				
Gnawing				
Hot–Burning				
Aching				
Heavy				
Tender				
Splitting				
Tiring–Exhausting				
Sickening				
Fearful				
Punishing–Cruel				

Your Pain is:

On Most Days ......   No Pain   Mild
                       Discomforting Distressing
                       Horrible   Excruciating

At Its Worst ......   No Pain   Mild
                       Discomforting Distressing
                       Horrible   Excruciating

At Its Best ......   No Pain   Mild
                       Discomforting Distressing
                       Horrible   Excruciating

TODAY   No Pain   Mild
                       Discomforting Distressing
                       Horrible   Excruciating

How many hours of the day are you in pain? ....
How many days per week are you in pain?   ....
How many weeks per year are you in pain? ....
What Drugs Have You Taken Today? ....
....

Your Pain Today – Tick along scale below

No Pain [_____] Worst Possible Pain

PLEASE DRAW YOUR PAIN

xxx Burning	= = Numbness
!! Stabbing	** Cramping
00 Aching	## Other

Figure 26.2 Example of a chronic pain assessment tool

It focuses not only on the strength of the pain but also on the site, the intensity, the nature and the day-to-day variation of the patient's pain. This is only an example of one of the many assessment tools that are used with chronic pain sufferers. One of the most common is the McGill pain questionnaire, and numerous examples of this complex assessment tool can be found by using an internet search engine such as Google (www.google.com) or Yahoo! (www.yahoo.com).

Asking patients to keep a pain diary can also be useful in providing clues to activities that help or hinder living with a chronic pain problem. Such a strategy can also help to make the sufferer feel that they are working in partnership with their health and social care practitioners to manage their pain.

The social care aspects of chronic pain

The difficulties facing a person who suffers from chronic pain mean that the social care professions have a significant role to play. Advice about benefits and monetary support available for patients whose chronic pain has compromised their earning ability, return to work programmes, changes to housing to facilitate independent living can all help these individuals to regain some control over their lives.

Conclusion

This chapter has provided a general introduction into the complex subject of pain management but has taken as its focus the cause and assessment of acute and chronic pain. An understanding of the specific types of medication that can be used is the primary concern of registered care staff; however, issues such as assessment and acting upon patient self-reports of pain are the responsibility of any individual who comes into contact with a person in pain, regardless of cause. Health and social care practitioners should understand and manage pain in the light of a holistic view of the complexity of a person's circumstances and needs.

The important messages from this chapter are:

1. The person who knows best about their pain is the sufferer. Ask them regularly about their pain and believe what they tell you.
2. Act upon assessment results. If a person is reporting pain, ensure that they get their medication, record that they had it and then go back and check whether that pain medication was effective – if not, try something else.
3. Remember that anxiety and fear can make pain feel worse.
4. An individual can sleep, read, watch TV and so on and still be in severe pain.
5. Remember that many factors influence how a person perceives and interprets their pain.

REVIEW
QUESTIONS

1 What are the main causes of acute and chronic pain?

2 How does acute pain differ from chronic pain?

3 What are the major ways in which painkilling drugs can be taken?

FURTHER
READING

Carr, E. and Mann, E. (2000) *Pain: Creative Approaches to Effective Management*, Basingstoke, Palgrave Macmillan, Chapters 3 and 4

Davis, B.D. (2000) *Caring for People in Pain*, London, Routledge, Parts III and IV

27 Wound Management

JAN DARGUE

Learning
outcomes

By the end of this chapter, you should:

■ HAVE a grasp of the different kinds of wounds

■ UNDERSTAND how health and social care workers should respond to wounds.

The concept of wound management has evolved and developed over recent years, with ritualistic principles being challenged, and you will see from this chapter that numerous core elements of wound care have changed. In the early 1960s, Winter ([1962]2003) identified that wounds treated in a moist environment healed more quickly than those treated in a dry environment and, as a result, today's dressings are based on the principle of moist wound healing; consequently, it is advised that dressings are not changed too frequently (Ousey, 2005). Of equal importance to you is the notion of wound cleansing. Blunt (2001) suggests that wounds need only be cleansed if certain factors are present and that the optimal cleansing solution is sterile saline 0.9 per cent, as opposed to antiseptics that were used historically, as they do not promote wound healing. Equally, it is recommended that we do not touch the wound bed with gauze swabs or cotton wool because this slows down the healing process by disturbing delicate tissues (Cole, 2003). These factors are just a few of the evidence-based principles that you will witness being carried out by qualified nurses. In time, you will become familiar with them, so that you can promote effective, holistic, evidence-based care to your clients and as such this chapter will develop these principles to enhance your understanding of them.

In this chapter we begin by asking what a wound is and go on to examine how wounds heal or don't heal and how you, as a health or social care worker, may promote wound healing.

Activity 27.1

Think for a few minutes about what you would do if you were visiting Annie, an older person living on her own in a rural area remote from neighbours. You find her lying on the kitchen floor with a deep cut to her left leg, having caught it on the cupboard door. She fell two hours ago and her leg wound is almost covered with a blood clot and is now bleeding only very slightly. Annie states that she wants you to deal with her wound as she does not want to go to hospital.

- What might you do? In order to determine the best response to Annie's situation, you need to consider her general condition:
    - Is she in pain? If so, how severe is the pain?
    - What type of injuries has she sustained as a result of the fall?
- Afterwards, it should be possible to:
    - Summon help from a healthcare professional – the paramedics, district nurse or GP.
    - Avoid moving Annie or giving her anything to eat or drink until she has been assessed by a professional.
    - Stay with her until help arrives. Talk to Annie and reassure her that help is on its way and that she will only be taken to hospital if it is necessary.

Other questions may occur to you:

- How did she sustain the wound? What kind of wound is it and what condition is it in? How large is it? How much is it bleeding? Is there any bone coming through the wound?
- Has she received any other injury such as a broken bone, especially her hip or her leg? Can she move her limbs?
- How best should you treat the wound?
    - You should leave the blood clot in place.
    - You should apply a non-adherent dressing to the wound to cover it until help arrives.

What is a Wound?

A wound is defined as any break in the skin surface and can be due to many causes. Wounds can be deep, as in Annie's case, or superficial such as a graze or a scald. Once the skin surface is broken, there is a potential risk of the wound becoming infected. Infection will delay healing and may cause deterioration in a wound; it can also cause unpleasant effects for the patient and, in some cases, it may be fatal.

How Wounds Heal

Wounds heal by a complex chain of events following skin damage, and wound healing is explained here in three stages:

■ *Stage 1:* Initially, the body attempts to stop the bleeding by producing a blood clot at the wound site, which in turn enables essential wound healing cells to travel across the wound area, as was the case with Annie's injury.

■ *Stage 2:* Inflammation occurs due to special types of white blood cells that leak out of the blood supply onto the wound bed, and these white blood cells play a major role in clearing the wound of bacteria and debris. The blood clot from stage 1 is broken down by a complex process, and in some simple wounds, the healing process then involves covering the surface of the wound with new skin cells.

■ *Stage 3:* In deeper wounds, the body now has to act to fill in the defect. New blood vessels are formed so that the wound is supplied by oxygen and nutrients and these blood vessels are supported on a scaffolding-like matrix made up of collagen that fills in the defect. The skin then grows over the wound surface from the outer edges.

This healing process may take days, months or in some cases years, depending on the type and severity of the wound and the health of the patient, but to maximise wound healing, numerous factors need to be considered and these will be addressed throughout this chapter.

Types of Wounds

Wounds are generalised into two main categories – acute and chronic (Table 27.1). *Acute wounds* usually occur following injury or surgical procedures and, in otherwise healthy people, the wound heals in a predictable time. *Chronic wounds* are often defined as wounds that fail to heal within six weeks, and the delay to heal is often due to underlying causes/illnesses that will be discussed in the following section.

Table 27.1 Acute and chronic wounds

Acute	Chronic
Burns/scalds	Wounds that fail to heal within six weeks
Cuts	Pressure sores (bed sores)
Cuts	Leg ulcers
Grazes	Diabetic ulcers
Skin tears	
Skin flap	
Surgical wounds	

Acute wounds will heal in healthy individuals, providing they are dressed with an appropriate product that enables the body to repair itself. Some acute wounds, with the exception of burns, scalds and grazes, can sometimes be stitched, stapled or glued with a special adhesive, providing there has not been a lot of skin loss, thus aiding the healing process. Chronic wounds, on the other hand, are not quite so straightforward to manage and often pose challenges to health and social care workers; however, there are many things that you can do to promote wound healing in this instance. *Pressure sores*, or *bed sores*, as they are commonly referred to, *leg ulcers* and *diabetic ulcers* are chronic wounds, which are a particular problem especially in the elderly population.

Activity 27.2

Consider Annie's situation for a moment and write down the things you think of that may delay her wound healing. You may find it helpful to consider external factors such as social/lifestyle issues, internal factors such as age and disease, and your role as a healthcare worker.

Your answer for this activity may include many facets relating to Annie, such as poor diet and/or fluid intake, hazards in the home and social isolation; she may be depressed due to lack of contact with people, which may affect her motivation to get herself food and drinks. Her general condition could be poor, as she may have a long-term disorder such as diabetes, heart disease or arthritis, she may be on medication that delays the healing process such as steroids, or drugs that reduce mobility or sensation, for example sedatives or alcohol.

It is also possible that Annie may have suffered a deliberate injury or physical abuse, caused by another person. If you suspect this, or if there is evidence of it, you will need to take action to safeguard her (see Chapter 9 for discussion of this).

You might also have considered your role within this activity in relation to being skilled in the care of wounds, including wound cleansing, and the application and removal of dressings and bandages. You need to be aware of what changes to report to qualified staff, especially in relation to wound infections, a deteriorating wound and possible allergies to products.

In general terms, if these issues are not dealt with appropriately, then the healing process can be prolonged.

The Causes of Wounds

Acute wounds are caused by a number of things that are self-explanatory, as suggested in Table 27.1, but when we start to consider the causes of chronic wounds, they are usually more complex and are the result of underlying problems. If you recall, chronic wounds are pressure sores, leg ulcers and diabetic ulcers and all wounds that fail to heal within a six-week period.

Let's start by considering the risk to Annie of pressure damage, as she has been laid on the kitchen floor for a period of two hours. It is possible that she has already sustained some pressure damage from her fall that may, or may not, result in an actual pressure sore. Pressure sores occur as a result of three main factors:

- Pressure
- Friction (two surfaces rubbing together) and shear (tissues wrenched in the opposite direction)
- Moisture.

In Annie's situation, she may have already sustained some pressure damage due to being laid on the floor where her bony areas, for example hip, sacrum or heels, have been in contact with prolonged pressure from a hard surface; she may have tried to shuffle along the floor and that may have caused some friction and shear between her clothes, skin or the floor; and she may have been incontinent of urine and/or faeces and, if left in contact with the skin, this can cause the skin surface to break down.

Pressure sores cause untold suffering on behalf of the patient and they are a major financial burden to the NHS – it is estimated that they cost between £1.4–2.1 million annually (NICE, 2005, p. 26). In the main, pressure sores are essentially preventable, providing the cause – pressure, friction, shear or moisture – is removed. This can be achieved by using effective moving and handling procedures, where hoists and slide sheets are used to prevent friction and shear; special mattresses/cushions or frequent change of the patient's position prevent excessive prolonged pressure; and the effective management of incontinence minimises skin damage.

Leg ulcers and diabetic ulcers are other types of chronic wounds that occur in the lower limbs of patients and although these wounds can affect any age group, they are more common in the elderly population. The healing process in these wounds is slow due to a poor blood supply and sometimes poor nerve supply. If the blood supply is poor, the wound bed receives insufficient oxygen and nutrients to promote healing, hence the tissues cannot repair themselves. A poor nerve supply is a problem associated with diabetic patients who may lose the sensation to their feet, which means that foot ulcers develop without the patient's knowledge because the pain sensation is impaired due to the nerve damage.

In patients like Annie, if her injury fails to heal within six weeks, it would then be classed as a leg ulcer and so it would be a chronic rather than an acute wound. An added problem here is that leakage from chronic wounds tends to have factors in it that destroy healthy skin, so the management of these wounds is more complex than in acute wounds and will be addressed next.

The Principles of Wound Management

In order to promote healing, wounds need to be in a healthy state and free from infection, dead tissue (this may appear as a hard blackened area or soft yellow tissue that is stringy in appearance), debris and particles. A wound should ideally be maintained at body temperature and not cooled using exposure or cold cleansing solutions; it should also be kept moist to promote effective healing. Moist wound healing has been around since the 1960s, but it has taken many years for the concept to be adopted into everyday practice; it is now a well-proven fact that wounds heal much quicker in a moist environment than in a dry environment. As a result of this moist wound healing theory, there are many different types of dressings classed as ideal (Table 27.2) that are used in practice, for example foam dressings, hydrogels, hydrocolloids, alginates and vapour permeable films. It is not your responsibility to be familiar with all these dressings but you will become familiar with the ones you commonly use. One aspect that you do need to bear in mind is that dressings are prescribed for individuals and must only be used for the person for whom they are prescribed.

Table 27.2 The ideal dressing

■ Controls wound moisture
■ Is free from particles and toxins
■ Does not allow bacteria into the wound
■ Has low adherence – does not stick to the wound
■ Keeps the wound at body temperature
■ Allows the wound to breath
■ Can be left in place for a maximum of seven days

Not all wounds will require cleansing, but if cleansing is indicated, sterile saline 0.9 per cent is the solution of choice, using an irrigation technique as opposed to cleansing with gauze. Irrigation (using a flushing technique) gently removes debris and loose tissue and minimises damage to the wound. You will find that some chronic wounds, such as leg ulcers, are to be bathed in clean tap water, but again the actual wound must not be directly cleansed as this can slow down the healing process. Table 27.3 gives the reasons for wound cleansing.

Table 27.3 Wound cleansing

■ To remove debris
■ To make the wound socially clean (see below)
■ To prevent leakage damaging healthy skin
■ To clean before swabs are taken

The priority is to remove dirt and other matter from the wound. Socially clean means environmentally clean rather than simply being sterile. Managing leakage from chronic wounds is very important as the discharge contains enzymes that destroy healthy skin, so absorbent dressings are required to deal with this problem. These dressings will need to be changed before the leakage becomes too much for the dressing to handle, because if the wound becomes too wet, the surrounding skin breaks down and, as bacteria thrive in wet environments, an infection may develop. If a wound swab needs to be obtained, the wound must be cleansed so that removable contaminants do not affect the swab findings.

If you suspect the patient has a wound infection, you must seek help. The signs are increased discharge, offensive odour, redness around the wound, the wound may be hot and the patient may have a high temperature and feel unwell. The prevention of infection is an important principle of wound care and can be helped by carers practising several safety measures known as *universal precautions*. This means effective hand washing before and after dealing with patients and before and after changing wound dressings; also the wearing of aprons and gloves is essential when dealing with any body fluid, and in this instance relates to dealing with Annie's wound (Gould, 2000).

Factors that Delay the Healing Process

This brief section is divided into two main themes, the first dealing with the patient's health and the second related to wound care practice.

Patients' General Health Condition

To promote wound healing, the patient's health needs to be maximised, which involves an adequate fluid intake and a healthy diet because wounds need fluid and nutrients to enable them to heal. If the patient has an underlying medical condition, as is the case with many elderly people, this needs stabilising. For example, if Annie had heart disease and diabetes, it is possible that her circulation is impaired, which would result in a limited oxygen supply to her damaged leg that would slow down the healing process. If a patient's diabetes is poorly controlled, they are at risk of poor circulation and poor nerve supply, especially to the lower limbs, as mentioned previously. The management of these long-term conditions is the role of all health-care professionals from both community and hospital backgrounds, and it is essential that patients have regular checks and reviews, especially in relation to medication and monitoring of their conditions, as this will affect wound healing.

Wound Care Practice

As a care worker, you need to be skilled in the care and management of wounds that you deal with. You must not take on the responsibility for wound assessment, dressing choice or monitoring of the wound condition, as this should be carried out by a qualified person.

Activity 27.3

Here are some common factors that delay the healing process for some patients. How could you prevent or deal with these issues?

- Wound infection
- Poor nutrition/hydration
- Anaemia
- Poor patient compliance
- Poor dressing/bandaging technique
- Incorrect diagnosis/treatment
- Drugs such as steroids, sedatives, alcohol and nicotine
- Dead tissue covering a wound (hard black covering or soft yellow appearance).

Your responses could include any of the following:

- Prevent cross-infection by careful hand washing and the use of universal precautions (aprons, gloves)
- Report signs of wound infection to a qualified person

- Encourage a healthy diet and adequate fluid intake
- Educate the patient as to the importance of leaving the dressing in place
- Make sure that you understand how to apply the dressing/bandage and also how to remove it
- Make sure the patient is taking their drugs as prescribed. If you are concerned, inform a qualified person
- If the patient smokes and wishes to stop, you need to refer them to a smoking cessation nurse/adviser
- Report the progress of the wound on a regular basis to the qualified nurse and only dress wounds that you are skilled to deal with. You should not be expected to look after complex wounds, although you may assist in the care of such wounds.

The following list is a resumé of basic principles that you need to consider in your everyday practice when caring for people's wounds:

- Do not change a dressing too frequently as this will disturb the wound and slow down the healing process
- Do not dry out the wound bed as wounds heal quicker if they are kept moist but not too wet
- Only clean a wound if you are instructed to do so, as this can cool the wound bed temperature, disturb new cells and slow down the healing process
- Change dressings carefully as per manufacturers' instructions as inappropriate removal can damage healthy skin
- Do not cut dressings to size as particles may escape into the wound and slow down the healing process
- Avoid cross-infection, make sure that you wash your hands before and after each patient, wear a plastic apron for each patient and wear gloves for a wound dressing procedure.

Conclusion

This chapter has given you a broad overview of wound care and what you can do to promote wound healing. You may find the references/websites useful to further develop your knowledge in this area of healthcare.

REVIEW QUESTIONS

1 What are the main types of wounds?

2 What are the main features of wound management?

3 What are the main factors delaying healing?

FURTHER READING

European Pressure Ulcer Advisory Panel (1998) *Pressure Ulcer Prevention and Treatment Guidelines*, Oxford, EPUAP

Hoban, B. (2005) 'Wound Care: What Every Nurse Should Know', *Nursing Times*, **101**(12): 20–2

Kemp, S. (2001) 'The Vital Role of Nutrition in Wound Healing, *Primary Health Care*, **11**(1): 43–9

NICE (National Institute for Health and Clinical Excellence) (2005) The Prevention and Treatment of Pressure Ulcers: Quick Reference Guide, www.nice.org.uk

WEBSITES: www.epuap.com
The European Pressure Ulcer Advisory Panel (EPUAP) website contains some useful up-to-date information on the grading, detection and management of pressure ulcers.

www.worldwidewounds.com
This is an excellent source of research information covering all types of wounds and new types of dressings/innovations.

http://www.woundupdate.com
Another good website that gives up-to-date information.

Multidisciplinary Palliative Care for Dying and Bereaved People

MARGARET REITH

By the end of this chapter, you should be able to:

■ DESCRIBE what is involved in palliative care

■ UNDERSTAND the process of palliative care

■ APPRECIATE how a multiprofessional approach contributes to palliative care.

You may find it useful to reflect at the start of this chapter on the following statement and list the elements of palliative care that you feel it emphasises:

> Palliative care is the active, total care of patients and their families by a multiprofessional team when the patient's disease is no longer responsive to curative treatment. Control of pain, of other symptoms and of psychological, social and spiritual problems is paramount. The goal of palliative care is achievement of good quality of life for patients and their families. (Oliviere et al., 1998, p. 2)

Goals of the Palliative Care Team

Involving the multidisciplinary team is essential to achieving the goal of palliative care. The team consists of doctors, nurses and healthcare assistants who treat physical symptoms and provide daily care for patients and their families; physiotherapists and occupational therapists who work with patients to improve the ability to cope with activities of daily living and maximise functioning and mobility. Social workers and counsellors are also integral to the palliative care team, addressing many of the non-physical issues so crucial to the holistic care of patients and their families. The social worker's focus is on the effects of life-threatening illness on the family system (Sheldon, 1997; Watson et al., 2005).

Practice study

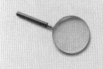

Richard

The following case highlights the roles of different health and social care workers working together as a team to provide the best possible end-of-life care to a patient, his wife, who is also his carer, and his family. The study demonstrates the importance of good communication between healthcare professionals as well as with the patient and his family.

Richard is aged 60 and is married with one son, Gerald. He was diagnosed with prostate cancer when he was 55 and more recently developed bone metastases or secondary bone cancer. His wife Gillian has her own health problems following a serious climbing accident many years ago, which left her physically disabled with impaired mobility. More recently, she has been diagnosed with diabetes. Gerald lives some distance away, is separated from his wife and has a daughter Sophie aged 9.

Assessment and Planning

Richard was first admitted to the hospice for two weeks for symptom control 13 months before he died. At that time his pain was not controlled and he required specialist palliative care to administer different analgesia. During this admission the hospice social work assistant saw Richard to ensure that he was receiving the benefits to which he was entitled (Richard is eligible for disability living allowance, and his wife is entitled to carers allowance). The social worker's assessment focused on exploring whether a care package was needed and to find out if any other social or emotional issues were causing particular difficulties. Richard did not want a care package but seemed depressed about his condition and was finding the adjustment to losing his independence, decreasing mobility and increasing fatigue difficult to come to terms with. He was immensely frustrated, having always been active, playing golf, walking and sailing. He had never been a person to stay at home watching television or reading. Not only was Richard suffering from physical pain, he was also in emotional and psychological pain. It was important to acknowledge his distress, frustration and also his fear of what lay ahead. Equally important was supporting Gillian – she was struggling with her own sadness but also her husband's low mood, anger and anxiety. Following Richard's discharge home, the social work assistant invited Gillian to attend a weekly carer's group at the hospice, run by another palliative care social worker and nurse. In the community, the hospice clinical nurse specialist remained in close contact with Richard and Gillian.

Richard was readmitted to the hospice 11 months later, having become paralysed because of the tumour growing and pressing on his spine. No further curative treatment was possible, so palliative care was offered to relieve the distressing symptoms and offer holistic care to both Richard and Gillian. On admission, Richard was in pain, had a chest infection and was generally unwell but the pain was soon well controlled by a new combination of analgesic medication. In addition, he had a good response to the antibiotics and so settled in the hospice, being nursed in bed. Before any plans for discharge could be made, he became unwell again, with a further chest infection and mouth problems. So not until a further two weeks had passed could plans be discussed. By this time Richard had been in the hospice for five weeks. It was the social worker's role to assess discharge options by discussing with Richard and Gillian their plans but also their hopes and fears. The information required from such an assessment could only be obtained through a series of interviews with Richard and Gillian and they were seen both separately and together. Assessment is a process rather than a single intervention.

Dealing with Strong Emotions: Anger and Frustration

In the course of this assessment, it became apparent that Gillian was troubled because Richard directed his anger at his situation at her, blaming her for him being stuck in the hospice, saying she did not want him home. Richard seemed unrealistic about his prognosis and his future. Gillian said she could not understand why he seemed not to know how ill he was. She thought it was obvious and that she would know that time was short if she was in this situation. He said he wanted to go home and see his dog again. The physiotherapist worked to try to enable Richard to sit in a wheelchair so that he could go home for a visit. However, he was unable to tolerate sitting for more than a few moments and was extremely uncomfortable, feeling unsafe. Therefore, nursing staff encouraged Gillian to bring Richard's dog to visit him.

However, when the social worker next saw Richard, he was still agitated, saying he could not stay in the hospice because he understood it does not provide long-term care and anyway he felt bored and trapped by his failing body, which was compromising his mobility, preventing him from walking. His frustration was compounded by feeling that he had lost his manhood by losing the use of his legs. For Richard, his expression of his sexuality was very important. Again Gillian, who visited him daily for periods of many hours, tended to find herself on the receiving end of his increasing frustration. Nursing staff arranged with the hospice complementary therapist for Gillian to have some aromatherapy to help reduce her stress and tension.

Gerald visited his father but did not bring Sophie with him. Gerald wanted to 'protect' Sophie and did not want her to be upset. The social worker helped Gerald to see that by 'protecting' Sophie, he was not doing her a service and that she also needed to say goodbye and tell granddad she loved him. With social work support, Gerald was able to bring Sophie to visit Richard before he died.

Dealing with Deterioration

The social worker discussed with both Richard and Gillian how best to try to find a way of coping with the present and future situation. Gently, she suggested that

Richard may be as well as he would be and the fact that he had deteriorated very quickly in the last few weeks may indicate that the disease process may be continuing to weaken him. She acknowledged with him how hard this was for him to face and that he did not want to leave his wife, son and granddaughter, but possibly nor did he want to continue being trapped in a body that was compromising his quality of life to this extent. The social worker went on to explain that the hospice had no plans to discharge him and that he was probably in the right place, but if he wished to look at alternatives, they could explore these together. Richard was still holding onto a belief that if he were at home, he would somehow be able to get out in a wheelchair. So the social worker tentatively suggested that the only way he could be at home would be if he was nursed in bed, as now. She also said she wanted to mention another possibility of considering a nursing home. She wanted both Richard and Gillian to know that this could be talked about in such a way that it would help to inform the decision and choice that he made. The social worker explored their doubts, concerns and fears of what this might mean for him.

Coping Strategies and Communication

It became clear to the social worker that they were struggling to communicate clearly about what lay ahead, because Richard was still clinging to a belief that he had many years left to live. For some people, denial works well as a coping strategy. However, it becomes a problem when it stops someone accessing the services they need, or from making realistic and appropriate plans or saying the things they need to say to those close to them. The social worker suggested to Richard and Gillian that they might be finding it difficult to make plans because they were unsure about what sort of time frame they were looking at and that, as a social worker, she was finding it difficult to help them with this, because she was not the right person to explain Richard's medical condition or prognosis to him. She suggested that if they were both agreeable, she would ask the doctor to talk with them both to help them through the fog.

The social worker was careful to emphasise that sometimes it was too painful for people to face the seriousness of their illness and that she would want to respect that, but if it was getting in the way of people being able to communicate with each other, then she might suggest that they do a deal and not talk about the illness and prognosis so long as they could make realistic plans and think about appropriate services. This session ended by setting a small goal, which was to see if a different wheelchair was available that would enable Richard to get outside the room in the hospice where he had been for five weeks. The social worker emphasised that she was not talking about home or anything longer than a short trip outside in the garden. She followed this up by discussing with the occupational therapist if it might be possible to borrow a different sort of wheelchair that might enable Richard to recline more and be more comfortable.

Review

The weekly multidisciplinary team (MDT) meeting took place the following day, attended by the occupational therapist, physiotherapist, doctors (specialist registrar and consultant), ward-based nurse, social worker, chaplain, pharmacist and the community clinical specialist nurse. Richard's medical care was reviewed but also his emotional and psychological turmoil and what the team could do to help him, as well as how they could best help his wife and family. The outcome was for the doctor and social worker to see Richard and Gillian together that afternoon.

Afterwards, reflecting on the interview, the doctor felt it had been difficult and at the point that Richard started talking about living far into his seventies, she felt stuck. The social worker explained that it was because she had been stuck the previous day that she sought her assistance and that perhaps this was about sharing this 'stuckness' and recognising this was part of Gillian's experience also. It is not unusual for people to experience conflict between facing the reality of a short prognosis and avoiding the pain this causes, and working with these ambivalent feelings needs to be understood and accepted.

Meanwhile, the occupational therapist explored wheelchair options and was disappointed to draw a blank for reasons beyond anyone's control. Therefore, the social worker talked to the nurses about what other options might be possible, including taking Richard's bed outside into the garden. This required a large amount of reorganisation but almost instantly the nurses were moving obstacles, opening doors and making preparations. Within a few moments, Richard was taken in his bed to a small, pretty garden area. A healthcare assistant made a tray of tea for Richard, Gillian and a friend who had by now called to visit. A second healthcare assistant commented to the social worker that the smile on Richard's face as he was taken outside was 'magic'. Her reply was that this is what palliative care is all about. Essentially, it is about looking holistically at a patient, his or her family and significant others and helping them to achieve the best quality of life possible and to be at peace with themselves and with each other. This can only be achieved by skilled listening and communication. It requires all members of the MDT to work closely together, responding appropriately to individual needs.

Practice study

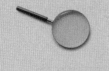

Richard (cont'd)

Several weeks passed and Richard's condition gradually deteriorated. Although at the weekly MDT review, there were times when some members of the team expressed the view that Richard should be transferred to a nursing home, the social worker was clear that unless his condition was stable, it would not be in the patient's best interests or his wife's for him to be transferred. The MDT accepted the social worker's opinion. Richard and Gillian were relieved that Richard's terminal care would be provided by the hospice. Although Richard's speech became increasingly difficult to understand, it was possible to communicate with him with time and perseverance. Towards the end, Gillian became very distressed because Richard was again saying some very hurtful

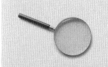

things to her. The team was concerned that these might be Gillian's last memories. So the social worker again intervened by talking to Richard about his life, his marriage and more specifically Gillian, her feelings and her future without him, acknowledging how sad this was for him to face. Slowly he reached a point where he could verbalise his love for his wife and was able to tell her he was sorry for the hurt he had caused her.

Gillian had always said that she wanted to be with her husband when he died, if at all possible. One day, as the social worker was sitting with Gillian beside Richard's bed, he was drifting in and out of consciousness and Gillian explained that she was planning to leave early because of a commitment she had made to attend the last class of the year for which she was the tutor. The social worker was concerned because she could see that Richard was dying and may die while Gillian was away. However, as the social worker, she did not feel it was appropriate to suggest she should stay. But as part of the teamwork that is so important in palliative care, she passed this information on to the senior nurse on duty, whose expertise in this area was much greater than hers. The nurse reviewed Richard and suggested to Gillian that she perhaps needed to stay. Richard died a few hours later with Gillian holding his hand.

Bereavement Services: Part of Good Palliative Care

One of the essential features of good palliative care is the bereavement service, which is offered to bereaved family members and friends including children and grandchildren. Richard had not wanted an overtly religious funeral but had made a strong relationship with the hospice chaplain who was asked by Gillian to conduct his funeral service. In the months following Richard's death, a volunteer bereavement counsellor from the hospice, trained and supervised by the social work team, supported Gillian. However, Gillian felt she did not need extended counselling because she had no unresolved issues or regrets. She found comfort from the fact that Richard had died with dignity and that they had both been able to share some very precious moments together. Throughout the last weeks of Richard's life at the hospice, despite his increasing burden of illness and times of profound sadness, he had demonstrated his very warm humour, sharing many lighter and funny moments with Gillian as well as hospice staff. Sophie attended a group for bereaved children at the hospice held on a Saturday where she could make a memory box and talk about her treasured memories of her grandfather.

Activity 28.1

Reflect for a few moments on what learning points this case study has highlighted for you.

Here are the learning points it raises for me:

- Understanding issues relating to loss and dying
- Dealing with powerful emotions linked to coping with terminal illness
- Importance of working as a team, communicating with all MDT members, and attention to detail
- Quality of life issues
- Importance of hope – it may be helpful to suggest a strategy such as hoping for the best but planning for the worst
- Importance of working directly with the patient but also with other family members who may or may not be carers – all are service users, have different needs and different coping strategies
- Value of bereavement support
- Importance of addressing the needs of children both before and after bereavement.

Conclusion

A holistic approach to end-of-life care requires health and social care professionals from several different disciplines to work together with patients, their carers, families and significant others. Social workers make an important contribution to the multidisciplinary team by enabling patients and their families to retain or regain control and promoting empowerment and choice, to help people find inner strength and confidence. Setting realistic goals helps families to feel less powerless and enables them to plan for and enjoy the time that is left.

REVIEW QUESTIONS

1 What is palliative care?

2 What does palliative care set out to achieve?

3 Why does palliative care depend for its effectiveness on a multidisciplinary approach?

FURTHER READING

Currer, C. (2002) 'Dying and Bereavement', in R. Adams, L. Dominelli and M. Payne (eds) *Critical Practice in Social Work*, Basingstoke, Palgrave Macmillan
A good brief introduction to practice with people experiencing death and bereavement.

Ellershaw, J., Foster, A., Murphy, D., Shea, T. and Overill, S. (1997) 'Developing an Integrated Care Pathway for the Dying Patient', *European Journal of Palliative Care*, **4**: 203–7
This article introduces the 'Liverpool care pathway', accepted nationally as a good standard of care for people in the last few days before death, and is also a good account of how a healthcare innovation is tested and introduced.

Monroe, B. (2004) 'Social Work in Palliative Care', in D. Doyle, G. Hanks and N.I. Cherny (eds) *Oxford Textbook of Palliative Medicine* (3rd edn) Oxford, Oxford University Press, pp. 1005–18
The best short account of social work practice in palliative care.

Picardie, R. (1998) *Before I Say Goodbye*, London, Penguin
  Ruth Picardie was a woman with young children and a newspaper columnist who wrote about her experiences of breast cancer and approaching death; this book contains the collected columns, with some contributions from other family members.

Sheldon, F. (1997) *Psychosocial Palliative Care: Good Practice in the Care of the Dying and Bereaved*, Cheltenham, Stanley Thornes
  The best general book on psychosocial work in palliative care.

RESOURCE FILE: Attachment and Loss: Death and Bereavement, below

Resource file

Attachment and loss: Death and bereavement

Although I have separated the headings below and linked each with different stages of the life course, I have done this to clarify the ideas. Bringing them together in this single Resource file emphasises the links between research and theories about infant and child attachment and loss and death and bereavement in adult life.

Attachment, separation and loss: the child's world

Dr John Bowlby studied infant and young child attachment to significant adults, especially mothers, for 30 years from the 1950s. He researched the separation of children from adults with Robertson (Robertson and Bowlby, 1952), looking at three phases of response by children to separation: *protest* (linked with separation anxiety), *despair* (linked with grief and mourning) and *denial* or *detachment* (linked with defences such as repressing upset feelings). For example, when the child goes to hospital and the parent rings and asks 'How is she?' and the nurse answers, 'Fine, she's stopped crying now and is quite quiet', the question is whether she's contented or resigned to unhappiness. Bowlby's research led to his great trilogy of books on attachment (Bowlby, 1969), separation (Bowlby, 1973) and loss (Bowlby, 1980).

He was influenced by Sigmund Freud and Melanie Klein (see Chapter 43), although eventually he broke with stricter psychoanalytic theorists and practitioners, arguing that interviews with the parents could shed crucial light on the child's behaviour, because this could not be explained simply as a response to the child's inner conscious and subconscious world. He also argued that grief and mourning are present where the child has no attachment parent figure. The mother–child relationship is unique, since the bonding between them fulfils the biological function of providing protection for the vulnerable infant. Deprivation of contact with the mother can be uniquely devastating for an infant or child, leading to feelings of loss similar in quality to adult bereavements.

Bowlby worked with Colin Parkes (well known for research on adult bereavement) to expand the phases of separation response in the child into four phases of grief in adult life – *numbness*, *yearning* and *protest*, *disorganisation* and *despair* and *reorganisation* (Bowlby and Parkes, 1970). Bowlby worked with Mary Ainsworth who in the early 1950s began some long-term studies of infants' attachment to mothers (Ainsworth, 1967). This gave Bowlby clues as to how patterns of children's attachment persist when children grow into adults. He also met Elisabeth Kübler-Ross, and exchanged ideas from his work with Robertson with her, before she published on the five stages of dying (see below). Bowlby also met Cecily (later Dame Cecily) Saunders, founder of the world-wide hospice movement.

Death and bereavement: the adult's world

Elisabeth Kübler-Ross (1970) describes a process whereby the bereaved person goes through a series of stages: *denial*, *anger*, *bargaining*, *depression* and possible eventual *acceptance*. Other writers since then have suggested this is too rigid. Not everybody passes through these stages; some people remain at one stage, while others move back and forth between stages (Corr, 1992; Sheldon, 1997). We should be wary of adopting the assumptions of rigid checklists of stages that everyone is assumed to go through, either when dying or as a bereaved person after a death. These may have looked good in essays 20 years ago, but they do not match up to many people's experiences. Death and bereavement should be regarded as particular instances of loss, which people may experience to a greater or lesser degree in many circumstances, such as losing a job, moving to another part of the country, migrating whether voluntarily or as a refugee, or making a transition involving leaving a person to whom one is attached. Having said this, the notes below focus on death and bereavement.

Jane Littlewood (1992, pp. 60–75) selects seven models of bereavement for particular discussion:

1. *Illness and disease models*, which relate to grief as though it is a disease
2. *Biological models* focus on how grief affects and is affected by physical factors
3. *Psychodynamic explanations* of grief are in terms of psychological factors (Sheldon, 1997)
4. *Attachment theories* focus on grief as a response to a disturbance to instinctive patterns of attachment and responses to it (Bowlby, 1980)
5. *Personal construct* and *cognitive models* focus on how the person constructs and gives meaning to the processes surrounding the bereavement
6. *Crisis intervention models* interpret grief as a crisis of coping
7. *Phenomenological* and *existential models* view a person's experience and meaning attached to the experience as the basis for understanding it.

According to Fiona Marshall (1993, p. 66), how the person feels about the loss is affected by four main factors:

1. How the person died
2. What the relationship was with the dead person
3. What support is available during the grieving
4. Previous experiences of loss.

Dent and Stewart (2004, p. 217) have devised a simple list of questions as a basic bereavement assessment tool for a sudden death in childhood, which I have summarised and generalised below, using the term 'relatives' instead of 'parents':

■ *About the death:* How were the relatives told? Were they present, fully informed throughout, satisfied with the hospital and other caring services?
■ *After the death:* Were the relatives given the chance to stay and attend to the person and were others allowed to say goodbye without being hurried?
■ *Postmortem and coroner:* Was any necessary contact, if it occurred, handled with full explanations and how did close relatives feel about it?
■ *Information and follow-up:* Were the relatives informed about the cause of death and the practical steps afterwards and given a follow-up appointment with the doctor to talk about the death?
■ *Funeral:* Was the funeral director and spiritual leader helpful? Did children attend the funeral? How did those who attended feel about the funeral?
■ *The media:* Did the media cause any problems for the relatives?
■ *Relationships with relatives:* Can the relatives and other family and friends talk about the death and are they able to stay in touch and close at this time?

FURTHER READING

Ainley, R. (1994) *Death of a Mother*, London, HarperCollins

Bowlby, J. ([1980] 1991) *Attachment and Loss*, vol. III, *Loss, Sadness and Depression*, Harmondsworth, Penguin

Bright, R. (1996) *Grief and Powerlessness: Helping People Regain Control of their Lives*, London, Jessica Kingsley

Child Bereavement Trust (2003) *Understanding Bereaved Children and Young People*, London, Child Bereavement Trust, www.childbereavement.org.uk

Dent, A. and Stewart, A. (2004) *Sudden Death in Childhood: Support for the Bereaved Family*, Edinburgh, Elsevier Science
A very full sourcebook with useful appendices of sources of further support.

Faulkener, A. (1995) *Working with Bereaved People*, Edinburgh, Churchill Livingstone

Holliday, J. (2002) *A Review of Sibling Bereavement: Impact and Interventions*, Ilford, Barnardo's

Hollins, S. and Sireling, L. (1989) *When Dad Died*, London, Gaskell/St George's Hospital Medical School
This little book contains much that is true in simple words that can be read and shared and talked about with people who are experiencing loss.

Lascelles, R.V. (1985) *Coping with Loss*, Birmingham, Pepar
A concise handbook of loss counselling.

Littlewood, J. (1992) *Aspects of Grief: Bereavement in Adult Life*, London, Routledge

Marshall, F. (1993) *Losing a Parent*, London, SPCK

Murray Parkes, C. (1972) *Bereavement: Studies of Grief in Adult Life*, New York, International Universities Press

Pennells, M. and Smith, S. (1995) *The Forgotten Mourners: Guidelines for Working with Bereaved Children*, London, Jessica Kingsley

Sheldon, F. (1997) *Psychosocial Palliative Care*, Cheltenham, Stanley Thornes

Thompson, N. (ed.) (2002) *Loss and Grief: A Guide for Human Services Practitioners*, Basingstoke, Palgrave Macmillan

WEBSITES: www.attachment.edu.ar/outline.html
www.attachmentdisorder.net
www.attachmentnetwork.org

Working with People

Part IV
Working with People

▌ Introduction

All work with people takes place in the context of relevant policies, legislation and standards. Here are some examples of laws that apply almost universally to practice: Data Protection Act 1998, Human Rights Act 1998, Race Relations Act 1976 and Race Relations (Amendment) Act 2000, NHS and Community Care Act 1990, Children Act 1989 and Children Act 2004. Relevant standards in each area of practice govern the assessment, planning and delivery of services.

The second foundation of effective work is ethics and values. Ethics are more general statements about what practitioners should and should not do, based on beliefs about what is right and wrong (see Resource File: Ethical Tensions in Practice, at the end of Chapter 5). These ethics shape the statements of principles and values embodied in practice. The tendency for official statements is to use terms such as 'principles' and 'values' interchangeably. In everyday life, people do not talk like this. They give their views about what they want. Carers and people who use services have reported what they want. According to these views (CSCI, 2004, pp. 7–8), they should:

■ have the choice to decide where, how and with whom they live

■ have independence, giving them maximum control over their lives

■ be treated with dignity and respect

■ be offered consistent and competent services

■ be able to feel safe in the services they receive

■ know that there will be frequent, unannounced inspections of the facilities they use, with inspectors spending more time talking to service users.

We can make a more general list of values, based on what our health and social care agencies and national bodies have drawn up. People who use services and their carers should:

■ be valued as individuals

■ be respected as people

■ have their cultures, religious beliefs and racial differences respected

■ have their differences celebrated

■ have their age and gender appreciated, with the purpose of developing equality-based practice.

A draft statement of five principles for self-care by health and social care service users and carers has been drawn up for national consultation in 2007 by the government's workforce development agencies, Skills for Care and Skills for Health, in the light of the White Paper *Our Health, Our Care, Our Say* (DoH, 2006a). The five principles are:

1. empower people to make more informed choices to manage their condition and care

2. communicate effectively so people can develop their self-care skills

3. enable people to use technology in their self-care

4. enable people to develop self-care skills

5. enable people to take part in planning services and to benefit from support networks (www.skillsforhealth.org.uk; www.skillsforcare.org.uk).

Part IV is based on the final assumption that the work should be purposeful and progressive, so as to benefit the people with whom we are working. That is, it should deal with the linked but distinct processes of assessment, diagnosis and planning, implementation and intervention, and review and evaluation. We begin this part by examining this idea of processes in some detail.

FURTHER READING

Thompson, N. (2001) *Anti-Discriminatory Practice* (3rd edn) Basingstoke, Palgrave – now Palgrave Macmillan

---

Resource file

Approaches to the job: Traditionaliser, utiliser or professionaliser?

What kind of practitioner are you? Research (Habenstein and Christ, 1963) into how nurses go about their work and the roles they adopt divides them into three main groups. These are sociological not psychological, so they do not describe the personalities of the nurses, but concentrate on how they construct, that is, interpret, their jobs and what they believe about what they do at work.

Traditionalisers tend to relate back to health and nursing, to the ideal of Florence Nightingale, basing their actions on the accumulated wisdom of previous generations, which they believe form a fixed body of knowledge. Suspicious of the benefits of massive changes, in the face of new, as yet unproven methods, they tend to fall back on established, familiar approaches. These are an extension of traditional arts of healing in the home and the community. At the same time, the nurse is unquestioningly deferential to the doctor, an unselfish aide, dedicated to the patient.

Utilisers are pragmatic, motivated by immediate needs and not dedicated to any further or higher goals. The job begins with the shift and ends when the nurse leaves. The nurse works efficiently but has no interest in the job beyond that. Each task is evaluated in terms of what it achieves, not in terms of any wider context of personal values. The nurse as a person is not engaged beyond what is expected in the workplace. The profession is just a job and the person is *in* the workplace but not *of* it.

Professionalisers are committed to using the best evidence available as the basis for carrying out the care. They base their practice on knowledge, relying on the tools provided by scientific, medical and social scientific research to enable them to work efficiently. The professionaliser believes in accepting responsibility for carrying out the services and in return expects society to recognise the validity of the training and the professional identity and status of the group to which she or he belongs. In return for the nurse being given responsibility for benefiting people, he or she expects trust not only from the individual person – the patient, the service user, the carer – but from society as a whole.

Activity Part IV Introduction

Having read the above, reflect on your attitude to your health and social care role. Then find a partner. If you are in health, find a social care partner, and vice versa.

Each spend five minutes telling the other which of the three you most closely resemble: traditionaliser, utiliser or professionaliser. Discuss the pros and cons of your views.

Processes of Work with People

ROBERT ADAMS

Learning outcomes

By the end of this chapter, you should be able to:

■ GIVE an overview of what we mean by the process of health and social care practice

■ OUTLINE what happens during each of the four stages.

This part of the book deals with the major stages of work with people and in this chapter we give an overview of the process of this work, before breaking the task down in the four chapters (Chapters 30–33) which follow. We begin by examining the meaning of this word 'process' and then discuss how we understand 'processes' of health and social care work.

What do we Mean by Process?

The word 'process' has different meanings in different circumstances. It is one of those words in everyday use that we also use in professional work in health and social care. By visiting different places where we encounter the word 'process' being used, we can identify some of the main ingredients that make up its meaning.

The first is passing time. It is often used in everyday life to refer to time passing. 'I waited in the dentist's surgery, but found the process tedious.' The second is a sequence of events. To this idea of process as simply the passing of time we can add the idea of change, for example when the manager of the car factory talks about the process of production, or the editor of this book refers to the process of publication.

This view of process involves adding the metal and plastic parts together and linking components to make them into a vehicle, or transforming data on computer disks into printed sheets and integrating them with an illustrated cover to create a published book. In health and social care we use the word 'process' in a different way from this, as we shall see below. In medicine and nursing, too, the term 'the nursing process' has developed a specific meaning to do with problem-solving. The doctor and nurses try to find out what is wrong with the patient – assessment, reach a view – diagnosis, come up with ways of tackling the problem – treatment plan, test it out on the patient – implementation, and review progress – evaluation.

The classic book by Helen Yura and Mary Walsh (1988) reduces this 'nursing process' to four words: *assessing*, *planning*, *implementing* and *evaluating*. In therapeutic work from psychiatry to art therapy, social work and social care, a quite specialised meaning of the word 'process' is used, *interpreting* what is going on, beyond the events, as we see below (Adams, 2002, pp. 255–8). In work with people, the additional ingredients of *using theories and research* to improve the health and wellbeing of people in the diversity of their lives are added to make an already complicated process even more complex. However, health and social care work sometimes involves supporting people rather than curing them. In other words, the process is based on the notion of *maintenance* in some situations and *change* in others. Whatever its aims, the process should be *purposeful*. More than this, the process of change has the capacity to *integrate* theory and practice and is capable in some circumstances of being a *transforming* one.

We shall make use of these different ideas in different chapters, notably Chapter 37 where we discuss theory and practice.

The Nursing Process

As noted above, Yura and Walsh (1988) applied the term 'the nursing process' to the four stages of the work that nurses did with patients: assessment, planning, implementation and evaluation. Over the following decades, as Aggleton and Chalmers (2000) demonstrate, different views about these processes developed, so that there is not one agreed list of the detailed processes which applies to all aspects of the work. In the 1980s, much of the work nurses did was still based in hospitals and the medical model of treatment of patients was dominant. Also, despite the many thousands of words written about the nursing process, there is surprising agreement about its basic components: assessment/diagnosis, planning, implementation and evaluation (Christensen and Kenney, 1995). Since the 1990s, many nurses have been practising in the community in a variety of settings – attached to GPs as health visitors or community nurses in what used to be called doctors' surgeries and are now grouped in Primary Care Trusts (PCTs) and to schools, factories, prisons and the armed services. More nurses work outside hospitals than in them and their practice increasingly is influenced by social rather than medical models of health and wellbeing. The professional distance between some nursing roles and some social work and social care roles has diminished and healthcare assistants and social care workers, for instance, often carry out similar tasks, working side by side in the community.

Process in Therapeutic Work

When therapists, particularly psychotherapists, discuss what is going on between the therapist and the client, they often talk about 'process' in a very specialised way. For example, Mrs and Mr M have had three meetings with the therapists. On each occasion, Mrs M does most of the talking while Mr M is almost silent. Mrs M takes every opportunity to blame Mr M for their problems and Mr M finds it necessary to go to the toilet two or three times during each meeting, complains of the airlessness in the room and opens a window and takes out his handkerchief and laboriously polishes the lenses of his glasses. Towards the end of the third meeting, the therapist points these things out and asks Mr and Mrs M to suggest what they think is going on. The therapist suggests that the underlying 'process' involves Mr M, for whatever reason, taking every opportunity to avoid joining his wife's conversation with the therapist. This is a way of viewing process as something real, but which may be in some way less immediately obvious, deeper, inside or beyond the events or actions of people.

Understanding Processes of Health and Social Care Work

In health and social care work, we find that the word 'processes' means more or less the same as 'stages'. When people talk about what stage of the process they have reached, they are normally referring to the sequence of procedures in care planning, from devising the plan to reviewing its implementation. It refers to an administrative sequence or set of procedures. Doing the work entails going through a number of stages, from the beginning to the end. It may seem an obvious task, but it is worth setting out at the start what we think it entails.

Activity 29.1

Spend no more than 10 minutes writing a list of the 'headline' actions you believe are involved in carrying out the process of health and social care work, in any particular piece of work with a carer and a person using services. A 'headline' is a heading covering an activity such as having the first meeting with the person receiving services. Our heading for this would be 'First meeting'.

You may like to compare your own list with the checklist below of 11 typical actions. The obvious point to make is that in contrast with the broad headings of assessment, planning, intervention and evaluation, actually doing the work involves many more activities: pre-meeting planning; making initial contact with the person; first meeting; communicating and engaging with the person; collecting information – from different agencies; analysing the information; making an assessment; planning – deciding what to do; refining assessment; intervening; reviewing.

We could add to the list, because after the review we may decide that more work is needed. We may return to the assessment and add further needs, which generate fresh tasks to be carried out. Here are three additional headings suggested by this: more refining of assessment; more intervention; more reviewing. In theory, this could go on indefinitely, as new needs constantly may be identified during the further work. The important findings from this are, firstly, that the list of stages may be much longer and more detailed than we anticipated and, secondly, a significant chunk of the sequence is circular rather than linear, that is, we can envisage that it may loop back after the review stage to reassessment and through further work.

Values, Principles and Practice

We have reached the point where the entire process is about to become cumbersome and formless, through being spelt out in so much detail. It is helpful to remind ourselves of what is important, the values that translate into guiding principles for our practice. Let us try to clarify these. Two key values are respecting the people we work with and taking proper account of the needs and wants generated through the diversity of people. These translate into statements of principles guiding practice. We could create a list of several dozen principles, but this would be meaningless and, in any case, unlikely to be used in practice. Instead, we have written four. The process of health and social care work necessitates:

- *Involving patients, carers and service users:* It is necessary to involve the people who use services at every stage of the work, from assessing, through planning, implementing and reviewing.
- *Making creative and purposeful decisions:* It is important that our practice is based on well-thought-out, imaginative decisions. Many of the people we work with will have had experience of bad decisions in their lives and it is necessary to give them a good experience of decision-making in practice (see Chapter 51).
- *Going beyond procedures:* Health and social care work would not deliver a quality service to carers and people using services if it just involved carrying out procedures according to an administrative set of rules. We have to recognise the necessity for our work with people to be based on values of respect for persons, valuing diversity, upholding rights and preserving dignity, choice and independence. We have also to work creatively with people to understand their circumstances, clarify their wishes and empower them through the process of our interaction with them, while also carrying out our responsibilities. This complicated set of tasks involves a delicate balancing act. We have to manage tensions between our duties and accountability to the agency employing us and our accountability to the carer and person using the services.
- *Exercising continual critical awareness:* We need to draw on our experience and knowledge and subject our work to continual critical reflection (see Chapter 34).

Now it is time to use a practice example so you can check what you have learnt in this chapter.

Practice study

Yuri and Kirsten

Imagine you are a health visitor working with a community care practitioner, visiting a young couple, Yuri and Kirsten, significantly overweight for no other reasons than poor diet and lack of exercise. Yuri has a heart condition diagnosed as hereditary as well as high blood pressure made worse by his lifestyle. Kirsten stays in their flat all day, every day, and suffers from mild depression.

Put practicalities of laws and procedures to one side. Spend no more than 10 minutes setting down brief notes detailing the kind of health and social care work which needs to be done with them at each stage, under the four headings: assessment, planning, implementation and evaluation.

Here is our brief checklist. We have only selected two key items to illustrate each stage.

	Healthcare	Social care
Assessment	Yuri needs lifestyle change to enable him to survive.	Kirsten needs to be empowered to engage with the world outside the flat.
Planning	Plan dietician's help for Kirsten, plus cooking class.	Plan for Yuri includes new diet, cookery advice and exercise.
Implementation	Conduct classes on nutrition. Maintain frequency. 'No excuses.'	Work with Yuri on self-monitoring blood pressure.
Evaluation	Check weight loss and blood pressure.	Ask Yuri and Kirsten to say how they have experienced it and whether they've benefited.

Conclusion

We have seen in this chapter the seemingly simple idea that the process of health and social care work can be summarised under the four headings of assessment, planning, implementation and review/evaluation. We have seen that the process linking these four broad headings can be complex, because of the complexity of the tasks when working with people. In the four chapters which follow, we deal with each of these four general headings in turn.

REVIEW QUESTIONS

1   What different meanings can you think of for the word 'process'?

2   What are the four main stages of health and social care work?

3   What is the actual sequence of activities in the course of the work?

Part IV

FURTHER READING

Adams, R. (2002) 'Social Work Processes', in R. Adams, L. Dominelli and M. Payne (eds) *Social Work: Themes, Issues and Critical Debates*, Basingstoke, Palgrave Macmillan, pp. 249–66

Christensen, P.J. and Kenney, J.W. (1995) (eds) *Nursing Process: Applications of Conceptual Methods*, St Louis, MO, Mosby

Compton, R.B. and Galaway, B. (1994) *Social Work Processes*, California, Brookes/Cole

Coulshed, V. and Orme, J. (1998) *Social Work Practice: An Introduction* (3rd edn) Basingstoke, Macmillan – now Palgrave Macmillan

Gates, B. (ed.) (2006) *Care Planning and Delivery in Intellectual Disability Nursing*, Oxford, Blackwell

Kenworthy, N., Snowley, G. and Gilling, C. (eds) (1999) *Common Foundation Studies in Nursing*, Edinburgh, Churchill Livingstone, pp. 369–72
A concise, readable summary of the nursing process.

Payne, M. (2005) 'Social Work Process', in R. Adams, L. Dominelli and M. Payne (eds) *Social Work Futures: Crossing Boundaries, Transforming Practice*, Basingstoke, Palgrave Macmillan, pp. 21–35

Yura, H. and Walsh, M.B. (1988) *The Nursing Process: Assessing, Planning, Implementing, Evaluating*, Norwalk, CT, Appleton & Lange, pp. 185–353
An extensive, detailed list of examples of the nursing process in practice.

Assessment **30**

ROBERT ADAMS

Learning outcomes

By the end of this chapter, you should be able to:

■ UNDERSTAND what is meant by assessment in health and social care

■ GRASP the essentials of the three main models of assessment

■ DEMONSTRATE basic knowledge of the single assessment process (or single shared assessment, in Scotland)

■ CONTRIBUTE to the assessment process.

Assessment is the foundation of good practice and the single assessment process (SAP) should be a seamless activity, across the health and social care spectrum, and should include the medical practitioners. Department of Health guidance is unequivocal. It stresses the necessity for practitioners across health and social care to

> reach an understanding of how medical diagnosis fits within the single assessment process. Medical diagnosis is the identification of a specific health condition, how it arose and its likely course. As such medical diagnosis can be seen as distinct from the assessment of wider health and social care needs. However, the inter-related nature of specific health conditions (such as stroke or a fractured neck or femur) with social, physical and mental health needs makes separation in practice unhelpful. (DoH, 2002b, p. 5)

The Carers (Equal Opportunities) Act 2004 and *Community Care Assessment Directions* (DoH, 2004f) require local authorities to involve service users and their carers in the processes of assessment and care planning. In theory, service users and carers have the right to choice in their services, although in practice they may need to be assertive to exercise this right. Social care practice should encourage service users to choose (see Chapter 39). The implications of the SAP and the Carers (Equal Opportunities) Act 2004 are that agencies and professionals should work together, in partnership with service users and carers, to ensure that they assess, plan and deliver appropriate services. Effective working together depends on many things, not least an understanding by care managers of the opportunities and pitfalls of teamwork. The way assessment is carried out – with full participation by the person using services as well as carers – is as important as the resulting assessment (DoH, 2001f). This chapter deals with this emphasis on *how* the work is done, which reflects the values underlying practice and is what distinguishes good practice from mere form-filling. Reliance on procedures as a crutch for practice can be nothing more than a deficiency in practice expertise. It is not realistic to try to manage uncertainty and risk out of existence. Uncertainty in practice results from the unpredictability of people's lives. This chapter focuses on the assessment of adults. Assessment of children in need and their families is referred to in Chapter 49.

What is Assessment in Health and Social Care?

We might expect a simple answer to this question, but this is not the case. The assessment of need is not a single, agreed idea that translates into a simple guideline for practice. There are three main complications. First, we can regard needs from different viewpoints. Jonathan Bradshaw (1972) clarified four main kinds of needs:

1. *normative need*, as defined by professionals
2. *felt need*, amounting to the person's wants
3. *expressed need*, that is, a felt need acted upon
4. *comparative need*, when compared with different groups in different areas.

Good principles of effective work with service users and carers necessitate that ways are found of discovering what people's felt needs are and agreeing with them ways of meeting them.

Second, assessment can be viewed in different ways. There are different emphases in the process of assessing, some being more concerned with gathering information, others with sharing information, back and forth between the carer, the service user and the practitioner. Some would argue that assessment should always be a participatory process, on the basis that service users and carers should be empowered and should participate in the process. However, it is important to recognise that, on occasions, assessment may not involve much participation by the person who uses the services, as he or she may be vulnerable, extremely ill or suffering from advanced dementia. Whatever the circumstances, at the heart of assessment are the skills we use in communicating (see Chapter 41).

Third, assessment may be a single event or carried out over a period of time (see the example of Richard's assessment and planning in Chapter 28).

Aim of Assessment

The aim of assessment is to make a judgement about a person's situation and needs. We achieve the assessment by tackling a number of questions, which, therefore, become our objectives.

Activity 30.1

Maria, 62, moved from Poland five years ago. Her husband Karl, 68, drinks heavily and stays at home, complaining that his legs let him down when he walks. Maria does all the shopping, housework and caring for him. Her only outings are to the grocer and off-licence a few yards down the street. Maria's English is poor and she is becoming forgetful. Over the past three months, she has had several accidents in the kitchen of their small, rented flat. On the last occasion, her neighbour saw smoke coming from the window and rescued her from a fire in the flat, which had started in the chip pan. She phoned social services and mentioned that from time to time she heard shouting and screaming, late at night.

Spend about 10 minutes drawing up a checklist of questions to guide you through the assessment process.

This is our checklist, extended to take in all the anticipated aspects:

- What do Maria and Karl think, feel and want?
- What are Karl's circumstances as a service user?
- What are Maria's circumstances as a service user?
- What are Maria's circumstances as a carer?
- What are Karl's felt needs and what is our view of his needs?
- What are Maria's felt needs and what is our view of them?
- What statement of their needs have I agreed with Karl and Maria?
- How can the agency best respond to those needs and, if possible, tackle them?
- Can we agree on a time by which the agency will have met those needs?
- Can we agree on how to judge whether the agency has met the needs?

This is quite a lengthy list of questions because at every stage we have to take care to involve the person and, where there is one, the carer in the assessment. The above situation is complicated because Maria is both the carer for Karl and a service user in her own right. It is a process of negotiation, in which the carer and the service user have the right to play a full and active part as participants. A visitor to the agency, who does not know how central this partnership is between practitioners and people receiving services, may ask 'When you already know what people want, why not complete the assessment on their behalf?' We do not because it is a basic principle that we do not do people's assessing for them. They have the right to assess their needs for themselves, in negotiation with us, the practitioners.

There are many different kinds of assessments. Assessment may be statutory or non-statutory, formal or informal. For instance, formal assessment of adults for social (community) care is carried out under section 47 of the NHS and Community Care Act (NHSCCA) 1990. It is extremely important for assessment to be carried out with thoroughness, efficiency and to a high standard. This is because the standard of the work which follows depends on the quality of the assessment.

For the assessment to be sound, it has to be based on administrative efficiency, that is, a systematic approach to gathering information. Department of Health (1991b) guidelines emphasise the importance of two particular points. First, it is necessary to clarify expectations, by ensuring that carers and service users understand the nature and implications of assessment as the key, first stage in the process of care planning. Second, it is crucial that the assessor possesses the communication skills (see Chapter 41) to develop a rapport with the person, so as to ensure the assessment is rooted in a real appreciation of the experiences and perceptions of the service user and carer.

Single Assessment Process (SAP)

The SAP (in Scotland, the concept is slightly different, empowered by s.12A, Social Work (Scotland) Act 1968, under the label 'single, shared assessment') contributes to National Service Frameworks (NSFs), for example the NSF for older people (DoH, 2001a) (see Resource File: Assessing Needs, at the end of the chapter). It is intended to:

- reduce administrative work
- ensure different agencies improve their joint working
- minimise duplication of effort and recording
- be person-centred
- systematically gather the views of carers and service users
- function at four levels of assessment: contact, overview, specialist and comprehensive.

Different disciplines should contribute to the assessment, which, in theory, is an integrated health and social care assessment bringing together the NHS Care Record Service and the electronic social care record (ESCR), forming the basis for care planning for all adult social care. The assessment draws on a variety of sources: any procedures and assessment tools the worker uses; the views of the service user and carer; the worker's previous experience; theories, perspectives and approaches relevant to assessment; agency guidelines; and legal duties and powers. In practice, this means prioritising three aspects:

- Assessment should be needs-led rather than service-led and person-centred rather than dictated by the demands of the agency.
- Assessment should involve finding out what a person's needs are, rather than looking to fit the person's needs into what the local authority already provides.
- Assessment should find out about people's problems, needs and wishes and note their strengths and capabilities. Assessment should be as much about the capacities of people to do things as about their incapacities. It should be a positive, holistic process, concerned with the whole person in the family and community environment in which he or she lives, rather than cut off from this and taken as an individual in isolation.

Models of Assessment

Assessments may be service-led, which means putting the needs of the agencies commissioning and providing services before the needs of the service user. In preference, they should be needs-led, which means putting the person's needs first. Even more important, they should be *person-centred* (sometimes called user-centred), which means:

■ putting the service user at the centre of all decisions
■ taking the service user's view as the decisive one.

Activity 30.2

Here is a summary of three main models of assessment of people: questioning, procedural and exchange, described by Smale and Tuson (1993). Read the summary and jot down one main strength and one main weakness of each model.

■ *Questioning model:* This assumes that the worker is the expert, that is, he or she knows more than the service user or carer and has the sole or main right to identify the right questions and ask them.
■ *Procedural model:* This assumes that the policy-makers and managers are the experts and the worker simply needs to follow the guidelines and procedures in gathering the information, so as to decide the person's eligibility for services.
■ *Exchange model:* This is a partnership model in which the service user is considered the expert in his or her own problems and the assessment involves an interchange of views with professionals. Under this model, all those involved in the person's situation have equally valid perspectives on assessing the circumstances and all are able to make a contribution to planning the services.

There is no one 'best' model of assessment in all circumstances, although the exchange model is usually advocated, as it promotes service user and carer participation in the assessment process. The strength of the questioning model may be when information is needed quite quickly as when assessing risk in an emergency, or when the person may be unwilling to give information which, however, should be provided, as in the case of a sex offender. A weakness of the questioning model is that it leaves the service user less scope to volunteer information and views outside the questions being asked.

The strength of the procedural model is in situations where information needs to be gathered systematically, covering a range of different aspects, without omitting any of them. Its weakness is its inflexibility and the tendency to contribute to mechanical assessment processes and a lack of imagination in the conclusions of assessment.

The main strength of the exchange model is that it empowers the service user to take a leading part in providing information on what he or she feels is important and relevant. Its main weakness lies in its tendency to create expectations which, where resources are rationed, may not be met.

Choice of Model of Assessment

Throughout the process of assessment, the service user's view should be paramount and the carer's views also should come close behind. This means that in most circumstances, the exchange model will be the most appropriate choice for workers, service users and carers.

Let us examine the *exchange model of assessment* in more detail. It entails:

- treating the service user as the expert on her or his situation
- empowering the service user and the carer
- drawing out the service user's perceptions, views, preferences and priorities
- exploring options with service user and carer/s
- summarising assessment
- specifying desired outcomes.

Person-centred Assessment

The assessment process should be person-centred, according to the NSF for mental health (DoH, 1999a) and older people (DoH, 2001a) as well as person-centred counselling (developed by Carl Rogers; see Chapter 45). It could be argued that a person-centred approach to assessment is more likely to lead to person-based services rather than service-led provision. The kinds of questions you would use in this approach could include the following:

- What do you as a service user/carer feel?
- What is your experience as a service user/carer?
- What are your needs as a service user/carer?

You may assess needs against a standard, such as the well-known hierarchy of needs developed by Abraham Maslow (1908–70) in the early 1940s (Maslow, 1943), based on a five-level pyramid (see Figure 11.1) from people's most basic physical 'deficiency' needs to the most fulfilling 'growth' needs, the satisfaction of each making possible the progression to the next. Starting from its base and moving to the top, the pyramid includes:

1. *biological and physiological needs*, for air, food, drink, sleep, shelter, warmth and sex
2. *safety needs*, for protection, security, boundaries
3. *affection and belonging needs*, for loving relationships in the family and satisfaction at work
4. *esteem needs*, for appreciation by others, status, reputation and recognition of achievements
5. *self-actualisation needs*, for personal development and fulfilment. Three more levels of growth needs were added in the late 1960s (Maslow, 1987)
6. *cognitive needs*, for knowledge and understanding
7. *aesthetic needs*, to create or appreciate beauty and harmony
8. *transcendence needs*, enabling people to achieve self-actualisation.

Maslow's hierarchy of needs may be criticised for implying that it is a hierarchy, with 'higher', more valued needs and 'lower' needs and stating that the individual moves from one level to another, whereas a person simultaneously may have needs, unsatisfied or satisfied, at several different levels.

Strengths-based Approach to Assessment

The strengths perspective, developed by Dennis Saleeby (2002), involves assessing people's needs from their strengths and potential rather than simply deficits, building on their existing knowledge, skills and resources to enable them to cope with challenges and difficulties. It identifies the positive qualities, skills and activities that the person receiving services and the carer possess, which can contribute to the work with them. For instance, it is important to identify what can be done to enable a carer and a service user to change, improve or at least maintain their continuing situations. The goal of change may involve the services being tailored to objectives that are beyond the immediate circumstances of the service user and carer.

Carrying out an Assessment

Assessment is not just one action. It involves a series of actions and involves preparing, collecting information, weighing it up, perhaps collecting more, weighing up again and analysing, and finally using the analysis. It necessitates the different practitioners from different agencies sharing their work in the SAP.

Assessing Carers

Assessment has to include the right of carers to an assessment. Carers are entitled to assessment under the Carers (Recognition and Services) Act 1995, provided the person for whom they are caring is receiving services under the NHSCCA 1990. The Carers (Equal Opportunities) Act 2004 aims to promote cooperation between local authorities and gives:

- local authorities the duty to inform carers of their right to an assessment
- carers the right for the local authority to take into account their outside interests – their work, leisure activities and education, including lifelong learning – when doing their assessment, that is, maintaining a balance between personal life, employment and caring responsibilities.

Under the Carers and Disabled Children Act 2000, people are entitled to an assessment if they are offering a substantial amount of care. For example, if a service user's son or daughter is providing a significant level of care, he or she is entitled to an assessment of their own needs and their ability to care, under section 1 of this Act. The NSF for older people (DoH, 2001a) also refers to carers' needs. The work, leisure and education needs of the carer are subject to assessment, to ensure that the carer is able to achieve fulfilment, as are financial circumstances. Financial assessment has to take into account the service being provided and the means of the service user. Charges are made by the providing local authority in the light of the financial assessment, where this applies. The service user can refuse to undertake a financial assessment, in which case the standard charges apply.

Risk Assessment

Department of Health guidance (DoH, 2003a) ensures that risk assessment is carried out as part of the consideration of a person's eligibility for services, pointing out that risks should include not only risks to independence but also health risks (DoH, 2003a, p. 2). Risk should be perceived and dealt with positively. A positive approach to risk management goes beyond simply looking for the hazards and risks in a person's life in a negative way. It uses risk management as a way of empowering service users and carers and maximising their potential (see also Chapter 11). Procedures should be used as a guide to practice and not rule it to the exclusion of other principles, such as the right of the service user and carer to be empowered. The overriding principle should be that the practitioner should not adopt procedures of risk management as a way of trying to eliminate risk. Risk is part of reality and needs to be lived with.

Risks are of many different kinds and often the many uncertainties in a person's life make it difficult or impossible to conduct a simple risk assessment which holds for any length of time. A person's circumstances can change and health and moods can vary on a daily or even hourly basis. It is common for risks to be assessed in terms of whether they are critical, substantial, moderate or low. There is an inevitable tension in everybody's life between enjoying life and taking risks. We take a risk whenever we get out of bed and go into the kitchen to make a cup of tea. The kitchen is the part of the home where most accidents occur. We take a risk when we walk down the street and cross a busy road to buy a newspaper from the local shop. However, we may judge that these risks are worth taking in order to live everyday life the way we want it. The main purpose of risk assessment should not be to reduce the person's chances of living a full and active life, but to identify only those hazards or possible accidents which threaten an unacceptably high level of harm to us or others. The question is who should judge this risk, us as service users, our carers, relatives or friends, or the professionals? The positive way of managing this entails work with service users and carers so that joint decisions can be arrived at, respecting their wishes.

Bringing the Assessment to a Conclusion

In bringing together the assessment, the worker draws on his or her own sources and also on the perceptions, experiences, judgements and wishes of the service user and carer. Their preferences and choices are central to the entire process of assessment and should not be forgotten at the point of finalising the initial assessment. At this point, the worker needs to summarise the assessment and develop recommendations for use at the planning stage. While service users' and carers' views are taken into account, professionals are accountable for their recommendations and agencies are responsible for allocating the resources which enable health and social care services to be delivered. Table 30.1 lists the main aspects.

Table 30.1 Headings of initial assessment: Anyborough

Name
Date of birth
Address
Next of kin
GP
Name of person making referral
Profile and social circumstances
Health (physical/mental/emotional) (medical treatments/alcohol use/drug use)
Communication
Personal care (washing/bathing/dressing/preparing meals/eating/drinking/medication)
Mobility
Accommodation and home management (shopping/laundry/heating/housework)
Social networks (informal)
Financial situation
Risks
Support services
Eligibility level (refer to eligibility criteria)
Assessment summary
Plan
Care manager (name)
Signature
Date of completion

Practice study

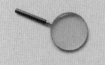

Maria and Karl (cont'd)

We have arrived at the point where we can bring together our assessment of the circumstances of Maria and Karl in Anyborough.

Staff now check their needs against the relevant legislation (National Assistance Act 1948, Health Services and Public Health Act 1968, Chronically Sick and Disabled Persons Act 1970, National Health Service Act 1977) and use the criteria below to judge the level of their eligibility for services: critical, substantial, moderate or low. Clearly there are risk and safety needs to both Maria and Karl, and Maria also has her own needs as carer. It would help to provide respite care for Karl, so Maria can seek opportunities for leisure (attending the Polish club and meeting other women) and education (day class in creative writing) outside the flat. There is a need to prevent

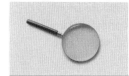

future abuse of Maria. Maria has a need to become empowered to the point where she can assert herself and say 'no' to Karl. Staff now have to assess how far the needs of Karl and Maria qualify them for services. The decision about which band of eligibility for services their needs fall into is based on stated criteria (Table 30.2).

Table 30.2 Eligibility criteria

Critical
■ Life is threatened
■ There are significant health problems
■ There is serious abuse or neglect
■ There is an inability to carry out vital domestic routines
■ There is a lack of vital family, social, education or work relationships and/or support systems
Substantial
■ There is only partial choice and control over the immediate environment
■ There is, or has been, abuse or neglect
■ There is an inability to carry out the majority of personal care or domestic routines
■ Vital family, social, education or work relationships and/or support systems will not be sustained
Moderate
■ There is an inability to carry out several personal care or domestic routines
■ Several vital family, social, education or work relationships and/or support systems will not be sustained
Low
■ There is an inability to carry out one or two personal care or domestic routines
■ One or two vital family, social, education or work relationships and/or support systems will not be sustained

SOURCE: adapted from DoH, 2003a, pp. 3–4

Conclusion

We have seen in this chapter that assessment is not merely a procedural task carried out to minimise risk to the agency, but a complex activity on which to build sound practice. In the following chapters, we follow the sequence of assessment through in order to illustrate how it is used and may be added to and modified in the light of subsequent practice.

Part IV

REVIEW
QUESTIONS

1 Why does it matter *how* assessment is carried out, as long as the information is gathered?

2 What are the main uses of the three models of assessment?

3 What is a person-centred, strengths-based approach to assessment?

FURTHER
READING

Milner, J. and O'Byrne, (2002) *Assessment in Social Work* (2nd edn) Basingstoke, Palgrave Macmillan

Parker, J. and Bradley, G. (2003) *Social Work Practice: Assessment, Planning, Intervention and Review*, Exeter, Learning Matters

Sharkey, P. (2006) *The Essentials of Community Care* (2nd edn) Basingstoke, Palgrave Macmillan

Resource file

Assessing needs

The single assessment process is intended to be carried out by all health and social care staff working together, in health settings including GP surgeries, hospitals, community health services and other NHS facilities, as well as children and families services, adult social services offices and Care Direct access points (DoH, 2002b). There is some merit in comparing the English, Welsh and Scottish systems.

Single assessment process (England and Wales)

The single assessment process (SAP) in England and Wales follows from section 22 of the NHS Act 1977. Although the guidance for the SAP sets out to put the person using services at the centre of the processes of assessment and care management, the guidance for single shared assessment in Scotland emphasises empowerment and self-assessment by carers and people who use services.

Single shared assessment (Scotland)

This takes place under section 12A, Social Work (Scotland) Act 1968 giving local authorities the duty to assess any person over 18 whom they believe needs community care services. Guidance indicates (Scottish

Executive, 2001) that the principles of single shared assessment are as follows:

1. People who use services and carers should be able to participate in the assessment.
2. The assessment should meet people's needs.
3. The most appropriate professional should carry out the assessment.
4. The assessor should be appropriately qualified and skilled.
5. Information about the person should only be shared with their informed consent.
6. Assessment must enable access to all community care services.
7. Other practitioners and agencies must accept the conclusions of the assessment.

Guidance on the single assessment process

Essential guidance is available in a Department of Health publication (2002b). Further, more detailed guidance is available (DoH, 2001a, 2003a).

For people being assessed in the single assessment process and single shared assessment, the benefits should be that it:

■ meets their needs

- provides appropriate assessment
- avoids duplicating information
- provides a key practitioner – the lead assessor
- provides quicker, integrated care planning.

Assessing needs of children

The common assessment framework (DfES, 2006b) is based on 10 principles of assessments (DoH, 2000a, p. 10), which are:

1. child-centred
2. rooted in child development
3. ecological
4. based on equal opportunities
5. based on working with children and families
6. built on strengths while identifying problems
7. interagency in assessment and service provision
8. a continuing process not an event
9. carried out in parallel with other practice and provision
10. grounded in knowledge and research regarding practice.

Highlighting a few key details of this, we can see how the assessment takes into account three interrelated components: the development needs of the child; the adults' capacity to respond appropriately; and the nature of the child's family and environmental factors, including the resources and supports available in the community and the culture in which the child is growing up (DoH, 2000a, p. 17).

FURTHER READING

DoH (2000) *Framework for the Assessment of Children in Need and their Families*, London, TSO

DoH (2001) *National Service Framework for Older People*, London, DoH

DoH (2002) *The Single Assessment Process Guidance for Local Implementation*, London, DoH

DoH (2003) *Fair Access to Care Services: Guidance on Eligibility Criteria for Adult Social Care*, London, DoH

Scottish Executive (2001) *Guidance on Single Shared Assessment of Community Care Needs*, Circular No. CCD8/2001, Edinburgh, Scottish Executive

Planning **31**

ROBERT ADAMS

Learning outcomes

By the end of this chapter, you should be able to:

■ UNDERSTAND what is involved in health and social care planning

■ CONTRIBUTE to developing and writing an effective plan

■ IDENTIFY issues relating to the planning process.

In the planning stage of the process of working with people, the worker negotiates realistic goals with the person receiving services. This chapter looks in some detail at the components of planning, using a practice example that tackles the tensions between meeting individual needs and the pressures on rationing resources.

What is Planning?

Planning is the process entailed in translating the assessment into a feasible plan. Too often health and social care planning proceed separately because the assessment, in effect, has been separate and parallel rather than joint.

When the assessment is completed, the worker moves with the service user and carer into the planning stage. Fully involving the service user and carer should ensure that planning involves developing services to meet the person's needs rather than fitting the person's needs into existing provision. The key tasks are to decide *what* to do, *how* to do it, *who* will do which parts of it and *when* and how they will work together. The plan should specify this, breaking down the components into a list of who does what and when, probably on a daily, weekly and monthly basis. There is a need to state the goals and particular outcomes. The *Fair Access to Care Services* (FACS) guidelines (DoH, 2003a) ensure that:

- all statutory organisations operate according to a single set of criteria to judge a person's eligibility for services
- each service user has equal and fair access to service
- the stages of assessing and planning care are adequately linked.

We should think of health and social care planning as a creative activity and not as a procedural necessity. As we shall see in the example of Mr Khan below, it is possible to take an assessment of a quite difficult situation, with personal problems that are becoming progressively worse and creating higher dependency, and then to use, for example, direct payments to empower a person, that is, enable greater independence, autonomy, choice and control over their own lives.

Person-centred Planning

The Care Manager

The care manager has responsibility for:

- overseeing the development of the care package that forms the care plan
- coordinating the assessment for the care plan according to the single assessment process (SAP)
- making sure risks to the service user are assessed and appropriately catered for in the care plan
- ensuring agencies and professionals collaborate effectively to produce the care plan
- enabling service users and carers to participate fully in the assessment leading to the care plan.

The Care Plan

At the end of assessment, hopefully agreement will have been negotiated and agreed between all parties about the needs of the service user and carer/s. The views of the service user should be taken into account fully in this process of negotiation. Where possible, the views of the service user should not be overridden or ignored. There may be situations where the service user is distressed or unable for other reasons to contribute a rational and coherent view about his or her assessment and needs. The carer may have signed an agreement with the service user at an earlier date to take lasting power of attorney under the Mental Capacity Act 2005.

The care plan should specify:

- the agreed needs of the service user
- the expectations of the service user
- the expectations of the carer/s

- the agreed plan of action for each need
- who is involved in meeting each need
- what services will be provided in meeting each need
- what outcomes should be achieved when each need is met.

Outcomes may be of three different kinds. Some are more to do with maintaining the person at the current level of activity. Others may involve an element of change. A third type of outcome may involve the impact of the service on the service user, in terms of improving the quality of life, such as feeling more empowered, being able to make more decisions and living more independently.

We should be in no doubt that the planning process may not be as straightforward as this section seems to imply. In an ideal situation, the assessment will lead straight to the negotiation of the care plan with the service user. In reality, the complexity of the situation may mean that there is no single 'answer' that will ensure meeting the needs of the carer and the person using services. Since the end of the twentieth century, however, one positive development has been the spread of direct payments, which we will outline and then explore an example where the choice is open to the service user of taking direct payments instead of the services available and using them to tailor a care package to meet his needs.

Direct Payments

Direct payments are cash payments given directly to the service user, under the Community Care (Direct Payments) Act 1996, to spend on services she or he wants and needs. Department of Health guidance (DoH, 2004b) states that the purpose of direct payments is to enable people to take more decisions affecting their lives, increasing choice and flexibility and enabling them to match the services more nearly to their needs.

Service users and carers may employ one or more carers or personal assistants from direct payments. The one exception is that direct payments cannot be given for people receiving treatment under the Mental Health Acts 1983 and 2007. Direct payments are intended by the government to enable people to live independently and to increase their choice, control and flexibility in the services they purchase. Direct payments have three main advantages:

1. They empower the service user to make decisions.
2. They give the service user choice of what care to provide.
3. They give the service user control over whom to select as a carer or personal assistant.

In 2003–4 only about 13,000 people over 18 used direct payments, so they were still not part of the mainstream of social care services (CSCI, 2005a, p. 3). However, the rate of take-up is increasing each year, from 5,000 in 2000–1 to 24,000 in 2004–5 and 37,000 in 2005–6 (Hansard, House of Commons Debates, 19 Jan 2007, col. 1412W).

Mr Khan

Mr Khan is 71 and suffering from the early stages of multiple sclerosis. For the past three months, he has been living in sheltered accommodation near his daughter's house. He recently fell in the bathroom and at present is unable to walk far or feed himself. He has been in hospital and a mild stroke is suspected. The assessment has highlighted the vulnerability of Mr Khan and his high dependency on a daily basis to having his needs met with necessary help from other people. Mr Khan's daughter has begun to try to persuade him to go into a residential home, which he is adamantly refusing to consider. In support of his strong wish to retain his independence, the assessment has highlighted that provided certain needs – help with feeding and shopping – are met, he is able to cope. Although he lives alone, his daughter and son-in-law are able to call on him daily. He has been assessed as in need of help and support and, following discussion with the care manager, has expressed the wish to receive direct payments on a regular basis instead of certain social services.

The direct payments are negotiated with Mr Khan so that he employs a personal assistant instead of using services from the local adult and community care department of social services. This gives him independence and flexibility over the care services he purchases. Mr Khan's apprehension at employing a care assistant is settled by the information, training and support that the care manager organises through social services. This enables Mr Khan to meet his personal and legal responsibilities as an employer. It also ensures that he manages the direct payment through a separate bank account and keeps detailed records of how he spends the monthly payments. Although this involves him in extra work, he gets satisfaction from the fact that it maintains his independence and gives him control over his life.

Mr Khan looks back and is glad that he overcame his initial resistance to having his finances – income and capital – assessed, in the process of determining his contribution towards the direct payment he now receives. He had not realised that the direct payment is not a benefit such as disability living allowance or attendance allowance and does not reduce these allowances. He had not realised that he can live in sheltered housing or even with another family member and still qualify for a direct payment.

In practical terms, even though Mr Khan relies on his personal assistant, other services are still supplied by the health and social services. His medical needs continue to be met by the GP, district nurses and hospital staff. The GP would like Mr Khan to spend a day and a night in hospital within the next fortnight, for more detailed assessment of his medical needs. A nursing care plan is drawn up for this, which forms part of the main care plan. It covers the following headings: mobility and comfort, communication, activities, clothing, hygiene, diet, elimination, relaxation and sleep. It contributes to the all-round picture of how the different practitioners will contribute to meeting Mr Khan's health and care needs:

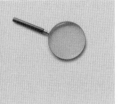

- Rehabilitation from the stroke is provided by an occupational therapist, a physiotherapist and a speech therapist from the NHS.
- Certain community resources and family support and care are available to Mr Khan.
- National and local organisations in the voluntary sector provide him and his relatives with help and information, notably Headway, the Brain Injury Association and the Stroke Association.

It may be useful to base your own planning on existing examples, hence this next activity, which rounds off this chapter.

Activity 31.1

In the light of the example of Mr Khan, devise your own care plan for Pat, who was a translator with a high level of office skills. She suffered a cerebral haemorrhage and her mobility is severely restricted, so she has given up her rented flat and moved in permanently with her sister. Assessment of her needs results in her stating her preferences:

- She would like to be able to follow her vegan, kosher diet at home with her sister.
- She would like to take an IT course, hopefully to enable her to use email to do some secretarial work at home, for an agency.
- She would like to have increased choice over her activities and to gain some independence through being able to work from home.

Issues for Practice

The key issues arising from the process so far are as follows:

1. The care plan needs to be devised with the people who use health and social care services and not simply devised with them in mind, consulting them when the details have been decided. Their feelings and wishes should be kept central to the planning process and they should be given copies in writing – or other appropriate formats, taking into account whether they are blind and need a translation into braille, whether their written language is other than English and need a translation, or whether they have a learning disability and need an 'easy to read' version – of all assessment and planning reports.
2. There are tensions to be managed between needs and eligibility for services, in light of the pressures on health and local authorities to set limits on spending. In particular, there are issues regarding the costs of drugs and the relative costs of different community and residential/hospital treatment options.
3. There is a need to determine the extent to which a particular person is eligible for free services, or what level of charges needs to be imposed, following means-testing. Some older people in particular are sensitive about means-testing and perceive it as stigmatising. There is also the question as to whether the person opts for direct payments (see Resource File: Charging and Direct Payments, at the end of Chapter 14).

Part IV

4. The risk assessment may need reflecting in the plan, particularly if there is a need for action, for instance under the safeguarding adults procedures (see Chapter 9).

Conclusion

This chapter has shown how planning has a vital part to play in providing creative health and social care services, in negotiation with the person using services, rather than handing out traditional services to the person, in a way that reinforces dependence.

REVIEW
QUESTIONS

1 What key feature of planning distinguishes it from assessment?

2 How can planning be creative and empowering?

3 How can direct payments contribute to an empowering care plan?

FURTHER
READING

DoH (2002) *The Single Assessment Process Guidance for Local Implementation*, London, DoH

DoH (2002) *Health Action Plans and Health Facilitation*, London, DoH
    Provides practical guidance on what needs doing.

Gates, B. (ed.) (2006) *Care Plannning and Delivery in Intellectual Disability Nursing*, Oxford, Blackwell
    This covers a wide range of settings where healthcare planning is necessary.

Parker, J. and Bradley, G. (2003) *Social Work Practice: Assessment, Planning, Intervention and Review*, Exeter, Learning Matters
    There are some good illustrations of practical tools for planning on pp. 62–83.

Payne, M. (1995) *Social Work and Community Care*, Basingstoke, Macmillan – now Palgrave Macmillan

Yura, H. and Walsh, M.B. (1988) *The Nursing Process* (5th edn) Norwalk, CT, Appleton & Lange, pp. 236–40
    Despite this book's age and publication in the USA, there are some excellent examples of how to write good, detailed plans to meet families' health and social care needs, rather than one or the other. The following text is an alternative source: Aggleton, P. and Chalmers, H. (2000) *Nursing Models and Nursing Practice* (2nd edn) Basingstoke, Palgrave – now Palgrave Macmillan

Implementation and Intervention

ROBERT ADAMS

Learning outcomes

By the end of this chapter, you should be able to:

- UNDERSTAND what is meant by implementation and intervention in health and social care
- CONTRIBUTE to the wide variety of different approaches and methods
- RECOGNISE some of the tensions and dilemmas inherent in practice
- CONTRIBUTE to the implementation process.

This chapter deals with the activities central to all work with people – actually carrying out the work. I visited an agency, where the staff, with some relief, described their role in community care as assessment and care planning, pointing out that it was far easier to assess people's needs than to work with them to tackle those needs. It is probably significant that the government's own guidance on eligibility for adult social care has a lot to say about assessment, planning and review and almost nothing to say about methods of implementation. This highlights a key feature of implementation – it is extremely challenging and probably demands more of our knowledge, skills and commitment than any other stage of the process. We will spend several chapters considering different approaches to implementation in Part VI of this book and refer to these at the appropriate points below.

What Implementing and Intervening Mean in Practice

It is vital, as with the other stages of health and social care work, that implementation and intervention are carried out with the full participation of the person using services. 'Their needs and their views and wishes must be at the centre of all decisions that are made' (DoH, 2002b, p. 5).

Implementing means carrying out. Implementation is concerned with the core activities of healthcare and social care – namely, carrying out the plans based on assessed need, agreed with patients, carers and people using services. These distinctive areas overlap to an extent, as some services such as community care span the entire field of health and social care.

It is important to recognise the centrality to the process of actually doing the implementation. Implementation and intervention should involve all parties to the care plan wherever possible. It is necessary for whatever intervention takes place to be agreed in advance with service users and carers. The assessment may be faultless and the care plan wonderful, but the providing authority may have a tendency to pay lip service to these at the implementation stage. The reasons may be quite understandable from the local authority's point of view. There may be resource constraints through lack of money in the budget and managers and practitioners may be pressurised to act as gatekeepers of scarce resources. In these circumstances, it is up to the care worker to ensure that the service does not fall short of what is required to meet the person's needs.

Practice study

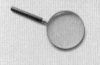

Lottie

Lottie, chronically physically disabled but wanting more control over her day-to-day life, overcame her fears about the complications and responsibilities of employing a personal assistant. She used the advice of the local adult services department and the support of a social worker to set up 16 hours of payment shared between two personal assistants five days a week, with her partner caring for her at evenings and weekends. Sometimes Lottie uses some of the hours during the week to give her partner some respite at the weekend. She has no doubts that the extra responsibility of managing the employment of her personal assistants is easily offset against the independence she has gained. After three years, she is pleased that she is able take part in local activities, including meetings of a service user and carer support network, rather than simply attending a day centre.

Intervention

Intervening has the additional meaning of using different methods to enable a person to change their life. Health and social care cannot simply be about 'help' and 'care'. In some cases, intervention means using the law to protect someone from harm or to protect somebody else from the risk that they will harm them. On the health side, surgical intervention, for instance to remove an ingrowing toenail or replace an arthritic hip joint, is likely to require the written consent of the person, in advance. In general, it is necessary for whatever intervention takes place to be agreed in advance with service users and carers, but there are exceptions. Sometimes decisions have to be made with which not all family members agree. There may be disagreements between a mother with Alzheimer's disease and her daughter who lives with her about whether the mother should be admitted to a care home. A person with a serious, acute mental health problem may be given residential or community treatment on a compulsory or voluntary order under the Mental Health Act 2007 for their own protection or the protection of others.

Intervention is inseparable from the assessment and planning which precedes it. A good assessment and care plan is essential to effective intervention and acts like a map, to guide the practitioner forward. There is an inbuilt tension in some interventions, between using the law to carry out work that imposes on the person using services and working in partnership with them. There are circumstances where we cannot do both simultaneously. Thus, there are tensions between:

- carrying out procedures and ensuring that practice is sensitive to the wishes and feelings of the service user and carer
- following custom and practice in the agency and developing informed, critical practice in the light of one's own reading and experience.

On one hand, intervention may consist of short- or long-term work with the individual or the family as a group, and may consist of providing services, managing care (care management), counselling or advocacy. On the other hand, intervention may be the process by which action is taken using legal powers, while the people receiving the services are being empowered to take control of their lives. These two may proceed alongside each other or actually may conflict.

Approaches to Intervention

A number of approaches and methods of working with people are particularly relevant to implementation, including cognitive-behavioural work (Chapter 42), various other forms of therapy (Chapter 43), counselling (Chapter 45), emergency, crisis and task-centred work (Chapter 46) and empowerment and advocacy (Chapter 40). Some approaches such as counselling focus on work with the individual. Others such as family therapy involve work with the family as a group. Such family work is one aspect of groupwork. Most work with people involves not only working with individuals but with groups (see also Chapter 54 on group living). Few people using services or carers have no other relatives, neighbours or friends with whom joint meetings occur during the work. Work with families is work with family groups, even though it may not always, or even often, be group-based work. Work may also be undertaken with so-called 'artificial' groups, for example, of people experiencing similar problems. When working with groups, it is good to be aware of the stages of such a group – from its formation ('forming'), through early negotiations between members ('storming'), to the point where norms are established ('norming') and finally to its work through to its ending ('performing') (Bion, 1968, and more recently, Douglas, 2000). There are many ways of working with and within groups and many types of group. A 'natural' group of family or household members is different from a group, say, of carers from different households coming together because of a common interest in issues for carers. Some workers are drawn towards working with individuals, even when a group is present at meetings. They will ignore others and focus on interacting with one person at a time. Finally, some groups are more therapeutic in orientation (Whitaker, 1985; Preston-Shoot, 1987; Douglas, 2000) and are led by professionals, while others, well described by Mullender and Ward (1991), are led by service user members.

Dealing with Tensions and Dilemmas

It is inevitable that work with the complexity of people's lives involves managing uncertainty and tensions. Uncertainty is inherent in many people's lives, so it is not surprising that it is a feature of health and social care work. Despite our best efforts to plan and insure against accidents, risks and unforeseen circumstances, none of us is exempt from the unexpected incident, situation or illness.

Tensions arise where the worker has to make a choice between two or more equally problematic options. The tensions may amount to *dilemmas*, that is, two choices, each of which resolves one problem while creating another or leaving the original one unresolved. In practice, the practitioner may need to accept the reality that just as tensions have to be managed, dilemmas must be accommodated. By definition, a dilemma is a choice, neither option of which provides a satisfactory outcome for everyone concerned.

Activity 32.1

Etta is a registered disabled lone mother of a daughter aged six, who was adopted because her mother was unable to cope. Etta has a history of heroin abuse, harming the child and self-harm. She is pregnant again to her current partner and is now working in an office, apparently no longer engaging in drug abuse.

■ Write notes on the various tensions and dilemmas facing professionals with responsibility for Etta's welfare and that of her unborn child.

Situations like this generate tensions and dilemmas that are by no means uncommon. Here are three of the main *tensions*:

1. There is a tension between following Etta's view of what is in her best interests and following the professionals' judgement of what is in her interests and that of the child under the Children Act 1989.
2. Etta has rights under the NHS and Community Care Act 1990 as a person who uses services and the agency has the right under that same legislation to determine how it delivers community care services to Etta, according to national standards.
3. There is a tension between Etta's rights and those of other people, including her partner and other mothers with whom she may come into contact.

Here are three *dilemmas*:

1. On one hand, Etta may be regarded as now mature enough to raise her child responsibly. On the other hand, it may be viewed as too risky even to allow her to stay in the maternity unit of the local hospital, quite apart from the longer term risk arising if she keeps the baby.
2. On one hand, Etta's welfare may be regarded as paramount. On the other hand, the health and wellbeing of the unborn baby may be viewed as paramount.
3. On one hand, Etta has a right as a woman to have and bring up the child. On the other hand, the unborn baby has the right to a stable, fulfilling family life.

There is no simple, clear-cut 'solution' to such a situation. The professionals have to discuss the different issues with Etta and her partner and try to negotiate a way through, taking due account of the views of others such as her partner.

Conclusion

This chapter has dealt with the contrasting activities associated with implementation and intervention. In the process, it has emerged that while implementation is a more neutral term covering the translation of any plan into practice, intervention is a term reserved for those situations where there is a compulsory element in the work the practitioner does with the person using services. It is clear from the example given that tensions exist in practice and that some of these may be expressed in terms of practice dilemmas.

REVIEW
QUESTIONS

1   What are the similarities and differences between implementation and intervention?

2   What are the advantages of direct payments over services provided by the local authority?

3   Can you give two examples of tensions that can arise in practice?

4   Can you illustrate a dilemma from practice?

FURTHER
READING

Cleaver, H., Walker, S. and Meadows, P. (2004) *Assessing Children's Needs and Circumstances: The Impact of the Assessment Framework*, Lyme Regis, Russell House

Long, B.C., Phipps, W.J. and Cassmeyer, V.L. (1995) *Adult Nursing: A Nursing Process Approach*, London, Kingsley

McFarland, G.K., Wasli, E. and Gerety, E.K. (1997) *Nursing Diagnosis and Process in Psychiatric Mental Health Nursing*, Philadelphia, Lippincott

O'Leary, C.J. (1999) *Counselling Couples and Families: A Person-centred Approach*, London, Sage

Walker, S. and Beckett, C. (2003) *Assessment and Intervention in Social Work*, Lyme Regis, Russell House

Part IV

33 Review and Evaluation

ROBERT ADAMS

By the end of this chapter, you should be able to:

■ UNDERSTAND what is meant by 'review' and 'evaluation' in health and social care

■ CONTRIBUTE to the processes of review and evaluation

■ RECOGNISE some of the issues to be tackled in practice.

We have reached what might be described as the final stage of the process of health and social care work, but to see it as final would be a mistake. It is true that review feeds into evaluation, but it is just as likely to lead to further questions about the assessment. Any modifications to the assessment will require adjustments to the plan and this will need implementing afresh. In fact, the sequence may more accurately be regarded as a cycle.

What are Reviewing and Evaluating?

Reviewing is arguably the most important aspect of practice because it is the stage where the worker stops and, with people using services and their carers, asks how effective the work has been to date. Yet in a busy day's work, many people find that reviewing is the activity most likely to be omitted or skimped. After all, it does not seem to be the highest priority activity, not moving us any further forward. Sometimes, it actually sets us back, because awkward questions arise. In a busy working week, it is easy to see the arguments for postponing asking questions such as 'How well are we doing?' or asking the carer or service user 'How well do *you* think we're doing?'

We can distinguish between review and evaluation as follows.

Review

Review is a constant, repeated process of appraising what we have achieved, adjusting our plans and restating what remains to be done. Clearly, reviewing is not just the review meeting itself, but is part of our frame of mind, our constant state of being a reflective, critical practitioner (see Chapter 34). We should state clearly at the start that reviews should be carried out with the full participation of service users and carers. Particular procedures govern different kinds of reviews. There are serious case reviews as part of child protection practice (see Chapter 10) (DoH, 1991c, 1991d) and case reviews as part of the work of adult services. We should remember that a review is an interim appraisal of where we have reached and we should be flexible and open to changes at all times. Implementation should be reviewed regularly, to see how far the goals of the care plan are being met. A review gives those taking part the chance to examine and discuss what has been achieved so far and to identify and discuss any issues that have arisen. Review is not necessarily a one-directional process. It is possible for the workers, the service user and the carer to revisit earlier stages. There is no reason why assessment and intervention should not be revisited in this way and gone through again, in whole or in part. This may have the advantage that this time the assessment will be richer and the intervention will be informed by what has been done previously.

In adult care, the Department of Health guidelines on care management set out standard procedures for recording reviews (DoH, 1991b, pp. 85–6), based on the original care plan, any particular achievements or failures, reassessments of the needs of carers and people using services, any cost implications and scheduling the next meeting.

Review may lead to revisions in the care plan, to take account of any changes in the person's circumstances. Revisions may take the form of new goals being put forward by one or more person present at the review meeting, or changes to existing goals. In all reviews, it is paramount to maintain the participation and empowerment of the service user and carer.

The following questions are integral to the review:

- What have the practitioners done?
- How are the service user and the carer feeling about what has been done?
- What do the service user and carer feel has been most effective?
- What do the service user and carer feel could have been done better?
- Did the actions of the practitioners lead to the objectives being met, totally, mostly, a little or not at all?
- If there were shortcomings, how did they arise?
- If there were shortcomings, what were they?
- Were the distinctive needs and wishes of the carer met totally, mostly, a little or not at all?
- If there were needs unmet, what were they?
- Should new goals be set?

■ Should one or more existing goals be revised and if so, how?

■ What should be done next?

In community care, a range of agencies are likely to be involved in delivering services: local NHS and social services agencies, associated voluntary and private organisations, neighbourhood and community groups, hospitals and Primary Care Trusts. Given that the single assessment process is used, the principle is to keep the service user and carer at the centre of the processes of assessment and care planning. Further aims are to achieve simpler and more accessible care services for service users and carers, achieve improved communication between agencies and practitioners and simplify working arrangements within and between agencies. A single, unified and integrated system of record-keeping would help this process, but in health and social care, this has not been achieved to date. There are moves towards single sets of agreed standards by which to judge the practice in particular aspects and joint sharing of all information.

Evaluation

Reviewing leads naturally into evaluating. Evaluation involves taking stock of all that has been done and what remains to be done, separating out the positives from the negatives and making a judgement about the worth of all of it, in its entirety. Because evaluation is wide-ranging, it is invariably complex and time-consuming, so it is relatively rare to find comprehensive evaluations taking place. However, all reviews of practice contain an evaluative element. The question 'how would you evaluate this?' is quite commonly asked and simply asks you to make a judgement. It does not prevent you making the judgement because you have not collected all the necessary evidence. Evaluation is a broader and more substantial undertaking than the kind of regular reviewing we have described above. Evaluation is the activity of making a judgement about the work as a whole. How useful was it? How well was it carried out? Did it meet the targets? What shortcomings were there?

People who use services and their carers should participate in evaluation. Their views and experiences should be at its core. Efforts should be made to ensure that the involvement of service users and carers plays a significant part and is not tokenistic.

Evaluation Skills

The skills of evaluation include gathering information, recording, exchanging and reporting information. These are skills shared to a great extent with reviewing. Exchanging information is an activity we may take for granted, but it often happens when, for instance, service users and carers ask for information. Examples of the kind of information include policies regarding charges for services, criteria for eligibility for services and procedures for claiming direct payments. On the worker's side, information may be sought from carers and service users about services, support, wants and preferences.

We need to note in particular the skills of recording, because it feeds into reporting. Good record-keeping is an essential foundation of writing good reports and is central to good practice. Effective review and evaluation both depend on good systems of recording, which itself is a prerequisite of good practice. It is essential to look back and note the assessment and planned goals devised at the start and set these alongside current assessments and planned targets, where these differ. At the same time, there will be information about implementation that has taken place.

While reading this section, you may find it helpful to read Chapter 35 and the Resource File: Quantitative and Qualitative Research, at the end of Chapter 34, because evaluation is an aspect of research. Like other forms of research, evaluation involves weighing up the evidence and reaching a judgement. This is a skill you can acquire through practice.

When you return to this chapter, hopefully you will feel able to consider some of the issues involved in undertaking evaluations of services. For example, following the government's principles of carer and service user involvement threaded through the past four chapters, we can argue that only evaluations involving them should be undertaken. Here is an exercise that tests your skills in weighing up the arguments for and against the related area of researching infant treatments.

Activity 33.1

Spend no more than five minutes jotting down the ethical and scientific arguments for and against trying out a new cancer drug for infants – which is expected to save thousands of lives worldwide – on groups of infants, some of whom are given the new treatment, while others are given a placebo and a third group are given no treatment at all.

You may find it helpful to discuss these arguments with a colleague or in a small group. There are strongly held views on both sides of the argument about whether infants should be used for research. Some people advocate that it is legitimate to do research on people to save lives, just as it is legitimate to use animals as part of laboratory trials to test life-saving drugs. Other people take the view that the permission of the person is necessary first. Obviously, infants cannot be asked to consent, so their parents or guardians will have to be asked on their behalf.

Strictly speaking, traditionalists argue that to be legitimate, the evaluation of practice needs to be based on experimental research methods. In medical research, this usually means random controlled trials (RCTs), which are experiments where patients are randomly allocated to different groups, some of whom receive the drug being tested, some receive a placebo (a neutral substance under the pretence it is the drug), while others are given no treatment and act as a control group. In the example we are considering, some of the infants suffering life-threatening conditions would be denied drugs in order to fulfil the requirements of medical research. There are clear ethical grounds to protest that human rights to treatment and care are being violated, but do the scientific arguments outweigh these?

There is no clear or easy answer to this question. It is a reminder that health and social care practice takes place in a problematic environment, where issues and questions constantly arise that cannot be 'solved'. They are life questions, touching on our own ethical and moral beliefs (see Resource File: Ethical Tensions in Practice, at the end of Chapter 5).

This has been a demanding chapter. Reviews and evaluations are among the most demanding tasks, because a good deal of information has to be collected from different people – colleagues, carers and service users – and because reviewing and evaluating involve making judgements which affect other people's lives.

Conclusion

This chapter has examined the linked but separate activities of reviewing and evaluating practice. We have explored the more restricted role of review and taken note of the wide-ranging character of evaluation. In each situation, it is essential that service users, patients and carers participate as fully as possible.

REVIEW QUESTIONS

1   How does a review differ from an evaluation?

2   What kinds of skills do you need to carry out an evaluation?

3   How may ethical considerations affect evaluation?

FURTHER READING

Cormack, D.F.S. (2000) *The Research Process in Nursing*, Oxford, Blackwell Science

Dempsey, P.A. and Dempsey, A.D. (2000) *Using Nursing Research: Process, Critical Evaluation and Utilization* (5th edn) Baltimore, MD, Lippincott

DoH (1991) *Care Management and Assessment: Practitioner's Guide*, London, HMSO

DoH (1999) *Working Together to Safeguard Children: A Guide to Inter-agency Working to Safeguard and Promote the Welfare of Children*, London, TSO

Uys, L.R. and Gwele, N.S. (eds) (2005) *Curriculum Development in Nursing: Process and Innovations*, London, Routledge

Becoming a Reflective and Research-capable Practitioner

Part V
Becoming a Reflective and Research-capable Practitioner

▌Introduction

Part V is short, but no less important for that. It encourages you to think about the research aspect of your role. It prepares you to be what is sometimes called 'the research-capable' or 'research-minded' practitioner.

Before dealing with research, Part V examines what we mean by reflective and critical practice, giving some examples based on the kinds of assessment tasks you are likely to encounter on a vocational or professional course. The final chapter in Part V deals with the core activity of assuring quality of services, to which the research skills of gathering and analysing information make a crucial contribution.

FURTHER READING

Allott, M. and Robb, M. (eds) (1998) *Understanding Health and Social Care: An Introductory Reader*, London, Sage
A valuable collection of extracts from the experiences of carers, people who use services, researchers and commentators.

Resource file

Evaluating research

In order to make a judgement about the quality of research evidence for practice, you need to be able to carry out a review of the research. Most commonly, the research will be written up in the form of a report or article in a journal. So your review will be what we call a *literature review*. Sometimes a review of the literature will take the form of a long piece of written work examining critically all the references the person can find on a particular topic. In this case, your literature review will be of just one article or report summarising the research. In order to evaluate the research, you need to follow a systematic procedure.

Your purpose

You are carrying out a literature review of one piece of research. You are assessing it from the point of view of its integrity, rigour and usefulness.

What makes a good literature review? It should:

- give a clear picture of what the research is all about
- explain the main features of the research
- analyse the ideas presented in the research report
- examine the strengths and weaknesses of the research.

Where do we start?

First, identify the kind of research it is. Karen Hucker's clearly written book on research in health, care and early years work distinguishes six main ones (Hucker, 2001, pp. 6–7), to which I have added an example in brackets:

- *basic* (researching a topic 'for its own sake'. This could involve writing a history of a voluntary agency, with a view to answering certain key questions such as why it developed in a particular way)
- *applied* (hoping to apply the results to improved practice)
- *strategic* (exploring a new area of policy)

- *scholarly* (examining the effectiveness of a new drug or therapy)
- *creative* (testing the contribution of interior design to recovery rates from illnesses and operations)
- *longitudinal* (following the development of a generation or 'cohort' of babies born on a particular day, or twins born in particular circumstances).

Ingredients of good research

Not all research is equally rigorous or helpful. Good research usually includes the following ingredients:

- *Introduction, summary, synopsis or abstract:* words referring to the brief statement of what the research is about
- *Aims, questions or hypotheses:* what the researchers are trying to find out
- *Methodology:* the theories, perspectives or ideas which underlie the methods
- *Methods:* the techniques used to collect the information, such as interviews or questionnaires
- *Results:* the description of what information was actually collected
- *Analysis or discussion:* discussion and interpretation or explanation of results
- *Conclusions:* a final statement of what has, or hasn't, been achieved
- *Recommendations:* suggested practice implications of the research.

Aims and objectives of the research

- Have you checked out the aims and objectives of the research?
- Have you clarified the actual focus of the research, as opposed to its stated focus in the aims and objectives near the start?
- Do these differ in any ways?
- Did the researchers admit that in some way the research fell short of achieving its aims and objectives?

Methods and methodology of the research

■ Summarise the methods used – were they wholly quantitative, wholly qualitative or a mixture of both? Discuss in your review the relative merits of these, in relation to the research you are reviewing.

■ Are the chosen methods appropriate to the aim of the research?

■ Have the researchers shown convincing evidence to you that they understand method and methodology issues?

■ Have the researchers taken into account the views of patients and/or people who use services and their carers?

Analysis of research issues

■ What limitations were identified by the researchers?

■ Did these undermine the usefulness of the research?

■ What were the findings of the research?

Evaluation of the research

To test the evidence base for practice, ask five questions:

■ Is the study *valid*? There are two aspects to this. *Internal validity* is achieved by the design, that is, the methods chosen. *External validity* means the extent to which generalisations can be made from the findings, that is, their generalisability.

■ Are the results *reliable*? Reliability means consistency, that is, if repeated in the same circumstances, the research would produce the same results each time.

■ Will the results improve practice?

■ Were the conclusions drawn appropriate to the research?

■ How significant and useful were the conclusions?

Remember, if you are a student presenting your review of the research report or article, you may need to show:

■ An understanding of the research process

■ An appreciation of how the research tackled ethical issues, such as researched people being exploited, taken for granted or not having the aims of the research explained to them properly and an opportunity to give, or withhold, informed consent. Informed consent is agreement freely given by the person after they have been given all the facts and potential risks and pitfalls of agreeing

■ You have examined issues of diversity and anti-discriminatory practice

■ You can state your conclusions clearly

■ You can present your bibliography correctly, by using the right convention, for example Harvard (see Resource File: References and Bibliography, at the end of Chapter 44), if you have referred to other publications.

FURTHER READING

Hucker, K. (2001) *Research Methods in Health, Care and Early Years*, Oxford, Heinemann

St Leger, A.S., Schnieden, H. and Walsworth-Bell, J.P. (1993) *Evaluating Health Services' Effectiveness: A Guide for Health Professionals, Service Managers and Policy Makers*, Buckingham, Open University Press

Reflective and Critical Practice

ROBERT ADAMS

Learning outcomes

By the end of this chapter, you should be able to:

- UNDERSTAND what we mean by practice
- DISTINGUISH between reflective and critical practice
- REFLECT critically on a piece of your own practice.

In this chapter we deal with the two words 'reflective' and 'critical', whose meanings often are taken for granted and are explored below. As we have found in discussing the process of the work (Chapter 29), once again we are using words – in this case 'reflective' and 'critical' – commonly used with an everyday meaning but with a more specialised meaning in health and social care work. We begin by defining practice, examining the meanings of the expression 'reflective practice' and go on to discuss its use.

You may find it helpful to refer to the Resource File: Ethical Tensions in Practice, at the end of Chapter 5, while reading this chapter.

What is Practice?

What do we mean by practice? The word has different meanings, some of which are more helpful to us at this point. Practice can have the connotation of doing something that is unfinished and provisional. When we are learning to play a musical instrument, our teacher will introduce us to a new piece which we take away to practise. There is a sense in which much of our work with people has this feeling of being provisional and needing practice. The expression 'practice makes perfect' comes to mind. When we are learning new tasks at work, our line manager or supervisor may suggest we try a new task, with the suggestion that we will learn by doing.

Effective practice involves:

1. *Being aware of the social and cultural context:* It is necessary to develop your awareness of the environment – housing, employment, community characteristics – and culture of the person with whom you are working. Are they from an ethnic group? Do they have particular cultural preferences and needs?
2. *Being aware of ethical issues:* It is necessary to have a developed ethical awareness, that is, an appreciation of connections between tensions, choices and decisions and your situation. For example, does the person's situation raise issues that leave you with some difficult decisions to make, because, whichever way you decide, there will be some gains and some losses?
3. *Being aware of the legal context:* It is important to be aware of the legal responsibilities, duties and powers of your agency or organisation, even though your personal legal obligations and powers may be limited. Do you have an appreciation of the legal basis for work with the person. Do you know the limitations of any legal powers of your employing agency?
4. *Ensuring your practice meets standards and requirements:* Are you sure your work with the person conforms to legal requirements, professional standards and local procedures? Are there any published codes of practice from a relevant professional body you should consider?

In this chapter, we shall be linking the word practice meaning 'doing' with a number of other words. First we introduce the idea of reflection.

What is Reflective Practice?

At its most obvious, reflection is what the silvered glass does when we look into a mirror – it throws our image back at us. Reflection on our practice is the process of examining our work as though we are another person seeing it from an independent viewpoint. Reflection is also a word summarising a complex series of activities, involving us in describing, analysing, interpreting and evaluating. These all feed into what we do next. All this happens more or less continuously while we are working with the person and, taken together, makes up our reflective practice.

As a student, you will be asked to write different pieces of work containing a reflective element. At least one will be a reflective commentary on your practice. This is a piece of writing in which you:

- consider the quality of work you have done
- examine its main features
- evaluate its strengths and weaknesses
- describe any aspect you would have carried out differently.

Here are two examples, not of the students' reflective commentaries themselves, but of the markers' notes on them. Read them through carefully.

Marker of weak student A
This reflective commentary shows:

- Poor use of material. Failing to make links between different forms of family violence and social policy, which shapes the situation the student was discussing.
- A tendency to regurgitate relevant facts and describe policies rather than make critical links with social work. A lack of application to practice.
- Lack of analysis in report despite 'wonderful' facts.
- Theories quoted but lack conviction and need embedding in the work. Lack of integration of theory with practice.
- A lack of detail in descriptions of the work done, so it is more difficult to judge claims of competence.
- Often, the descriptions of work done are very generalised, too descriptive and superficial.
- Little evidence presented of the process of assessment, planning, implementation and review of the case.
- A lack of critical analysis.
- A worrying tendency to write about the practice as though the 'care' role is about 'mothering' at the expense of professional work with the service user and carer.
- No self-awareness and no element of self-criticism anywhere in the reflective commentary.

Marker of strong student B
This reflective commentary shows that the student:

- Has brought together the complexities of the subject.
- Has drawn on policies, legislation, organisational settings and sociological as well as psychological perspectives.
- Appreciates the ethical and value components of the work.
- Can manage working with people within time constraints and in different practice settings.
- Can cope with the practicalities of the process of assessment, planning, implementation/intervention and review/evaluation.
- Has used supervision well.
- Has an active rather than a passive process of working with the service user and carer.
- Has gone well beyond descriptive work to analysis and linking ideas with personal and professional development issues.

Activity 34.1

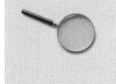

Having read the above, list the main weaknesses of student A and main strengths of student B highlighted by the two markers.

There is not space here to go through the notes and comment in detail, but hopefully, the comparison has enabled you to understand what reflective practice entails.

Being Reflective in our own Practice

Our prior learning and experiences influence how we work with people. We can use our own experiences to inform our work with other people.

Practice study

Kerri

Kerri's husband abused her for many years and, when she left him, he committed suicide after murdering their only son, aged 11.

■ Spend a few minutes reflecting on Kerri's circumstances.

Before proceeding, we need to discuss 'reflection'. The word reflection has many meanings and its use in health and social care is influenced by these. We may look in a mirror and see our reflection, but may look in a window or pool of water and find it distorted and fractured. Reflection is more than a reaction, which implies simply an immediate, gut response, and is probably more useful when it is informed reflection. By this we mean the reflective practitioner does at least three things:

■ thinks in a purposeful way about current work with the service user and carer
■ draws on previous experience of work with others
■ makes links with knowledge of theories, approaches and methods of practice.

We need to be clear about what reflective practice is not. Reflective practice may overlap with effective practice but the two do not necessarily correspond. After all, the worker may decide after careful reflection that the work done was not particularly useful to the service user and did not achieve the desired outcomes of either the service user or the worker.

In order to be reflective, we must have confidence in our ability to think. Thinking, as Yelloly and Henkel (1995, p. 8) note, is often avoided by filling one's time:

in such a way as to minimise the powerful and distressing impact of the work; indeed sometimes the organisational structures themselves seem almost designed to keep pain at bay and to prevent thought.

It is important to recognise that the worker may encounter distressing situations requiring a thoughtful appraisal and a caring, yet professional response. However, the agency may have put procedures in place which make it possible to avoid bringing one's uniquely personal response into the situation and using it to help to decide what to do and how to act. Yelloly and Henkel (1995, p. 9) point out that 'routinised responses and procedures (though an essential framework for action) can also lead to a rigidity which is inimical to the uniquely personal response needed in the caring professions'.

The implications of being reflective need to be faced. Reflection is a challenge. It involves challenging the service user and carer and it is challenging for the practitioner. The essence of the challenge lies in the implications of reflection for change. It is likely that the service user, carer and the practitioner will face changes as a consequence of interacting with each other. In one sense, we would expect change to be part and parcel of everyday work in health and social care. Yet we have to be realistic. Change is often uncomfortable at the very least and may often involve major disruption, as people's assumptions and beliefs are thrown into doubt and their daily practices questioned. Change is also likely to involve losses and these can heighten anxieties.

Practice study

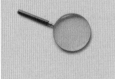

Kerri (cont'd)

When dealing with Kerri's response to her catastrophic bereavements, I draw on my own past grief when my mother and sister died at an early age. I recall how I tried to carry on working on a day-to-day basis, blocking out the feelings of loss and incomprehension.

Reflexivity

When we discussed using our emotional responses to the work situation above, we were referring to *reflexivity*. This is the process of using our own thoughts and feelings in response to the situation we are facing, to help us understand what the other person is going through. Hopefully, we can keep our response under control, because if it overwhelms us we shall not retain the necessary independence to be able to work effectively with the service user. For reflexivity to work effectively, we have to be able to maintain a balance between sensitive self-awareness and detachment.

Practice study

Kerry (cont'd)

Kerri came to the women's refuge, still suicidal herself. The shop where she worked refused to employ her after her story became newspaper headlines. The worker at the refuge engaged in advocacy, supporting her through the process of an industrial tribunal, thereby helping her to challenge the prejudice underlying this response to her.

Part V

Using Supervision

Supervision is a system enabling the practitioner to be supported in and receive critical feedback on the work by a line manager, colleague or other person.

In reflecting on the dramas of Kerri's life, I was even more aware than usual of my need for supervision. I benefit from it directly because it enables me to maintain independence and professionalism while remaining sensitive and aware. Indirectly, Kerri benefits because any emotional baggage in my head is cleared out to enable me to focus more objectively and yet creatively on her problems.

It is helpful to distinguish between informal and formal supervision. Informal supervision refers to all those ad hoc, accidental or off the cuff ways in which I chat on the phone or face to face with my supervisor about some aspect of the work. Formal supervision is a planned sequence of regular meetings, with a negotiated structure to enable both the supervisor and the person supervised to examine and evaluate the work and its implications for them and other stakeholders in it.

Activity 34.2

Jot down half a dozen ways in which formal supervision can help you.

Supervision can:

- help the process of reflection
- offer a regular place where you can request, receive and give feedback
- provide you with tools to help you reflect
- help your professional, and personal, development
- enable you to manage and monitor your own learning
- enable you to learn about yourself and where you are coming from
- enable you to set goals for where you are going.

Demonstrating you can Reflect on your Practice

It is difficult to teach ourselves how to make the jump from simply behaving in a particular way to reflecting systematically on it. On the other hand, it is possible to practise writing reflectively about your practice and this is more than halfway to the goal of becoming reflective. In this section, we explore how you can write reflectively about your practice.

This is an example of the first attempt of a student on a Foundation Degree in Health and Social Care to write reflectively about her practice:

I applied to take an evening class A level in sociology because I was interested in politics and wanted to know more about poverty. When I started the course, I realised it was more about inequality, the family and society. I became interested in social care and started to do voluntary work in a housing charity ... I have found work with homeless people very challenging ... I have questioned many of my beliefs and assumptions about homelessness and homeless people ...

Last year I decided to work full time for the voluntary organisation and applied for a paid position ... I registered to take the Foundation Degree in Health and Social Care.

Activity 34.3

Read the following checklist of the six stages involved in writing a reflective note about your practice and take 10 minutes to list what you think is missing from the above reflective note.

- Stage 1: Identify a piece of your practice
- Stage 2: Practise jotting down some brief notes about the practice
- Stage 3: Put your practice in its wider context. Briefly summarise details about the agency, its location, 'clients' and main working methods
- Stage 4: Give a brief description of your practice
- Stage 5: Write a reflective review of your practice
  - Illustrate how you have used supervision sessions
  - Discuss the interaction between your work and your values
  - Discuss your learning
- Stage 6: Show how you have integrated theory into your practice.

Critical Practice

Practice study

Daniel

Daniel is an African Caribbean man in his mid-twenties, who, having been abused by a neighbour in his early teens, ran away from home and lost contact with his parents. He became a male prostitute in London, eventually returning to Yorkshire after being seriously injured in one of a series of racist attacks in the neighbourhood where he lived. The police pursued inquiries and eventually charged him with sexual assault, leading to his conviction. Daniel became a schedule 1 offender, which entails him being listed on the sex offenders' register.

In working with him as a volunteer in a hostel, Len found his own responses required self-monitoring. He tended to be judgemental and to relate much of what happened to his feelings about his own teenage son. Also, the local press were running letters from residents complaining about the hostel, using the argument that 'these people shouldn't be allowed in the community'.

Len developed a more self-critical approach after several supervision sessions with his manager in the hostel, where he learned to be more critical about his practice. He learned that some aspects of the work raise issues that cannot be resolved but have to be coped with or managed. The most important of these for him was the tension between working supportively with Daniel, at the same time as monitoring his move-

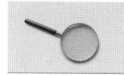

ments and behaviour, because he was regarded as potentially a threat to young males. Len found it challenging, as on the one hand Daniel was a survivor of abuse, while on the other hand he was an abuser himself.

Components of Critical Practice

1. *Contextualising:* This means the activity of relating Daniel's particular circumstances to his immediate family and environment and appreciating the cultural factors which are part of that unique setting.
2. *Ethical issues:* This entails taking account of any particular ethical tensions and dilemmas that arise in working with Daniel (see Resource File: Ethical Tensions in Practice, at the end of Chapter 5).
3. *Legal aspects:* This involves taking into account any requirements arising from legislation applying to the case.
4. *Standards and procedures:* This involves practising in line with national standards and local procedures.

Conclusion

When we work reflectively and critically, we think as we practise and we are prepared to admit continually that we have made mistakes and continue to make them. The important thing is not how many mistakes we make but ensuring we learn from them. It is important to use our reflective and critical skills to improve our practice, rather than carrying on doing more of the same, shrugging our shoulders and saying that because of factors beyond our control we are unable to do anything to change the way we are working.

REVIEW QUESTIONS

1 What are the main differences between being reflective and being reflexive?

2 What are the main differences between being critical and being self-critical?

3 What is contextualising?

FURTHER READING

Banks, S. (2004) *Ethics, Accountability and the Social Professions,* Basingstoke, Palgrave Macmillan

Brechin, A. (2000) 'Introducing Critical Practice', in A. Brechin, H. Brown and M.A. Eby (eds) *Critical Practice in Health and Social Care,* London, Sage, pp. 25–47

Bulman, C. and Schutz, S. (2004) *Reflective Practice in Nursing,* Oxford, Blackwell

Ghaye, T. (2006) *Learning Journals and Critical Incidents: Reflective Practice for Health Care Professionals,* London, Quay Books

Martyn, H. (2000) *Developing Reflective Practice: Making Sense of Social Work in the World of Change,* Bristol, Policy Press

Schön, D. (1983) *The Reflective Practitioner: How Professionals Think in Action*, New York, Basic Books

Schön, D. (1987) *Educating the Reflective Practitioner*, San Francisco, Jossey-Bass

Scrutton, S. (1999) *Counselling Older People*, London, Arnold

Taylor, B.J. (2000) *Reflective Practice: A Guide for Nurses and Midwives*, Buckingham, Open University Press

WEBSITES: www.iassw.soton.ac.uk/generic
www.scie.org.uk/publications/knowledgereviews
These are useful websites for international codes of practice.

Resource file

Quantitative and qualitative research

There are two main types of approaches to collecting research information or data: quantitative and qualitative.

Quantitative data is information collected by counting and calculating. So, quantitative data is in number form. This has the advantage that numbers can be totalled and various mathematical methods can be used to assess the trustworthiness of the data. This is called significance, a word with a precise mathematical meaning.

Qualitative data tends to be more descriptive. It is most commonly seen in case studies. We should remember that qualitative data can be combined with quantitative data. For example, it is possible to describe individual cases of financial abuse in a residential home and then total them, to distinguish between the people in terms of their age, gender and race and whether they are experiencing physical or sensory impairment, or learning disability.

In general, the *advantages of quantitative approaches* are that they enable us to:

- total up and measure data
- apply statistical tests which tell us whether the results are significant
- assume that, if they are significant, the results can be generalised to the population as a whole.

The *advantages of qualitative approaches* include enabling us to:

- delve into the detail of individual people's experiences
- reach a more profound understanding of complex situations
- study a single or small number of cases where it isn't important to generalise our findings.

FURTHER READING

Berg, B. (2006) *Qualitative Research Methods for the Social Sciences* (6th edn) Boston, Allyn & Bacon

Macnee, C.L. and McCabe, S. (2007) *Understanding Nursing Research: Using Research as Evidence-Based Practice*, Philadephia, PA, Lippincott, Williams & Wilkins

Part V

35 Research Perspectives in Health and Social Care

TONY LONG

Learning outcomes

By the end of this chapter, you should:

■ HAVE a basic knowledge of the nature of research

■ UNDERSTAND some of the main complications arising in doing research

■ APPRECIATE what is involved in carrying out ethical research.

What is Research?

How do we know what we know? Well, that may seem like a simple question, but it really isn't. Most of us can swim and ride a bike (not at the same time, of course), but how do we know how to do that? Well, these were things that we had to try in order to be able to do them. We might have had swimming lessons, but nobody ever learned to swim without getting in the water and thrashing around a little trying to stay afloat. Most of us learned to ride a bike by wobbling along with someone shouting that they were still holding on to us. Knowledge learned in this way is *experiential knowledge* – learning by doing.

Sometimes there are things that we all know. How? Well, we just know, that's all. How do you know that spiders are more frightened of us than we are of them? If anyone has ever asked them, they can't have received a reply. Such *mutual knowledge* is part of everyday life and it is something that we acquire through childhood and belonging to groups.

Another form of knowledge is *formal knowledge*, and this is where research comes in. We wouldn't want someone to design the plane we fly in to go on holiday by just having a go and seeing what happens. Nor would we be happy for a group of people to agree that wings should be designed in a particular way because they all think that it seems about right. (Try asking some friends to talk about something that you all know about, and see just how different your understandings are of what is thought to be common or mutual knowledge.) Experiential knowledge and mutual knowledge sometimes are not enough. We need to be more certain of the knowledge we apply in many instances – including in the application of health and social care. We need to be sure that an intervention will bring about a specific physiological or psychological reaction in a patient or client, and so we need to base our actions on stronger evidence and more convincing data. Formal knowledge, then, arises from research.

There are many definitions of research, but generally they all agree that research should be systematic and rigorous, add to a body of knowledge, answer questions, solve problems or guide changes in behaviour or policy. Sometimes research is designed to find specific answers to local problems, sometimes to bring about change on a grand scale through generalisable findings, or simply to add to a general field of science without any specific application in mind. Whatever the purpose, good research depends upon sound design, rigorous processes and clear communication of the findings.

Research Design

There are many methods used to collect data for research purposes, and there is also much academic debate on notions of research paradigms and the quantitative–qualitative debate – issues relating to the theoretical bases for research. On the whole, these need not concern us too much here, and a brief explanation will suffice.

Quantitative Designs

Many aspects of life, nature, science and the world generally can be measured, counted or otherwise quantified. We can count how many people smoke. We can measure the average height of 16-year-olds over succeeding years. We can record the blood sugar levels of diabetic patients at varying times during the day. We can also record numerical values for the degree of anxiety that clients may feel, or the amount of pain that someone feels after an operation. You may have realised that the last two cannot be measured directly (milligrams of pain or centimetres of anxiety, perhaps), but they are attributes that can be expressed and converted into measurements. One way, for example, is to ask a patient to draw a line on a scale from 0 to 9 to indicate the amount of pain they feel (see Figure 35.1). The distance from one end can then be measured and compared with a reading 30 minutes after the administration of a painkilling drug.

Circle or mark the box

No pain at all	0	1	2	3	4	5	6	7	8	9	As much pain as I can bear

Put a mark through the line to indicate the degree of pain

No pain at all		As much pain as I can bear

Figure 35.1 'Measuring' pain

Qualitative Designs

Sometimes and in varying circumstances we may be interested in understanding more about a client's perspective on their situation, for example how a parent copes with a baby who won't stop crying, or how looked after young people see their experiences of social services care affecting their offending behaviour. These things might be quantifiable, but it makes sense to gather more varied data, which is less given to measurement but allows for richer description of the issues and expression of the individual's thoughts and feelings in their own terms. It may be more difficult to find ways to work with such data (especially, for example, with children), but the results can be particularly worthwhile.

Activity 35.1

Reflect for a few minutes and jot down notes on two or three areas you would consider most appropriate to research using (a) quantitative methods and (b) qualitative methods.

Here are my thoughts. The fact is that both approaches have a place in health and social care research. The key is to know which to use and when, and this depends on what we are trying to achieve. To demonstrate most convincingly that one action or stimulus causes another, we should employ quantitative methods, for example to evaluate how two alternative drugs do, or do not, improve a person's health. To understand more about the context of a situation and learn more about people's reactions, thoughts and values, we will more often use qualitative methods, for example to explore what a person feels and experiences when caring for a close relative, 7 days a week, 24 hours a day.

Methods of Data Collection

There are as many means of designing a study and collecting data as our imaginations allow us to conceive. Traditional methods such as experiments, interviewing and questionnaires have been joined by the interpretation of paintings, sculpture and drama, and, in the electronic age, by surveys using texts and emails. There is space here for only a brief overview of some of these methods.

Interviews

Perhaps the most natural of all methods is to hold a conversation with someone else to ascertain their views about an issue. This is the basis of the interview and it is something that most of us need to be skilled at in order to fulfil our normal roles in health and social care. Interviews may be carried out with a single individual or a group – perhaps as a focus group. We may plan a series of interviews with the same respondent to check for changes in perception or reaction throughout the duration of an experience. Interviewing has the advantage of the researcher being able to pick up on non-verbal clues in the respondent's behaviour, expression and tone of voice.

These may all lend additional meaning to what is being said. Unfortunately, this can also be one of the weaknesses of interviewing. We often see and perceive things erroneously, misinterpreting these unspoken messages. If the respondent doesn't understand the question, we can rephrase it or repeat it, and the same choice is open to the researcher if they don't understand the reply. So interviews can be particularly varied in nature and purpose, addressing a wide range of topics. We often have the basic skills (although these need to be enhanced for sound research) and a great deal of rich data can be gained.

Questionnaires

Another method of data collection with which we are all familiar is the questionnaire – often as a form of survey. Questionnaires may take many forms – brief customer satisfaction cards in fast-food outlets, pages of close-typed questions in the paperwork delivered with new electrical goods, online surveys filled in on the internet or those completed by market researchers stopping us in the street. Whatever the form, the general aim is to attract a large number of responses, quickly, and often from far-flung geographical areas. There are several advantages to using questionnaires in research. They are easy to disseminate – postal questionnaires can be delivered to addresses almost anywhere in mainland Britain usually by the next day and only for the cost of a stamp.

A wide range of individuals and groups can be targeted, although a word of caution is needed here. We all have a habit of not returning at least some of the questionnaires we receive, and it is important that non-return is not a random process. We are more likely to respond to a questionnaire if we feel strongly about its content, for example. It would be a mistake to think that the responses are necessarily representative of the whole group to which they were sent. Other problems are that questions (and, indeed, answers) which appear ambiguous cannot be clarified, and however carefully we design a questionnaire to lead the respondent through in an orderly fashion, individuals often have a habit of disassembling the order before answering. Most of the work in using questionnaires lies in getting the design right, ensuring that questions ask what we mean them to ask, and amending ambiguous or leading questions. A classic mistake, for example, is to ask how many bedrooms there are in a house in order to establish something about the size of a house and the owner's wealth. Think about this. Does a bedroom converted into a playroom still count? How many newly built houses now have much smaller bedrooms than older houses? No wonder it has been said that the questionnaire is the hardest form of data collection instrument to get right.

Experiments

The classical way to conduct research is the experiment. Experiments are designed to test hypotheses or suggested relationships between variables. This leads to convincing evidence of causality: that a specific action causes a specific outcome to occur. Drugs are tested through experimental research in order to ensure that giving a drug (the stimulus) consistently causes another event, for example the alleviation of pain or the reduction of blood pressure. In such cases, it is vital to be as sure as possible that research findings could not have happened by chance, and statistical tests are used to check this. This usually implies that a large number of research subjects need to be included. Exhaustive efforts are made to ensure that only the chosen variables are involved and that a third factor could not have exerted an effect instead of the intended stimulus.

The strengths of experiments may be readily apparent, but there are weaknesses, too. It is difficult to measure human responses experimentally: human irrationality can simply be too strong, and our physical and psychological responses simply too complex to be reduced to variables that can be manipulated in the experiment. The results of experiments, necessarily undertaken away from the complexity of real life, may not translate effectively to the reality of health and social care situations.

Observation

While observation can be particularly difficult to do well, it is also an especially adaptable approach. In everyday life we rely on observation a great deal. We watch people and their reactions as well as listening to what they say. We take note of what is going on around a conversation or interaction and the circumstances in which behaviour is acted out. This complexity forms the reality of the situation, but also makes the objective collection of data rather more troublesome.

Some years ago there was a TV ad for a newspaper in which a city gentleman was seen apparently running away from a rough-looking thug. As the drama unfolded, the thug made a leap for the city gentleman – presumably to wrestle him to the ground and steal his wallet and briefcase. No. In fact, the 'thug' was pushing the other man out of the way of falling masonry, saving his life at considerable danger to himself. The caption was 'Things are not always as they seem.' How true that is. We may think that we observe an uncaring assistant forcing an infirm resident to make decisions and care for himself, yet what is actually happening is that the assistant is encouraging recovery and the gradual regaining of independence. It is always difficult in observational research to remain objective – to see what is there rather than what we interpret as happening.

Despite this, observation helps us to see past people's beliefs about their behaviour and to recognise what is actually done. Currently there is a major problem with MRSA in hospitals and other caring establishments. Effective hand washing is held to be the main strategy to overcome this. Ask doctors, nurses, porters and others if they wash their hands as often and as effectively as they should, and most will answer that they do (and they will believe it). Watch what actually happens. We often can't believe the things we do until, or even when, shown the evidence on film.

Mixing Methods

Some of the problems in health and social care require that we seek answers to different parts of the topic through different methods all within the same study. In a study examining the preparation of nurses to care for children with cancer, documentary analysis was used to establish how the competence of the nurses was intended to be assessed, then assessors and students were interviewed to find out what processes were actually used, and finally interactions between nurses and child patients were videotaped to be scrutinised by an expert panel to decide what attributes ought to be considered in future (Sanderson et al., 2004).

Research Governance and Ethics

Inappropriate behaviour on the part of researchers at various times (for example the Tuskegee study of black men with syphilis that ran from 1932 to 1972, or the more recent scandal of the retention of organs by Alder Hey children's hospital) has led to mechanisms to protect human research subjects.

Respect for Individuals

The key to acting in an ethically appropriate manner in research is to maintain respect for individuals. In large part this is based on accepting that people who are able to make decisions about themselves for themselves should be both encouraged and allowed to do so. Most adults (and many children, even though very young) are able to process information about their potential participation in a research study and come to a rational decision about their choices. This is known as *competence*.

Vulnerable People

Some individuals and groups are more vulnerable than others to having this right denied or to being unable to engage in the rational processes needed for competence. One of these has already been identified – children and young people. Others might include some (but not all) older people, some people with mental illness and some with degenerative or traumatic illness. Individuals from ethnic groups whose first language is not English may be more vulnerable, as might anyone in a subordinate position to the researcher (perhaps students as research subjects for their lecturer). Particular attention is needed to provide information in a form that is accessible to the specific group or individual and to ensure that sufficient effort is put into facilitating their understanding and expression of choice.

Informed Consent

Once potential research participants have received sufficient information about the study and any associated risks in a form they can understand, they are asked to confirm their consent to be included. Participants usually sign a consent form to provide evidence of this, but they are still free to withdraw from the study at any time without risking adverse changes to their care or services. Sometimes, when a study is conducted over a long period of time, the ongoing nature of consent has to be checked periodically by the researcher (see Resource File: Life Experiences and Biographical Research, at the end of this chapter).

Part V

Confidentiality

Respecting individuals also involves respecting their right to privacy. Details of participants in research studies usually remain confidential to the researcher, and to prevent accidental disclosure, these are stored separately from the data. In this way an individual's name or other personal data cannot be linked with what they have said or what was observed about them. This might be important, for example if disclosure of what one individual said were to be divulged to their employer. As more varied forms of data are collected (video, photographs and so on), researchers face additional problems of how to store data securely and how to dispose of it safely at the end of a study.

The Research Ethics Committee

Under many circumstances, research with humans in health or social care is now subject to approval by a research ethics committee. Such committees are made up of professionals and lay members, and they scrutinise proposals submitted by researchers before the study is allowed to begin. More information about this can be found at the website of the Central Office for Research Ethics Committees (COREC).

Research Governance

In addition to the attention of the research ethics committee, research in the NHS or social services is subject to review and ongoing monitoring through research governance procedures managed by NHS Trusts and social services departments. This ensures that accurate records are kept of the conduct of the study, the researchers themselves are screened before being allowed to access patients or clients, and appropriate insurance and other safeguards are provided in case of untoward incidents or unforeseen outcomes.

Activity 35.2

Spend a few minutes making notes on the particular benefits you think arise from practitioners using research into health and social care service.

| Conclusion

Research is an important means to enhance our knowledge and to find solutions to problems locally, nationally and even globally. It contributes to the improvement of services, enables us to find out which forms of practice give most benefit to people who use services and helps us to know how best to conduct ourselves as professionals in health and social care.

REVIEW QUESTIONS

1 What are experiential, mutual and formal knowledge?

2 How do the three sources of knowledge feed into your work?

3 How do quantitative and qualitative research differ from each other?

4 Which aspects of information about your patients, clients or residents can be measured?

5 What sorts of details or attributes about your patients, clients or residents cannot be measured and by what means can this data be gathered?

6 What could you learn about your colleagues' behaviour by observation, interviewing or administering a questionnaire?

7 What factors about your patient or client group would make them vulnerable as research subjects? What would the researcher need to do to protect them from harm?

FURTHER READING

Gerrish, K. and Lacey, A. (2006) *The Research Process in Nursing* (5th edn) London, Blackwell
   A good general introduction to the whole of the research process.

McLaughlin, H. (2006) *Understanding Social Work Research: Key Issues and Concepts*, London, Sage

RCN (2004) *Research Ethics: Guidance for Nurses*, London, RCN, www.rcn.org.uk
   Includes a wide range of electronic resources and further reading.

WEBSITES: http://www.npr.org/programs/morning/features/2002/jul/tuskegee/
   A brief resource about the Tuskegee research study.

   http://www.rlcinquiry.org.uk/
   The Alder Hey retention of organs inquiry.

RESOURCE FILE: Life Experiences and Biographical Research, below, and Chapter 40 on empowering approaches to research

Resource file

Life experiences and biographical research

It is easy to talk about collecting people's memories and experiences, but doing it properly is complex and raises serious ethical questions to be answered. We begin with the account written for this book by Dave Fountain.

My name is Dave Fountain. I am 40 years old. I was a former instructor in first aid weapons and drill in the army, when just over four years ago I had a cerebral haemorrhage. Before that, I've always

regarded myself as fit and kept myself fit. When I collapsed I was suffering from a 'nine-day-old headache'. I had my brain haemorrhage (subarachnoid anneurism) on 25 March 2000. I was in a coma for exactly (date wise) four months. Later, I had meningitis, peritonitis and I caught MRSA in hospital. Luckily I was fit and stubborn, which got me through.

When I first came here (Victoria House, Hull) four years ago, I didn't want to be thought of as disabled and I didn't want to be here at all. Then I thought it would be for a short time. I've accepted it now and am even able to help other people. For example, I help some with their art and so on. In the army, I was an instructor and when I left I got a report stating I'd be able to teach. At Victoria House lately I've been able to use what I learned. For instance, at a recent 'ability day' I demonstrated how to pot up plants.

I get a lot more satisfaction from things now. Before, I had a number of problems, including memory problems and 'temper tantrums'. Twelve months ago, I wasn't the hopeful person I am now. I used to have the 'why me' syndrome. It was like a bereavement. I'd lost my career in the army and my life. I used to go running every night before the haemorrhage. I drew a picture for Iris, the art therapist at Lincoln. I drew my dog, backwards. I don't know if this was a bit of autism. I wanted to say 'My best buddy Tex'. She spoke posh and she wrote 'Tex, a much loved friend'.

People who have helped me with my problems include the following.

My mum who came as soon as I was ill and still continues to visit me regularly and looks after my little dog Tex.

Merv my step-dad, who very sadly died recently.

My son Stuart, then aged 13, and daughter Sam, then aged 11, who ran for help when I became ill.

Pearl, the retired staff nurse next door, who threw me into the car and drove me to hospital at Barnstaple without waiting for the ambulance.

The air ambulance crew who airlifted me to Derriford Hospital, Plymouth.

The Italian brain surgeon who treated me for the cerebral haemorrhage and the abcess on the side of my brain, which I got after my operation.

The hospital staff at Plymouth and Nottingham, who also helped me subsequently overcome peritonitis, meningitis and MRSA.

Linda and Kelly, physiotherapists at Ashby Rehabilitation Ward, St George's Hospital, Lincoln. Instead of saying 'you've got to do that', they used humour with me. They helped me to walk again. When I lost confidence walking, Linda would say 'there goes your bottle, over there.' When she was trying to help me to straighten my arm, she'd say 'come on.' I'd say, 'I'm trying, I'm trying', and she'd say 'yes, very trying.' I've almost got full movement back in my arm now, whereas before it was almost impossible to move it.

The patient transport driver who brought me from Lincoln to Victoria House, Hull, four years ago and asked me to lie down rather than telling me. I agreed to it, for the sake of his peace of mind.

The care staff at Victoria House. They have helped me by being nice, even when I didn't want to be nice to anybody! There's Diane who's always straight and upfront, Esther who's straight in your face. They're what I need. I don't want people messing around. Clare and Andy, assistant managers, and Richard, general manager, at Victoria House. They chat to me and tell me when I have to do things. They tell me off when I get out of hand.

Julie, the activities coordinator at Victoria House. I was festering three years ago. I'd lost control of my life. I was under the impression I would only be at Victoria House for a short time. Then I broke my foot and was back in a wheelchair for six weeks. I more or less stayed in bed all day, because I felt very depressed. I was more or less nocturnal. Julie got me up and about again and helped to bring my feet back on the ground. She organised Changes Workshop, the IT learning shop. I had to get up for that, one morning a week. It was a struggle. We had one or two set-tos. Through that, I found out I was interested in animals and horticulture. Then we started going to Miresbeck. It's a nursery run as a charity. It was awesome. Julie went with me to the nursery at first. I go there and work at my own pace. We get silver and gold awards at various flower shows. All of us do what we need to do, but if someone doesn't feel too good, they can have time out.

I used to carry a walking stick when I went out. It was lack of confidence. My confidence has grown. I walk independently now and I can almost straighten my left arm. I feel more able to talk to people and I'm not so angry with people any more. I have tackled my problems by reading, listening to 'audio books' and talking to/with members of my family, members of staff and residents at my 'home'.

I still want to do more. I would particularly like help to gain the majority of my confidence back again.

I have completed a one-day course in food hygiene and hope soon to finish my 'seedlings' horticulture course. My next plan is to pass my computer literacy and information technology (CLAIT) course, which I am presently studying, and pass my horticulture NVQ (level one).

Since I wrote this in 2004, I moved into minimum assistance housing and am now living much more independently.

Preparing these life experiences

What is the story behind Dave's written experiences? Dave had expressed an interest to staff at Victoria House Hull, run by the Disabilities Trust and offering respite and permanent accommodation to 24 people with physical disabilities, in writing his life story. I visited him at Victoria House several times and offered to help him edit the work he had already done. He agreed and we worked together to produce the above account for this book. We had to discuss and decide how far we could identify real people he wanted to mention and whether he wanted his full name to appear alongside his life story. We met again in his bungalow after he left Victoria House, and he made final alterations to his written account. The entire process took 18 months. Last weekend he received the contract from the publishers and we met and talked about it before he signed it. He is very pleased with the result. I am relieved about this, mainly because I want him not to regret it.

Life experiences and biographical research

At a recent meeting of two university staff with a dozen service users and carers, we decided to go round the room with each person talking for two minutes about how he or she had come to be at the meeting. None of us planned or scripted our statement in advance. We planned in advance to tape record the meeting, using a digital recorder placed in the centre of the table. We asked permission from each individual to do this and to transcribe (type out) the tape recording for subsequent use in some learning materials on participation and empowerment, the contents of which the group are reviewing critically as they are developed. None of the materials will be used unless the person concerned is happy to give informed consent afterwards, having read the transcript and had a proper chance to alter or scrap it.

Apart from being meaningful in itself, this meeting was a learning experience for all of us and, with a lot of powerful emotions and memories recalled, was very moving. Afterwards we agreed that next time we should have the chance to prepare our thoughts before speaking.

Practitioners need to value the life stories of people who use services and their carers. They have many uses, not least in reminiscence work with people who are likely to benefit from journeying back into their past. The gathering of people's life stories (some people prefer the word 'experiences' to 'stories', because stories may not be real and may not be told adult to adult) relates to qualitative research methodology and draws on skills of oral history-taking and biographical research. Biographical methods can be used in health and social care to prepare autobiographies, anthologies and life storybooks and can contribute a 'bottom-up', 'grass-roots' or user perspective (Bornat and Walmsley, 2004, p. 223), as well as being empowering for the person offering the information. The technical sound of some of the above terms should not put off students and practitioners from trying these approaches, as long as we bear in mind that, like many powerful tools, they can be used with varying degrees of skill, with varying results. It is best to talk first to somebody – a colleague or tutor – who is experienced and who can suggest ways of preparing before gathering the story and can offer support or supervision. Often, we only have one chance to take a life story. With hindsight, we may greatly regret not having asked the person's permission to tape record it, or to use it and may regret not having planned in advance a list of areas of the person's life to prompt for further memories.

Biographical research

Neither of the above examples is 'pure' research. But what is 'pure' research? I would say these are two types of collaborative research. I responded to Dave's interest in writing and what he was writing fitted into this book. The group exercise with the group and the tape recorder was linked with producing learning materials but may or may not lead to this, depending on what individual group members decide. Normally, before research involving collecting biographical data about people begins, approval has to be sought from an ethics committee or similar body. One stage of this should involve seeking written permission from the subjects (people you approach for information). The ethics committee will need reassurance that:

- subjects have given 'informed consent'
- subjects understand what the data (information) will be used for
- tape recordings or notes will be stored in a secure container
- after a maximum of, say, five years, they will be destroyed.

FURTHER READING

On oral history

Thompson, P. (2000) *The Voice of the Past* (3rd edn) Oxford, Oxford University Press

On biographical methods

Bytheway, B. and Johnson, J. (2002) 'Doing Diary Based Research', in A. Jamieson and C. Victor (eds) *Researching Ageing and Later Life: The Practice of Social Gerontology*, Buckingham, Open University Press, pp. 155–74

Chamberlayne, P., Bornat, J. and Apitzsch, U. (2004) (eds) *Biographical Methods and Professional Practice: An International Perspective*, Bristol, Policy Press

Johnson, J. (ed.) (2004) *Writing Old Age*, London, Centre for Policy on Ageing

Quality Assurance of Practice

ROBERT ADAMS

Learning outcomes

By the end of this chapter, you should be able to:

■ DEFINE quality assurance

■ PUT quality assurance in health and social care in its policy and legal context

■ ILLUSTRATE how quality assurance operates

■ DESCRIBE how complaints and whistleblowing contribute to quality assurance.

You may like to refer to the Resource File: Making a Complaint/Whistleblowing, at the end of the chapter, and Resource File: Dealing with a Complaint, at the end of Chapter 52, while reading this chapter.

Since the early 1990s, through a succession of inquiries into incidents where patients and service users have suffered, increasing pressure has been put on the NHS and social services departments to rectify shortcomings in services. Methods of quality assurance imported from industry have been adapted to the health and social services and used to assess the extent to which they measure up to standards published by the Department of Health. This chapter deals with the procedures and processes of assuring the quality of these services. We begin with a definition:

> Quality assurance refers to the systematic process of verifying that the product or service is being delivered according to a specified benchmark or standard.

Legal and Policy Context

On 1 April 2004, the Commission for Social Care Inspection (CSCI), created under the Health and Social Care (Community Health and Standards) Act 2003, became the single inspectorate for social care in England. It incorporated the whole of the former Social Services Inspectorate, the SSI/Audit Commission Joint Review Team and the National Care Standards Commission (NCSC). The Healthcare Commission (HCC) replaced the Commission for Health Improvement, took over the Audit Commission's responsibilities for the efficiency, effectiveness and cost-effectiveness of healthcare, and took over the private and voluntary healthcare tasks of the NCSC. The HCC is responsible for assessing public and private health services in England and replaces the routine inspections of NHS Trusts with inspection where there is an evident problem, and requires providers to review their performance and publish statements of their performance.

The HCC:

- replaces the routine inspections of NHS Trusts in England with inspection, where an evident problem needs investigation
- assesses public and private health services
- requires providers to review how they have performed and publish statements of their performance
- deals with complaints about the NHS that have not been resolved locally
- assesses and reports annually on the performance of organisations providing healthcare
- gives NHS Trusts an annual performance rating.

It also produces reports based on surveys and inspections of particular aspects, such as the first independent inspections of hospital cleanliness in England and the census of hospital admissions showing that black African and Caribbean people are three times more likely to be admitted to hospital and more than 40 per cent more likely to be detained under the Mental Health Act 1983, both published in December 2005.

The powers of the CSCI are granted by the Care Standards Act 2000 and the Health and Social Care (Community Health and Standards) Act 2003 and include:

- promoting improved social care services (CSCI, 2004)
- registering and inspecting services against national standards
- inspecting social care for adults and children in the public, private and voluntary sectors
- inspecting local authority social services against 'value for money', giving star ratings
- taking enforcement action when services fall short of minimum standards in particular aspects (DoH, 1993)
- carrying out and commenting on research into social care
- investigating complaints
- reporting annually to government.

The CSCI inspects and registers the following services: adult placement, care homes providing personal care and/or nursing care, children's homes, domiciliary care agencies, nurse agencies, independent fostering agencies, voluntary adoption agencies, residential family centres, and schools accommodating pupils for more than 295 days per year. Inspection of local authority fostering services and adoption services takes place but registration of these is not necessary.

The three criteria for registration include:

1. Fitness of premises
2. Fitness of persons (staff managing and running the service)
3. Fitness of services and facilities.

In 2005, the management of magistrates, Crown and county courts was combined into one new organisation – Her Majesty's Courts Service (HMCS). Her Majesty's Inspectorate of Court Administration (HMICA) is an independent inspectorate reporting directly to ministers about services for people coming to court. The inspectorate checks that people attending court receive a good service. It does not inspect or comment on judicial decisions.

Standards for Services

The quality of services is regulated by central government through published standards, for example standards for work with older people (DoH, 2000b, 2002a, 2003c) and the NSF for treating coronary heart disease (DoH, 2000c), while others such as social care standards for adults are still being consulted on (DoH, 2005). In 1997, the government set up the independent advisory body, the Better Regulation Task Force (BRTF); in 2006, this was replaced by the Better Regulations Commission (BRC). The Better Regulations Executive (BRE), introduced by the government in 2005, adopted the five principles of good regulations developed by the BRTF, namely that regulations should be:

■ *proportionate:* intervention only when necessary and remedies proportionate to the risk
■ *accountable:* decisions open to public scrutiny and justification
■ *consistent:* rules and standards 'joined up' and implemented equitably
■ *transparent:* regulators and regulations clear, accessible and open
■ *targeted:* that is, minimising side effects by focusing on the problem.

On a day-to-day basis, the performance of NHS Trusts and local authorities is monitored through the gathering of detailed information on the main aspects of their work. These methods provide an ongoing check on quality and, in theory, ensure that any irregularities in performance show up. The performance of the NHS in England used to be assessed by a system of star ratings against targets set by the government, but has been replaced by 'annual health checks' (http://annual-healthcheckratings.healthcarecommission.org.uk) scoring a broader list of aspects including financial solvency and services to patients and the public. Criteria for monitoring healthcare by the Healthcare Commission include access to a GP and a primary care professional (PCP), waiting times for outpatients, A&E departments and GP patients, death rates from major diseases such as cancers and heart disease, immunisation, infant health and settings such as hospitals and services by independent providers.

Adult care by local authorities is monitored by the CSCI, using a system of star ratings – Serving people well: no: 0*, some: 1*, most: 2*, yes: 3* (CSCI, 2006b, p. 18). The scores for adult care and children's services are totalled separately and feed into the general performance ratings for social services in England (CSCI, 2005c).

Apart from these national frameworks for measuring performance, there are standards in specific areas drawn up by special interest groups. As examples, the NSF for work with older people (DoH, 2001a) gives a general standard, while the Residential Forum sets out specific standards for items to be included in quality assurance of any residential care home:

■ a clear statement of the home's purpose
■ requirements and criteria for judging success of the services offered by the home
■ means of meeting the requirements
■ staff procedures
■ training for staff in assuring quality
■ systems for recording and monitoring
■ procedures for auditing and mechanisms for corrective action
■ systems for evaluation (Residential Forum, 1996, p. 52).

Inspection

Inspection of services by the CSCI aims to put the people using services first, improve services and eliminate bad practice. The CSCI produces four different kinds of inspection report:

1. *Care services inspection reports:* the main means of raising standards of services, at least to the level of national minimum standards. Inspections may be announced or unnanounced, depending on whether specific concerns have been raised by third parties. Services are graded according to whether standards have been met:
   – Level 4: Commendable: standard exceeded
   – Level 3: No shortfalls: standard met
   – Level 2: Minor shortfalls: standard almost met
   – Level 1: Major shortfalls: standard not met
2. *Local council inspection reports:* these focus on the quality of care provided through local authorities
3. *Joint inspection reports*
4. *Secure training centre reports.*

The CSCI is responsible for ensuring that service users – often referred to as 'experts by experience' – are part of inspection teams visiting care services run by local authorities (in an anticipated total of about 100 inspections per year), as well as home care agencies, care homes and children's services, including residential homes and fostering agencies (5 per cent of an anticipated 2,000 plus inspections per year) (CSCI Consultancy Specification, 14 March 2006, unpublished document).

The CSCI also publishes research reports highlighting quality issues in particular areas. For instance, a research report of the CSCI (2006c, pp. 39–40) was critical of the management of medication practices in care homes for children, younger adults and older people. Compliance with medication standards varied widely in all three types of homes. The standards were not met in 1,500 (12 per cent) care homes for older people, 900 homes (11 per cent) for younger adults and 200 (15 per cent) children's homes (CSCI, 2006c, p. 40). The failings included incorrect storage of medicines, giving service users the wrong medications, poor recording of use and poor management of the home including untrained staff handling medications. Good practice was identified in 44 per cent of homes for older people, 46 per cent of homes for younger adults and 37 per cent of children's homes (CSCI, 2006c, p. 40). Adequate practice included good staff training and supervision, medications regularly audited, involving service users in planning their own care and good joint working with healthcare practitioners (CSCI, 2006c, p. 41).

Independent Research: An Important Contributor to Quality Services

Research is often used to evaluate the strengths and weaknesses of policy and practice. Research of this kind makes a crucial contribution to quality assurance. It is preferable for evaluative research to be carried out by independent bodies funded by government rather than by government itself. Independent researchers do not have the inhibitions of officials responsible for the services. An example of useful evaluative research is the study published by the Joseph Rowntree Foundation in 2006, which drew attention to the diversity of the profile of service users in residential care and to the need to rectify variations in the equity of services. For instance, the fact that the decline in the quantity of residential and nursing care places in urban areas meant that there were more unmet needs in those areas, as care homes were not necessarily sited where they were most needed (Banks et al., 2006, p. viii). In some areas, notably London, minority ethnic people were underrepresented in care homes (Banks et al., 2006, p. 54).

Audits of Services

Often there are reports about audits being carried out. Accountants carry out an audit and say the firm is about to go into liquidation. Government services cannot go into liquidation as such, but they are accountable for their spending. The government set up the Audit Commission in the early 1980s and it produces reports on different aspects of public services, based on carrying out financial audits of their work. In health and social care, a financial or clinical audit is a:

> Structured process of reviewing and evaluating services, checking what is actually happening against what should be happening and specifying where changes need making so as to improve the service.

Part V

In order to be useful, an audit requires:

■ A practical problem, issue or service being delivered
■ A statement of what should be happening in an ideal situation, sometimes called 'aims', 'outcomes' or 'purposes'
■ Opportunities to check out what those on the receiving end (patients, service users, carers) think should be happening
■ A way of measuring the standards being audited
■ Willingness of managers and staff to implement changes with a view to improvements, after the audit.

In health and social care, *benchmarks* are used to specify particular standards of service that should be met. These benchmarks or standards should be:

■ expressed in simple terms
■ measurable as the criteria for judging whether services are adequate.

Making a Complaint

Registered providers of health and social care services are bound by law to produce a complaints procedure, specifying how service users, carers or patients can complain about the service. The procedure normally involves the complaint being investigated or responded to first by the service provider, although if the complaint is made to the Commission for Social Care Inspection, the CSCI may decide itself to carry out an investigation. A complaint about an allegation of abuse against children or adults will be referred by the CSCI to the local social services department. A complaint about a non-care aspect such as hygiene of premises may be referred to the local environmental health officer to investigate. A complaint that suggests a criminal offence may have been committed will be handed over to the police (see Resource File: Making a Complaint/Whistleblowing, at the end of this chapter; Resource File: Dealing with a Complaint, at the end of Chapter 52).

Whistleblowing

Whistleblowing usually involves a person making public some aspect of a group or organisation which they feel is wrong, dangerous, deficient or otherwise needing putting right through public attention. It is the activity of telling a third party, apart from colleagues or the employer, about malpractice. It will be unusual if any worker in the health and social care services does not come across some aspect of whistleblowing. This can arise directly or indirectly in three major ways, where:

■ you are the whistleblower: you notice practice you feel is not acceptable and you consider telling a third party, outside the line management, about it

■ a colleague is the whistleblower: you see another person 'blowing the whistle' on practices they consider unacceptable

■ the whistle is blown about practice involving you: where someone complains about, or 'blows the whistle' on, some practice with which you're connected.

Each of these will involve you in stress, in one form or another.

The Publication Interest Disclosure Act 1998 section 43B(1) seeks to prevent, or at least tackle, corporate and institutional malpractice. Employees who make a *protected disclosure* about some failure, injustice, criminal offence or health and safety issue they believe is arising in the workplace are offered protection from being dismissed or disciplined by their employer as a consequence of the disclosure. It also requires agencies to designate a senior manager to give guidance to staff on whistleblowing. Whether or not staff who blow the whistle always feel protected and supported is more problematic. Doubts about this often lead to staff not having the assertiveness and confidence to blow the whistle. Any staff who want to make a disclosure can do so through the National Audit Office (see Appendix 2).

Conclusion

This chapter has referred to the policy and legislative basis of the government bodies that have been created since the 1980s to promote quality assurance in health and social services. It has introduced the main features of quality assurance, including inspections and audits. Finally, it has drawn attention to the ways in which people, including carers, patients and people who use services, may complain and employees may 'blow the whistle' on shortcomings in services. We should note as a postscript that the government has announced the intention to merge the CSCI and the HCC.

REVIEW QUESTIONS

1 By what criteria does the CSCI judge the services it inspects?

2 What are clinical and financial audits and what do they need to contain in order to be useful?

3 What legislation supports whistleblowers and what are the arguments for and against blowing the whistle on extreme malpractice in the organisation?

FURTHER READING

Bury, T. and Mead, J. (1998) *Evidence-based Healthcare: A Practical Guide for Therapists*, London, Butterworth Heinemann

Cooper, P. (2002) *Delivering Quality Children's Services: Inspection of Children's Services*, London, DoH

DoH (2001) *Assuring the Quality of Medical Practice: Implementing 'Supporting Doctors Protecting Patients'*, London, DoH

Ellis, R. and Whittington, D. (1992) *Quality Assurance in Healthcare: A Handbook*, London, Edward Arnold

Government Accountability Project (2002) *The Risks and Costs of Whistleblowing*, www.whistleblowers.org

Hunt, G. (1998) *Whistleblowing in Social Services: Public Accountability and Professional Practice*, London, Edward Arnold

Marr, H. (1994) *Quality Assurance in Nursing: Concepts, Methods and Case Studies*, Edinburgh, Campion Press

Scrivens, E. (2005) *Quality, Risk and Control in Health Care*, Buckingham, Open University Press

WEBSITE: http://www.publications.doh.gov.uk/complaints/toolkit/index.htm
A good practice guide for people working in the complaints area in the NHS.

RESOURCE FILE: Making a Complaint/Whistleblowing, below

Resource file

Making a complaint/whistleblowing

There are organisations which regulate health and social care professionals, such as:

- *in health:* the General Medical Council (doctors), General Optical Council (opticians), Nursing and Midwifery Council (nurses, midwives and specialist community public health nurses)
- *in social care:* General Social Care Council (England), Care Council for Wales, Northern Ireland Social Care Council and Scottish Social Services Council.

Providers of health and social care services normally will have a complaints procedure. For example, every care home registered with the CSCI must have a complaints procedure. The CSCI helpline for people wanting to make a complaint is 0845 0150 120.

Complaints about NHS treatment usually are directed through the NHS organisation or primary care practitioner concerned. This is called *local resolution*. Complaints normally have to be made within six months of becoming aware you have something about which to complain.

If unhappy about the 'local resolution', you can complain further orally or in writing. You should receive a response from the chief executive of the NHS organisation within 25 working days or the primary care practitioner within 10 working days.

If unhappy with the response, you can ask the Healthcare Commission for an *independent review* of your case (Healthcare Commission, FREEPOST NAT 18958, Complaints Investigation Team, Manchester, M1 9XZ, complaints@healthcarecomission.org.uk). If unhappy with the response, you can complain to the health service ombudsman (OHSC.Enquiries@ombudsman. gsi.gov.uk). You can also receive advice and support with your complaint from the Independent Complaints Advocacy Service (ICAS), which was set up in 2003.

Under the Local Authority Social Services Act 1970, incorporated into the NHS and Community Care Act 1990, social services authorities were required to have a complaints procedure for adult services.

Complainants in England who are unhappy with the response to their complaint can complain to the local government ombudsman (LGO). The annual report of the LGO for 2005–6 shows that 18,626 complaints were received, a decrease of 0.4 per cent on the previous year, although the general trend is up by 15 per cent over the previous eight years. About 1,500 of the complaints were about social services (LGO, 2006, p. 13).

Whistleblowing is the term generally applied to people who publicise shortcomings from within the organisation in which they are working. The code of practice for social care workers (GSCC, 2002, para 3.2, p. 13) requires social care staff to use 'established processes and procedures to challenge and report dangerous, abusive, discriminatory, exploitative behaviour and practice'.

FURTHER READING

Government Accountability Project (2002) *The Risks and Costs of Whistleblowing*, www.whistleblowers.org

Hunt, G. (ed.) (1998) *Whistleblowing in the Social Services: Public Accountability and Professional Practice*, London, Edward Arnold

Hunt, G. (ed.) (1998) *Whistleblowing in the Health Service: Accountability, Law and Professional Practice*, London, Edward Arnold
These two books by Hunt are critical studies written from the perspective that there is widespread failure on the part of employers to rectify shortcomings in services and abuses which are not dealt with adequately by employers.

Approaches, Methods and Skills

Part VI
Approaches, Methods and Skills

Introduction

Part VI of the book deals with what some people regard as the heart of the matter: the different approaches and methods that practitioners tend to draw on when they work with people.

The fact is that without the preceding chapters providing the knowledge base and laying out the stages of the work, Part VI would be of little use. This is the appropriate moment to introduce it, since with it we bring a considerable body of theory and illustrations from practice. This requires you, the reader, to make some hard choices, selecting approaches and not attempting to take on too much.

Part VI also deals with some other essentials. First, there is the integration of theory and practice. This is much discussed on courses and Chapter 37 is written with this in mind. I have built into it my experience of the past 20 odd years as an external examiner of professional courses in higher education, hopefully enabling you to grasp more of what is required. Chapter 38 emphasises that the different components of theory and practice apply holistically to the health and wellbeing of the patient or person using the services with whom you are working.

Another essential aspect discussed in Part VI is the participation of patients, service users and carers in the actual process of the practice.

Working with particular approaches requires particular *qualities* – which I regard generally as inbuilt in us and not able to be changed much, in the short term at least – and *skills* – methods and techniques – about which we can always improve our knowledge.

By qualities we mean such aspects as sensitivity and self-awareness. By skills we mean such aspects as the ability to communicate effectively, to listen and to learn. With these hints in mind, read on.

Integrating Theory and Practice

ROBERT ADAMS

Learning outcomes

By the end of this chapter, you should be able to:

- ■ UNDERSTAND different facets of the meaning of theory
- ■ EXPLAIN what we mean by practice
- ■ WORK THROUGH the process of integrating theory and practice.

A long-time manager of a joint residential and nursing home used to say something on the following lines whenever she came on short courses: 'I'm not one of those head in the clouds people full of airy fairy theories, but a down-to-earth, practical person, living in the real world with her feet on the ground.' There are some assumptions in this statement, namely that to be practical is better than to theorise and that practical work does not have anything to do with theory. This chapter is based on quite different assumptions that underlie all professional courses in the health and social care field, as well as youth work, community work, teaching and many other professions involving working with people. These assumptions are that:

1. There are theories embedded in all practice. This means that our theories about us, our interaction with others and the wider environment are embedded in all our feelings, thoughts and actions.
2. In good practice, the practitioner is conscious of how the theories are integrated with the practice.

What is integrating theory and practice? Before going further, we can attempt a preliminary statement of what integrating theory and practice means. It means developing our awareness of the ideas embedded in our work with people.

What do we Mean by a Theory?

Theory is a broad term covering the ideas and assumptions that influence our practice. Payne (Payne, 2005b, p. 5) distinguishes three aspects of theory: explanatory theories, models and perspectives. *Explanatory theories* are used to understand why something happens in the way it does. They are like predictions: 'If you do this, that is likely to happen.' For example, theories about how groups develop may be drawn on by group workers to explain how new groups go through several fairly predictable stages (for instance, forming, norming and performing) in their early life. *Models* offer a general pattern that fits particular circumstances. For instance, the Department of Health (DoH, 1991b) developed a number of different models to enable practitioners to improve their skills in assessing people's needs (see Chapter 30). *Perspectives* are quite removed from practice yet still may be used to understand a practical question. For instance, Goffman (1961) studied total institutions such as prisons, monasteries and mental hospitals from a sociological perspective called 'interactionist' because it relied heavily on analysing how people interacted with each other to build up a picture of how the institution functioned. He theorised that total institutions displayed most or all of a list of characteristics (treating people in large groups or blocks, tightly programming each day). For instance, Goffman used his interactionist perspective to analyse the admission procedures in these total institutions, concluding that they invariably involved stripping new arrivals of their previous status and roles and humiliating them.

Brown and Harris's (1978) research into how some women become depressed led them to conclude that social factors, rather than just individual problems, bring this about. We could develop a theory to explain this, by stating that some women's depression arises from the way their lives – their domestic tasks, their isolation – are organised.

What do we Mean by Integrating Theory and Practice?

If we did our work unthinkingly, we would be just behaving. Behaviour is a word psychologists use to describe things done, without reference to thoughts, feelings or experiences. *We can distinguish observing behaviour from understanding actions.* Actions are things we do, where actions are understood because we take the time to find out what the person doing them is thinking, feeling, deciding and experiencing. In health and social care work, we use the word *practice* to refer to these actions. Practice goes beyond what we do. It refers to how we consciously relate what we do to various ideas, theories, perspectives, frameworks and approaches which inform what we do. In other words, we develop the ability to think about these while we are doing and reflect critically afterwards on how well we have practised. We can see from this that in health and social care work, the words *theory* and *practice* have particular meanings they do not have in everyday speech.

Integrating is another word which needs explanation. It implies making links between theory and practice, but is more than just connecting. The implication is that the two components of theories and practices are interacting because the connection between them is live.

Socially Constructed Practice

We have one more ingredient to add – the idea that practice is not a given fact but is socially constructed. What do we mean by *socially constructed*? It is not as difficult as it sounds. Imagine a situation where you have spent several hours making preparations for some visitors to your residential establishment, whom you have not met previously. They are due to arrive simultaneously in two minibuses. Unexpectedly, the first minibus arrives early, with the news that the second will be two hours late, after a breakdown. You go ahead with the tour of your establishment and subsequent discussion with the first group of visitors and have completed this before the second group arrive. The first group are very impressed and compliment you and your staff.

By the time you begin the tour with the second group, you are tired. Also, various difficulties with the residents have arisen and you are trying to deal with these behind the scenes, without them interrupting the progress of the visit. This irritates you. By the mid-point of the visit, you are impatient, exhausted and have run out of the welcoming spirit. The second group of visitors have seen exactly the same things, so you hope, but the discussion with them after their tour goes very differently to the first group. They are not impressed and you do not handle their questions and comments with your customary care and skill. They go away concluding that there is much room for improvement in your establishment.

Clearly, there is not one, objective reality in your establishment about which all these different people would agree. The different versions of reality are constructed by different circumstances and different people's experiences and are perceived differently, depending on who you are and how you took part that day.

Before going further, we can state what is necessary if we are to integrate theory and practice. It requires that we develop our awareness of the values, assumptions, concepts and approaches embedded in our work with people. This involves stating or restating our principles on which the work is based: our commitment to respecting the person, empowering the person, appreciating diversity and adopting an equality perspective, including trying to follow the principle of enabling adults and children to remain at home with their families wherever possible. It also involves being aware of our duties under relevant legislation, to safeguard and protect the person and promote her or his welfare. We also need to follow through the process of assessment, taking into account service users' and carers' views and perceptions and any other relevant views, such as those of professionals, relevant research evidence and our own practice wisdom. In all of this, we will be:

- weighing data
- analysing and using data
- assessing as a continuing process.

An Example of an Integrative Practice Study

We are now going to work our way through an integrative practice study. It simply accumulates the sequence we have been through into one set of linking activities.

This is quite a long example, but it is worth following it through, as all professional education and training uses some form of test to assess whether you can carry through this process. As you will see, it is simply a matter of not panicking, keeping on track and, from start to finish, asking the right questions at the right time.

Practice study

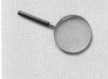

Selina

Selina is in her mid-thirties and has three children under eight. Selina is black and her partner is a white, respected member of the local community, whom she says nobody would suspect of regular and sustained violence towards her. Selina is also registered disabled, as a deaf person. She states that her previous partner also abused her over a long period and this is destroying her relationship with her current partner. She has referred herself to the Family Support Service (FSS) funded from a domestic abuse government grant, which, because much family violence is directed at women, works almost exclusively with women. You are the support worker with Selina.

Activity 37.1

Write a practice summary of your work with Selina, using the following questions as a checklist to guide your writing. You can then check what you have written with my notes below.

- Have you made a preliminary assessment of the situation?
- Have you related your handling of the situation to current research in this area of practice?
- Have you ensured that your practice is consistent with current legislation and local procedures?
- Have you given clear and sufficient evidence of planning, assessing, communicating, intervening and reviewing the work?
- Have you given clear and sufficient evidence of value requirements?
- Have you demonstrated that you have reflected on and critically analysed your practice?
- Have you related what is going on in Selina's life to theories about how people cope?
- Have you demonstrated that you have applied relevant knowledge to your practice?
- Have you demonstrated that you have transferred values and skills to your practice?

Have you made a preliminary assessment of the situation?

You could use the exchange model of assessment (see Chapter 30) to find out why Selina has referred herself and whether she has had contact with other agencies.

Have you related your handling of the situation to current research in this area of practice?

You could draw on research evidence of the negative effects of domestic abuse on the quality of women's lives, their self-esteem, self-confidence and their relationships, as well as on their children. You could add examples of particular pieces of research.

Have you ensured that your practice is consistent with current legislation and local procedures?

The work with Selina needs to conform to the Race Relations Act 1976, Race Relations (Amendment) Act 2000, Disability Discrimination Act 1995, Children Act 1989, Data Protection Act 1998 and Human Rights Act 1998.

Have you given clear and sufficient evidence of planning, assessing, communicating, intervening and reviewing the work?

You use the preliminary assessment to do your own pre-meeting planning before the first proper meeting and discussion with Selina. At the first meeting, you are able:

- to ensure that Selina is relaxed
- to confirm confidentiality and its boundaries where child protection issues arise
- to avoid jargon and patronising attitudes
- to be aware of both Selina's and your own non-verbal cues and body language
- to begin by explaining your role and that of the agency
- to carry out the assessment, using the exchange model
- to do some planning with Selina.

At subsequent meetings, you are able to use counselling techniques (see Chapter 45) and task-centred and other problem-solving approaches (see Chapter 46) to enable Selina to identify, take control of and work on her problems.

During these meetings, you get to know a good deal about the long-standing pattern of low self-esteem and abuse through childhood into adolescence and adulthood that Selina has experienced. You use your wider knowledge of this to help your work to empower Selina to deal with her problems. This is done by balancing the knowledge you have gained of Selina's history of being abused against the need to pass on to Selina some skills in coping strategies, by using a strengths-based and solutions-based approach (see Chapter 30) to assess and build on her strengths.

At the conclusion of 12 weeks, you review with Selina and her children the work done, both alone with Selina and with the children present.

Have you given clear and sufficient evidence of value requirements?

You are careful to demonstrate to Selina in meetings and discussions that you *respect* her as a person and are committed to *empowering* her to find ways of tackling her problems. You also *challenge any discrimination* against Selina and are keen to enable her to arrive at a way of coping which both *protects her* and *promotes her independence and wellbeing.*

The aspects of values linked with what is often called the value base of practice are highlighted in italic above.

Have you demonstrated that you have reflected on and critically analysed your practice?

The most useful ways of reflecting critically involve questioning the way you have worked. The best way of doing this is to ask two further questions:

1. What did you do well?
2. Was there anything you would do better, that is, differently, next time?

Have you related what is going on in Selina's life to theories about how people cope?

There are many ways of doing this. One useful theory, developed by Bartlett (1970), is called *social functioning theory.* This is a way of understanding how people may manage demands from their environment by pulling together enough support within themselves and from other people, or may find themselves unable to cope when the demands from others in their environment exceed the available supports. One way of overcoming the stresses people feel when they are not coping is by encouraging them to seek support and opportunities to change their circumstances so as to reduce their problems. In Selina's situation, this may necessitate her taking charge of her life, joining a self-help group of women in a similar situation, who are determined not to be treated as victims, but to become assertive, proactive and empowered. Selina benefits from the boost to her confidence through this.

Have you demonstrated that you have applied relevant knowledge to your practice?

This is the place to note that you have drawn, for example, on knowledge of human growth and development and the life course (see Chapter 8 for details of what this entails).

Have you demonstrated that you have transferred values and skills to your practice?

You can refer briefly here to examples of values you have demonstrated in your work with Selina and specific skills you have used. For instance, under values, you might give an example of how, when Selina made a comment that you might have disagreed with, you avoided intervening by criticising her view. In other words, you were *non-judgemental.* Under skills, you might refer to how you put Selina at her ease at the start, by using various communication skills (see Chapter 41 for details).

Looking back

It is possible to extend at great length any discussion of such a broad topic as the integration of theory and practice. What counts, though, is the actual content, the meat, of the discussion and not how lengthy it is. By working through the above questions, you will ensure that you tackle the right aspects.

Conclusion

This chapter has shown how you can use a step-by-step approach to build up to work with people that integrates theory and practice. It is not too difficult to write about this, as long as you keep up your confidence and try to express what you feel and think in words, using as a guide a checklist of key questions, such as the one put forward above. Let us try to draw out some of the implications of the work we have done in this chapter, recognising that it is one of the most difficult in the book. There are three points to make:

1. We have noticed that it is easier to talk about theory on its own and practice on its own than to bring them together. Perhaps the connection between theory and practice is difficult to make because the move from knowing to doing requires strong links in the form of expertise in learning how to learn and how to reflect.
2. Learning skills are necessary to enable us to acquire new knowledge and skills and we need skills in reflection to keep our practice on track, as we deal with uncertainty – the unexpected – and tensions – conflicts of interest and other differences between people.
3. We have talked about what constitutes practice. As we saw in Chapter 34 dealing with reflective practice, that word 'practice' contains such richness of meaning, it needed a chapter to itself.

REVIEW QUESTIONS

1 What is theory?

2 What do we mean by integrating theory and practice?

3 What is socially constructed practice?

FURTHER READING

Berger, P.L. and Luckmann, T. (1979) *The Social Construction of Reality: A Treatise in the Sociology of Knowledge*, Harmondsworth, Penguin

Burr, V. (2003) *Social Constructionism*, Hove, Routledge

Parton, N. and O'Byrne, P. (2000) *Constructive Social Work: Towards a New Practice*, Basingstoke, Palgrave – now Palgrave Macmillan

Thompson, N. (1995) *Theory and Practice in Human Services*, Buckingham, Open University Press

RESOURCE FILE: Writing a Case Study/Integrative Study, below

Resource file

Writing a case study/integrative study

A case study (some courses use the term 'integrative study') is a demanding piece of work in which you need to bring together three ingredients:

- material from practice
- evidence from what you read
- your own critical reflection.

Think of the case study as a meal you're cooking. The practice material is the ingredient you already have. Your search for relevant reading is your shopping around for extra vegetables and spices. The dish needs the magic of your own creativity to turn the ingredients into a fabulous dish on the plate. To do this, you sit down, turn the pages of your cookery books and jot down ideas and inspirations. The actual cooking is the stage of writing the case study. You need to allow time and take care over the choice of ingredients to achieve your special effect. That is how your case study should take shape. You should think of it as a piece of creative writing. We shall take the three elements in turn and then discuss how you bring them together when you write the study.

Practice

You should choose a case that will meet the assessment criteria. I often prefer to use the word 'situation' rather than case. Think of it as a piece of practice. Check the choice of case with staff if in doubt. In general, choose a case that interests you and clarify in your mind why this is before finally deciding. Reject cases that offer you nothing to write about at one extreme, or are too demanding and complex at the other. If critical reflection on what you did is one of the assessment criteria – and it invariably is – choose a case that enables you to illustrate work you did well and work you would do differently next time. This gives balance to your presentation and shows your ability to demonstrate a self-critical approach.

Evidence from what you read

You will need to back up what you write with selected evidence from what you read.

Your critical reflection

By the time you come to write the main critical contents of your case study, you should find that you are weaving these three components together – illustrations from your practice, evidence from your reading and, most important, your reflections which bring these together.

Final product: your finished case study

You should read this through carefully before submitting it, to make sure it *meets the assessment criteria*, refers to *everything* you have been asked to mention and does not contain any *mistakes* in basic spelling, punctuation or presentation.

FURTHER READING

Basford, L. and Slevin, O. (2003) *Theory and Practice of Nursing: An Integrated Approach to Caring Practice*, Cheltenham, Nelson Thornes

Hewison, A. (2004) *Management for Nurses and Health Professionals: Theory into Practice*, Malden, MA, Blackwell

Smith, L., Coleman, V. and Bradshaw, M. (eds) (2000) *Family Centred Care: Concept, Theory and Practice*, Basingstoke, Palgrave – now Palgrave Macmillan

Thomas, N. (2005) *Social Work with Young People in Care: Looking After Children in Theory and Practice*, Basingstoke, Palgrave Macmillan

Promoting Health and Wellbeing

ROBERT ADAMS

Learning outcomes

By the end of this chapter, you should be able to:

■ RELATE health promotion to the factors such as disadvantage and health inequalities influencing the health of people, including barriers to health and wellbeing

■ IDENTIFY several of the main health promotion models and approaches

■ DISCUSS relevant health promotion issues for health and social care workers.

In 2004, the White Paper *Choosing Health* (DoH, 2004c) was published. This set out the government's strategy for encouraging people to live healthier lives by making better informed and healthier choices about their diet and lifestyle. The White Paper signalled a broad approach, not only encouraging individuals but also aiming to shape the commercial and cultural environment. It put health promotion firmly on the social policy agenda for national and local government, but the government was criticised for not acting earlier to compel food manufacturers to reduce levels of saturated fats and salt in 'instant', frozen meals such as pizzas and burgers.

Changing Constructions of Health

A glance at the latest line-up of film stars from Hollywood may suggest that there is consensus about the appearance of the ideal beautiful woman, but a quick tour of different continents over the past couple of centuries will reveal the true diversity of ideals about what is health and beauty. Ideas about what people should eat and drink in order to stay healthy, and how they should look, change from era to era and, nowadays, from country to country.

Spend a few minutes jotting down some notes on how you think ideas about the healthy woman who also looks good may have changed since Victorian times.

In the past, the illness of an unhealthy child might have been regarded as visited on the family by God as a punishment for some previous wrongdoing. Ideas about health have often connected with ideas about how people should look. In previous centuries, women were required to confine their bodies in corsets that were so tight they damaged their internal organs. Some eating disorders of women in particular may be worsened by pressure from the mass media for them to conform to an idealised body shape. You could select some men's and women's magazines and go through them to pick out images and articles that give messages about what so-called 'healthy' and 'desirable' young men and women should look like. In parts of the world nowadays, it is acceptable for women to diet to the point of dangerous thinness in order to maintain an elegant body shape. In other parts, plumpness to the point of obesity is considered a sign of fertility and desirability. In Western developed countries such as the UK, stemming the rapid increase of obesity among children and adults alike has become a major target for public health planners and policy-makers (Crawford and Jeffery, 2005).

Health, Healthy Living and 'the Body Beautiful' are Social Constructs

Just as beauty is in the eye of the beholder, health is a social construct, that is, the product of people's beliefs and values in a society. Healthy living is not a scientific fact, a set of agreed statistics and ways of staying healthy, any more than health promotion is simply a list of rules that workers simply hand out to people. There are general endorsements by the White Paper (DoH, 2004c) of promoting healthier lifestyles through smoke-free workplaces, cutting unhealthy food promotion for children and better labelling of food, but it is also the case that advice on safe and healthy foods is sometimes controversial and subject to debate between researchers, rather than the product of a general consensus between them. Wellbeing is a notion associated with the subjective question of how a person feels rather than with objective measures of health or illness. Wellbeing also could be associated with holistic approaches to health. In 2001, the National Institute for Mental Health set up a spirituality and mental health project, studying the importance to people of the spiritual dimension and examining how to build constructive relationships with faith communities and faith-based organisations (Gilbert, 2006, p. 36).

Health Promotion in an Unequal Society

Health promotion does not take place in a vacuum. Nineteenth-century philanthropists, such as Robert Owen (who built New Lanark), Cadbury (who built Bourneville in Birmingham), James Reckitt (who built the garden village in East

Hull) and Titus Salt (who built Saltaire), designed model communities to cater more holistically for the housing, education and leisure needs of workers in the factories and their families. Many measures to improve the health of the working classes in Victorian Britain were taken as much as anything to ensure the continuance of a steady supply of labour, necessary in the factories and heavy industries of the rapidly growing industrial towns of London, the Midlands and the north. It was the poor physical condition of the soldiers called up to fight in the Boer War around 1900 that contributed to the demand in Parliament half a dozen years later for free school meals and milk to be provided. This ensured that the recruits shot down in their thousands in the First World War were far fitter and better fed.

Health, like food and water, is unequally distributed. Globally, more than half the world starves and goes thirsty, while the rich countries of the West suffer from diseases caused by lack of exercise, overconsumption and overindulgence. Within the UK, just as the concept of health is socially constructed, people's health and ill-health varies geographically and through the different strata of society. Despite the above points about overconsumption, within the UK, people who are better off have better life chances – they live longer – and enjoy better health – they suffer less from chronic conditions such as heart disease and chest complaints – than poorer people (Black Report, 1980).

Health promotion in the late twentieth century became not just an issue about the provision of public services through the NHS and local authorities, but also a privatised commodity that people could buy as part of a lifestyle choice, through choosing the healthy eating – low fat, low salt – options at the supermarket and becoming members of a gym. This has been reinforced through keep fit programmes on television and in lifestyle magazines. These developments have helped to:

- Maintain the construction of health promotion as the responsibility of the individual, diverting attention away from the fact that for years governments have benefited from tax revenues from tobacco. Only since 2000 have they considered contributing to reducing the incidence of smoking-related conditions treated in the NHS at a high public cost by eventually banning smoking in enclosed public places in Scotland from 2006 and in England and Northern Ireland from 2007.
- Hide the contribution by public services to ill-health through the provision of poor quality school meals, meals on wheels, hospital meals and meals in day services and residential care.

Advertising, Children's Diets and Childhood Ill-health

The early twenty-first century has seen growing concern among politicians and policy-makers about increasing rates of child and adult obesity. However, it would be a mistake to target campaigns for healthier eating and greater exercising at individuals, while neglecting the role played by the producers of fast foods, supermarkets and contracted-out school meals services in reinforcing poor eating habits in younger people.

The Hastings Report (Hastings et al., 2003) indicated that what children choose to eat and drink is influenced by advertising, especially that of junk foods and heavily sugared drinks. This fed into the debate about how to reverse rapidly rising rates of obesity and diabetes among children and adults alike. There was recognition that exercise and lifestyle were also significant related factors affecting health, but concern over children's diets rose even more when Jamie Oliver, a 'TV chef', led a popular campaign in 2004–5 against junk food in school meals.

Models of Health Promotion

The many different models and approaches to promoting health relate to two perspectives on health – the medical and the social. Medical perspectives focus on treating the illnesses and conditions of the patient, while social perspectives deal with the person in the wider context of the factors affecting their lives. We can relate this to the division of health promotion strategies by Tones and Tilford (2001, p. 30) into three categories of educational, preventive and empowerment approaches.

According to the *medical perspective on health*, held by many medical practitioners, good health coincides with the absence of disease, illness, symptoms of illness or abnormality (Kelly, 1996, p. 5). Linked with this are many medically based models of health promotion, such as the prevention schemes referred to by Tones and Tilford and the *knowledge–attitude–behaviour (KAB) model* (Kemm and Close, 1995, p. 29). This outdated and largely discredited model may be allied with an individualised medical model of diagnosis–treatment–cure and is based on the assumption that professionals telling people will be sufficient to change their attitudes and behaviour.

Social perspectives on health emphasise the interaction between a person's health and the wider social environment and relate closely to the educational and empowerment approaches identified by Tones and Tilford. The World Health Organization *Constitution* (WHO, 1948) defines health as 'a state of complete physical, social and mental wellbeing and not merely the absence of disease and infirmity' (Nutbeam, 1998, p. 12).

Among many models of health promotion derived from a social perspective on health, the somewhat idealistic *empowerment model* (Kemm and Close, 1995, p. 29) suffers from the weakness that it is rather detached from the surrounding political and social realities of society and healthcare provision. It focuses on empowering individuals to enable them to make life choices that improve their environment and health, by providing them with the relevant knowledge, skills and resources.

The *community action model* (Kemm and Close, 1995, p. 30) emphasises social action and encourages people to join forces and campaign to demand environmental improvements that promote their health. In this connection, Pike and Forster (1995, p. 45) talk of a radical model that owes something to empowerment and community action.

Integrated Model of Health Promotion

The WHO definition of health promotion emphasises empowering people to direct their own wellbeing (see Nutbeam, 1998, p. 12; Resource File: Health Promotion (3) Understanding Health, at the end of this chapter). Kelly (1996, p. 5) points out that, at both extremes, the medical and social models have limitations, in that they need to be based on sound research evidence on what works and not to take resources from other, more effective approaches. A way forward is the *integrated model*, which brings together aspects of both medical (clinical) and social (empowerment) perspectives on health. Contemporary health promotion uses an integrated model (Pike and Forster, 1995, p. 39), which draws on a range of sociological and psychological disciplines and professions, combines treatment and education-based approaches, is pitched at the individual, group and community levels, and works with a range of organisations in the public, independent and private sectors. It does not rule out the previous models such as empowering people, but recognises their complexity and locates them in the broader context of attempts to change people's lifestyles.

Activity 38.2

Summarise the strategy you would adopt when planning a campaign to promote healthy living among adults or children.

Ethical Principles of Health Promotion

Health promotion should be built around ethical principles. Kelly (1996, pp. 26–7) puts forward six principles for ethical health promotion:

1. To have the prime aim of meeting the health needs of individuals and populations
2. Not to withhold information contradicting conventional wisdom about health gain
3. Not to harm people
4. Not to make false claims or provide damaging information
5. Not to permit practitioners to engage in practice in which they are untrained
6. Not to permit practitioners to discriminate or practise unfairly.

Two core activities flow from these principles:

■ Promoting social justice
■ Promoting individual awareness and action.

As described above, the second of these receives most attention, while the first requires most strategic development and resources, in terms of government intervention. Health promotion work needs to take account of inequalities in health in order to lessen the likelihood of perpetuating, or even reinforcing, those inequalities (McLeod and Bywaters, 2000).

At the strategic, long-term level, governments need to examine ways of ensuring that children establish healthy styles of eating and parents have the financial resources to buy healthy food and the knowledge and motivation to prepare it. The barriers to these initiatives, in terms of the pressures on adults in households to work and the lack of a culture of families sitting down together to eat meals, are apparent. It is also clear that, in city centres and venues where people come together for public entertainment, the options in terms of healthy eating are severely limited.

The second area involves the provision of awareness-raising, information and support services concerning healthy living, which enables individuals and communities to make rational and informed choices about improving their lifestyles and health (DoH, 2002c). Health promotion in a locality involves adopting a coordinated approach, based on a mixture of prevention and early intervention, with the NHS leading local authorities and other partners in a multiagency Healthy Care Partnership.

Some approaches to health promotion focus on the setting, such as the urban environment, the school, the workplace or the family. Other approaches focus on an aspect of people's lives, such as the life cycle, illnesses such as type 1 diabetes, habits such as smoking or problems such as obesity.

Stages in health promotion

Chambers (2005, pp. 22–3) spells out the stages in health promotion as follows: initial audit, action planning, implementing action plan, monitoring and evaluating progress.

Auditing

The first stage in health promotion is to carry out a healthy care audit. This has three components:

1. views of patients, service users and carers
2. information from the multiagency partners
3. information from reports and reviews of health in the locality.

Action planning

The partnership:

1. shares and discusses views of the local situation
2. examines additional information
3. collates additional information
4. identifies priorities emerging from the audit
5. takes note of patients, carers' and service users' priorities
6. defines objectives and the means to achieve them.

Implementation

Hopefully, the partnership will have been clear about objectives and realistic about the resources required. A long enough timescale will have been allowed to enable the implementation to get underway.

Monitoring and evaluation

These activities will need to focus not only on immediate targets, but also on longer term goals. It will be essential to include the views of carers and health and social care service users in the process of evaluation. The key question to ask them is: 'What difference has this [specify the particular initiative] made to you?'

Promoting Children's Health

Government policy since 2000 on the health and wellbeing of children seems somewhat reactive rather than proactive, in the sense that it has responded to the Hastings Report (see above) and Jamie Oliver's school meals campaign, rather than incorporating these into an existing proactive strategy. However, the NSF for children, young people and maternity services was already being worked on when these initiatives took place and it sets out standards for promoting children's and young people's health and wellbeing (DfES and DoH, 2004). It builds on previous government initiatives for children with particular needs, such as implementing the recommendations of the Healthy Care Programme for looked after children, which is funded by the DfES and developed by the National Children's Bureau (Chambers et al., 2002).

The National Healthy Care Standard is a national programme intended to help looked after children and young people achieve the five objectives outlined in *Every Child Matters* (HM Treasury, 2003, p. 14): to be healthy, stay safe, enjoy and achieve, make a positive contribution and achieve economic wellbeing.

Areas of health promotion

These include healthy eating and physical activity, mental health, sexual health, substance and alcohol use, smoking, and play and creativity (for details see www.ncb.org.uk/healthycare).

Activity 38.3

Spend a few minutes jotting down all the ideas you have about possible projects under each of the above six areas for promoting the health of children and young people.

Here are some examples of health promotion initiatives, under the six headings:

1. *Healthy eating and physical activity:* drop-in health assessments in discreet rooms at local supermarkets and leisure centres; dieticians visiting schools and youth

clubs; training courses available on local radio and cable television linked with the internet; sports promotion in schools during holidays; free dietary advice and support advertised in local clubs, pubs and other places where young people congregate; free 'cook and eat' groups at adult education classes.

2. *Mental health:* employment of a community therapist at a drop-in centre run by a local voluntary organisation; anger management courses run by therapist at the centre; self-help groups for stress relief and depression; drama therapy.

3. *Sexual health:* outreach sexual health worker with young people; free condom distribution scheme; teenage pregnancy helpline offering information and support; support group for young mothers and fathers; helplines for sexually transmitted diseases; leaflets on sexual health available in local coffee bars, boutiques and schools.

4. *Substance and alcohol use:* individual and group counselling on alcohol abuse; leaflets on local self-help and therapy resources; drama workshops and travelling plays developed by young people with support from local drama group; drug education sessions for schools, youth clubs for looked after children; training for residential care staff, adopters and fosters carers.

5. *Smoking:* combination of individual and group support; Smoke Free Home projects; working in partnership with other practitioners; identifying and reducing stress factors that discourage giving up; linking with advice on healthy living and raising self-esteem and confidence building; targeting particular groups and lengthening period of support (Sure Start, 2006, pp. 73–5).

6. *Play and creativity:* leisure clubs attached to schools, residential homes and youth clubs; drama, dance and music projects for all children, with particular emphasis on attracting looked after children and young people and those with physical impairments and special needs; play therapy for looked after children.

Practice study

Alex and Tamsin

Alex, a black woman suffering from the early stages of multiple sclerosis who becomes periodically depressed, lives in a small village and has a younger partner Tamsin, who has always been brought up to remain independent and never to ask anybody for help, who is trying to care for her. She struggles for a couple of years, refusing all help and, having been to the doctor for something to help her with the stress, is eventually persuaded by a friend to approach social services, who appoint you to assess her needs as carer. You are aware of how structural discrimination affects some carers and service users and how it contributes to prejudice and direct and indirect discrimination. You use feminist theory to examine how Alex's and Tamsin's needs and relationship are invisible. They are excluded as a couple from much village life and through Alex's slowly developing condition are losing confidence to continue to assert their need for a social life in the community. One of the comments they often make to each other is about how male-dominated agricultural activities in that area are and how disadvantaged they are by not being able to draw power from the presence of a man, who would make their household respectable in the view of some local people.

Activity 38.4

Identify the main healthy living issues for Tamsin and Alex. Tamsin is finding it increasingly stressful trying to keep Alex fit and active while holding onto her own part-time secretarial job at the village school. Specify what you would like to see in the assessment of Tamsin's needs as a carer and in the plan for her.

Conclusion

This chapter has noted that ideas about health are a social construction. Nevertheless, inequalities in health provision persist and, when there are health concerns, they make it more complex for policy-makers to try to devise ways of improving people's health. On the whole, the least healthy people in Britain are those with the least means and motivation to do anything to improve their health. The chapter has considered health promotion campaigns, bearing in mind their limitations.

REVIEW
QUESTIONS

1 What are the main differences between a medical and social model of health?

2 What are the main findings of the Hastings Report?

3 What would you prioritise in a health promotion campaign focusing on children?

FURTHER
READING

DoH (2004) *Choosing Health: Making Healthy Choices Easier*, White Paper, Cm 6374, London, TSO

Health Education Authority (1995) *Health-related Resources for People with Learning Disabilities*, London, Health Education Authority
A useful collection of practice-related health promotion resources.

Healthy care leaflets for young people *Staying Healthy; Feeling Good: A Young Person's Guide* ref: DfES/0528/2004 and for staff healthcare ref: DfES/0850/2004 from: DfES Publications, PO Box 5050, Sherwood Park, Annesley, Nottingham NG15 0DJ, tel. 0845 6022260, dfes@prolog.uk.com

Kemm, J. and Close, A. (1995) *Health Promotion: Theory and Practice*, Basingstoke, Macmillan – now Palgrave Macmillan

NCB (National Children's Bureau) (2005) *Healthy Care Training Manual: A Health Promotion Training Programme for Foster Carers and Residential Social Workers*, London, NCB

Pike, S. and Forster, D. (1997) *Health Promotion for All*, Edinburgh, Churchill Livingstone

Tones, K. and Tilford, S. (2001) *Health Promotion: Effectiveness, Efficiency and Equity* (3rd edn) Cheltenham, Nelson Thornes

WEBSITES: www.dfes.gove.uk/qualityprotects (under Work Programme, then Health Issues)
www.ncb.org.uk/healthycare

RESOURCE FILES: Health Promotion (1) Children, Young People and Maternity Services, at the end of Chapter 17
Health Promotion (2) Stopping Smoking, at the end of Chapter 19
Health Promotion (3) Understanding Health, at the end of Chapter 38

Part VI

Resource file

Health promotion (3) Understanding health

What is health?

When we consider how much money is poured into health services in different countries across the world, it is surprising that there is no agreement among researchers, commentators and experts on what health and health promotion are.

Different ideas about health exist. The WHO *Constitution* (1948) defines health as 'a state of complete physical, social and mental wellbeing and not merely the absence of disease and infirmity' (Nutbeam, 1998, p. 12). The *Ottawa Charter for Health Promotion* (WHO, 1986) defines health promotion as 'the process of enabling people to increase control over and to improve their health' (Nutbeam, 1998, p. 12).

The Ottawa Charter specifies three strategies for health promotion:

1. Advocacy for health: combined action by individuals and groups 'to gain political commitment, policy support, social acceptance and systems support' for particular initiatives (Nutbeam, 1998, p. 5)
2. Enabling everyone to achieve their full health potential
3. Mediating between different societal interests with the aim of improving health (Nutbeam, 1998, p. 13).

The *Jakarta Declaration on Leading Health Promotion into the 21st Century* (WHO, 1997) confirmed the above and identified the following five combined strategies as most effective to:

- promote social responsibility for health
- increase investments for health development
- expand partnerships for health promotion
- increase community capacity and empower the individual
- secure an infrastructure for health promotion (Nutbeam, 1998, p. 13).

Health promotion model

The transtheoretical model of Prochaska and DiClimente, sometimes known as the stages of change model, is used in health promotion to enhance the value of interpersonal work between health practitioners and people. The essence of this model is the view that people move through several stages before they leave an unhealthy, health-damaging habit and adopt a healthy one. The two implications of this are that:

1. health educators need to recognise and capitalise on those times when people are ready to change
2. when people relapse, opportunities, guidance and skills should be provided to enable them to try again (Prochaska and DiClemente, 1984).

FURTHER READING

Nutbeam, D. (1998) *Health Promotion Glossary*, Geneva, WHO

Prochaska, J.O. and DiClimente, C.C. (1984) *The Transtheoretical Approach: Crossing Traditional Boundaries of Therapy*, Homewood, IL, Dow Jones/Irwin

WHO (World Health Organization) (1948) *Constitution*, Geneva, WHO

WHO (World Health Organization) (1986) *Ottawa Charter for Health Promotion*, Geneva, WHO

WHO (World Health Organization) (1997) *Jakarta Declaration on Leading Health Promotion into the 21st Century*, Geneva, WHO

Involving Patients, Carers and Service Users ROBERT ADAMS and WADE TOVEY

Learning outcomes

By the end of this chapter, you should be able to:

■ PLACE in its policy context the move towards patient and public involvement

■ DEFINE what is meant by involvement and participation by carers and people who use services

■ IDENTIFY the main issues and tensions arising in the practice of participation.

Policy Context

Since the early 1990s, health and social care policy and practice have moved towards empowering carers and people who use services, among other things by increasing their participation in the organisation and delivery of health and social care. These shifts in policy and practice have been driven by two factors:

■ pressure from carers and people who use services themselves. People with disabilities have been among the most vociferous critics of how they have been treated by staff in health and social care

■ legislation such as the NHS and Community Care Act 1990, the Carers (Recognition and Services) Act 1995, which gave carers the right to an assessment, provided the person for whom they are caring is receiving services under the NHS and Community Care Act 1990, the Carers and Disabled Children Act 2000, which entitles people to an assessment if they are offering a substantial amount of care, and the Carers (Equal Opportunities) Act 2005, which gives local authorities the duty to inform carers of their right to an assessment and to have their work, leisure and learning needs taken into account (see Chapter 29 for more details).

Since the late 1990s, the goal of increasing participation by patients, carers and people who use services (often called service users or users) in the delivery of health and social care services has formed part of the government's modernisation agenda for public services.

Involvement and Participation

The NHS Improvement Plan (DoH, 2004d) assumed that the health services would empower people by increasing their choice of services. The Green Paper *Youth Matters* (DfES, 2005a) proposes empowering young people. The Green Paper *Every Child Matters* (HM Treasury, 2003) puts forward the priority of greater involvement of children and their families. However, there may be a gap between the user empowerment and patient-centred emphasis of much government policy and the reality of people who use services feeling powerful and exercising that power. Empowering people and ensuring their active participation in services is a long, slow process rather than a simple task to be achieved overnight.

The Longman Dictionary defines 'to involve' as 'to engage as a participant'. This does not inform us about the crucial element – the degree of involvement. We can clarify these ideas about involvement and participation in the following way. There is a continuum of involvement, from being barely involved at all to being highly involved. At the same time, we may refer to a continuum of participation, from low to high participation. Although the two terms seem synonymous, the continuum of participation seems to be located at the top end of the continuum of involvement.

Arnstein (1969) wrote about a ladder of participation. Arnstein compares different levels of participation with climbing a ladder, from the person being controlled or manipulated at the lowest rungs, through to fully participating on the top rung. Roger Hart (1992) envisages eight rungs in a ladder of children's participation, the highest offering the greatest participation and the lowest three being non-participative:

- Rung 8: shared decision-making between young people and adults
- Rung 7: action initiated and led by young people
- Rung 6: action initiated by adults and decisions shared with young people
- Rung 5: adults consulting and informing young people
- Rung 4: adults allocating young people to a particular role and informing them about how they are involved
- Rung 3: *tokenism:* young people apparently having a say but in reality having little power over how they participate
- Rung 2: *decoration:* young people being used indirectly to boost a project or campaign
- Rung 1: *manipulation:* adults pretending to use young people in order to boost a cause.

Hart points out that we should not regard rung 4 as less desirable than rung 8 and we should not set out the aim that people on lower rungs should be aiming for higher ones. In each area of the organisation's work, different levels of involvement will be appropriate and desirable.

Wilcox (1994, p. 4) adopts Arnstein's ladder but reduces the number of rungs to what he calls five 'stances': giving information, consulting, deciding together, acting together and supporting independent community interests. His argument is that they are not arranged in a hierarchy of preferences, but each is appropriate in different situations (Adams, 2007, Ch. 2).

It may be difficult to judge how far an involved person actually is participating. A service user invited to a case review is involved in the sense of attendance, but this does not necessarily mean participation in making the decisions. It may be tokenism – putting on the appearance of participation where the reality is different. Some other words often used in this connection are consultation and collaboration. *Consultation* is asking people's views with no necessary connection between that and any future decisions. *Collaboration* is about people working in partnership together and sharing some of the responsibility and power to make decisions.

Carer Involvement

Defining a Carer

This is not straightforward, because of the complication created by the statutory, voluntary and private sectors 'employing' so many people, paid and unpaid, in different caring roles. The Equal Opportunities Commission (EOC, 2005, p. 1) defines a carer as an unpaid person looking after or providing help for a sick, disabled or elderly person in their own or another household, as partner, other family member, friend or neighbour. Our definition is as follows:

> A carer is a person giving social care to another person informally, that is, including carers receiving direct payments, but not including carers who are employees of health or social services, or paid care workers or personal assistants.

Payne (1995, p. 127) describes informal care as

> care provided to individuals by people in contact with them through links which have not been created in order to provide that care. Usually, informal care is provided by relatives, friends and neighbours of the individuals cared for, through links which come about through kinship, common interests or the fact that the people involved live close to one another or work or have worked together' (Payne, 1995, p. 127).

There is general recognition that *caring is a feminist issue*. Although men have begun to take on more of the informal caring roles than formerly, women still form the majority of the workforce in both health and social care. In medicine and social services management, in many Western countries since the Industrial Revolution, men have held the majority of the highest paid and most powerful positions (Achterberg, 1990, p. 168). In many societies, it is considered normal that women should stay at home and do the caring. Despite the evidence that when the burden of caring falls on women it often blights their chances of leisure, relationships outside the household, educational advancement and progressive paid employment, this caring is often invisible in society. This is one reason why the Carers (Equal Opportunities) Act 2004 is so welcome, because among other things it attempts to tackle this inequality. Traditionally, the wider context is that care has been viewed predominantly as something women do 'naturally' and men do exceptionally, when nobody else is available. In part, this is because there are gender inequalities in society.

How Many Adult and Young Carers Are There?

According to the 2001 UK census (*Social Trends* 34), 10–12 per cent (5.9 million) of people in England and Wales are informal carers. About three-fifths of these are female. The feminist view that caring is mainly woman's work has been softened slightly by evidence that men are involved significantly in caring. Of the third who are caring for 50 hours or more a week, the majority are women. Of the fifth who are caring for less than 20 hours a week, most are men. There are 179,000 carers over 75 years old. However, among the over 85 group, more male carers are likely to be caring for more than 50 hours a week.

We should not forget the reality of young carers. It is even more difficult to estimate their numbers, but there may be as many as 150,000 young carers (HM Treasury, 2003, p. 43). Carers cross the policy divide between adult and children's services, in the sense that children's and adult services in England are part of different 'skills sectors' (children's through the Children's Workforce Development Council and adult care through Skills for Care) and are provided through different local authority departments. Ideally, child and adult carers should be dealt with as part of one seamless service (Dearden and Becker, 2000).

Situation of Carers

Carers have long felt that they are a distinct group with their own needs, but these have seldom been recognised. They have been tacked on to the needs of people who use services. The phrase 'service users and carers' usually means, in effect, 'service users', especially where they are very vocal and influential. However, since 1990, carers have become increasingly organised and this has enabled them to use self-help to become more involved. Legislation has been passed giving carers rights. The Carers (Recognition and Services) Act 1995 entitles them to assessment, provided the person for whom they are caring is receiving services under the NHSCCA 1990. Despite this, at the turn of the twenty-first century, four out of five carers did not know they were entitled to an assessment (Seddon and Robinson, 2001). The Carers and Disabled Children Act 2000 gives carers the right to an assessment if they are offering a substantial amount of care. The Carers (Equal Opportunities) Act 2005 gives carers certain rights regarding their employment, health and lifelong learning and gives local authorities the duty for care managers to inform carers of their right to an assessment.

Carers' Organisations

Carers have formed a number of powerful national organisations, including the Princess Royal Trust, Carers UK and Crossroads. However, these are coordinating organisations and tend not to have direct responsibilities for caring. At a local level, carers have organised themselves effectively into groups and networks. In some areas these are very numerous. In Leeds, for example, the directory of carers' support groups for 2004 lists 59 carer support groups (Princess Royal Trust, 2004). These include 9 for all carers, 4 for children, 5 for dementia, 8 for learning disability, 13 for mental health and 6 for older people. Some carers offer mutual help and support. For example, Oasis, the Carers' Centre, Hull, East Yorkshire provides information, advice, support for the person cared for and respite for the carer.

Payment for Informal Caring?

In part, social care workers work in settings where care has been constructed and defined in male terms, so the informal caring they do becomes even more complex to describe (Orme, 2001). For instance, where does a woman's responsibility as daughter, sister, mother, aunt and neighbour end and her activity as informal carer begin? This is only one example of the difficult questions that arise when we begin to discuss how to cost the participation by carers. Another is how do we continue to ignore the low status and appalling pay and working conditions of the *paid* workforce of largely women carers, let alone the low status of *unpaid, informal* carers? Pringle's critical analysis of adult care includes a key quote from the work of Finch and Groves, when he talks of the inescapable intertwining of gender with adult care as a 'women only' activity, or 'low status services delivered to elderly women by low status women workers of a younger generation' (Finch and Groves, 1995, quoted in Pringle, 1995, p. 106).

There is a debate about whether to pay women for caring work, summarised by Lister (1997, pp. 168–94). There are arguments against giving any payments if they are not on the basis of equality with other paid work. On balance, it appears that the balance lies in favour of rewarding women in financial terms, even if this is inadequate, symbolic rather than realistic and still reflects the gendered inequalities in society's undervaluing of caring (Lister, 1997, pp. 186–7).

Service User Involvement

Defining a Service User

It is easy to come up with a simple definition: a service user is a person using a service. There is more of a problem about what to call 'service users', which is an indication, perhaps, of a difficulty with their identity, as viewed from agencies who have traditionally held all the power. In the past, words such as client and consumer have been used in health and social care. Other words such as customer, service consultant or adviser and 'expert through experience' have been suggested and some government agencies use the latter. In this book we use the words 'service user' or 'person using services' to refer to people receiving adult care services, whether from one or more professionals or through direct payments enabling them to buy services themselves.

People Who Use Services: Increasingly Assertive Stakeholders

People who use services are an increasingly assertive interest group, or 'stakeholder' interest. A stakeholder means somebody who has a stake in something, in this case the delivery of quality health and social care services. One contrast between carers and people who use services is that the latter have developed considerable influence over policy since the early 1990s. They have developed more power through organising themselves in groups and organisations, such as survivors' groups and self-advocacy groups. Some individuals and groups of people who use services do advocate very effectively on their own behalf. On the whole, it is the case that people who share an experience of disability are more vocal and organised than some other groups. The expression 'hard to reach' is used by agencies to refer to people who use services in some other less accessible categories of need. The term 'seldom heard' is preferable because it is framed from the viewpoint of the service user rather than the agency. Many agencies have developed policies and practices more friendly to people who use services. For example, they can benefit from bodies such as NHS Direct, which offers confidential advice from a nurse over the telephone, if a person feels unwell and is uncertain what to do.

Survivors' groups, self-advocacy groups and 'experts through experience' are examples of users taking power, and more information about the first two of these is in the next chapter. The CSCI, as the body responsible for coordinating inspections of care provision, has contracted consultants to recruit sufficient people who use services, known as 'experts by experience', to take part in inspections of care homes, home care agencies and children's services including fostering agencies and residential homes (see Chapter 36).

Activity 38.3

Spend no more than 10 minutes listing all the words you think might be used to refer to a service user.

Here is our list:

- client
- consultant
- contributor
- customer
- consumer
- member
- partner
- service adviser
- service consultant
- service member
- service user
- supporter.

Note: Some people use the word 'ambassadors' for people in self-advocacy for physical impairments. This may be a good word to use for advocates for participating people who use services or people who use services themselves.

Involving Children and Young People

Government guidance (DoH, 1991d) is clear that children should be involved as fully as possible in decisions being made in review meetings about their welfare. The problem is how to encourage them to make their contribution. In wider groups, it is noteworthy that young people have become vocal in some areas. Youth councils and community and social action groups exist in some local authorities and encourage young people to participate in a variety of ways, from social activities such as leisure and creative projects at one extreme, to raising issues and becoming involved in campaigns at the other extreme. In some areas, there are Young Person's Customer Panels, operating through distributing questionnaires and involving teenagers in focus groups and forums.

The Healthy Care Programme is run by Healthy Care Partnerships of agencies and organisations in different areas. It grew from the National Healthcare Standard, a national initiative to develop healthcare standards for looked after children, and incorporates the principle that looked after children and young people should participate throughout the entire process of healthy care – from initial audit and action through to reviewing and evaluating progress – with their carers and have their rights and responsibilities respected (Chambers, 2005, p. 19). This involvement, as Chambers acknowledges, is more than young people's 'reluctant consent' (Chambers, 2005, p. 19).

The stages of young people's participation are as follows:

1. Informing them of the issues
2. Stimulating them to form opinions
3. Providing opportunities to express opinions to decision-makers
4. Providing feedback on outcomes of opinions in shaping services
5. Ensuring children from diverse backgrounds, abilities, ages and cultures participate (Chambers, 2005, p. 19).

Two points are particularly important:

1. Feedback should be given to children and young people on the views they express, so that they can see the effects of their participation.
2. Healthy Care Partnerships should ask what different children will actually see resulting from any particular action.

Conclusion

This chapter has examined different shades of meaning between involvement and participation by carers and people who use services. It has discussed definitions of the terms 'service user' and 'carer' and has compared their situations relative to health and social care services. It has looked at some of the practice issues in relation to enabling them to participate more meaningfully in those services.

REVIEW
QUESTIONS

1 What is the ladder of participation?

2 What are the main similarities and differences between a service user and a carer?

3 What is a survivors' group?

FURTHER
READING

Beresford, P. and Croft, S. (1993) *Citizen Involvement: A Practical Guide for Change*, London, BASW/Macmillan – now Palgrave Macmillan

Carr, S. (2004) *Has Service User Participation Made a Difference to Social Care Services?* Position Paper 3, London, Social Care Institute for Excellence (SCIE)

Chambers, R. (2000) *Involving Patients and the Public*, Oxford, Radcliffe Medical Press

Nelson-Jones, R. (2007) *Life Coaching Skills: How to Develop Skilled Clients*, London, Sage

Stalker, K. (ed.) (2003) *Reconceptualising Work with 'Carers': New Directions for Policy and Practice*, London, Jessica Kingsley

Turner, M. and Balloch, S. (2002) 'Partnership between Service Users and Statutory Social Services', in S. Balloch and M. Taylor (eds) *Partnership Working: Policy and Practice*, Bristol, Policy Press, pp. 165–79
This may help to develop the capacity of some carers or people who use services to become more active participants.

Wilcox, D. (1994) *A Guide to Effective Participation*, York, Joseph Rowntree Foundation

WEBSITE: www.invo.org.uk (INVOLVE is a national advisory group promoting and supporting the active involvement of the public in the NHS and social care research)

Resource file

Participation by carers and people who use services

What works best in attempts to engage service users and carers in more meaningful participation? Carr's (2004) authoritative review of relevant research is based on six specially commissioned literature reviews of participation in the major service areas (Danso et al., 2003; Janzon and Law, 2003; Williams, 2003; Barnes et al., 2003; Rose et al., 2003; Crawford et al., 2003). The report makes four important points:

1. We should regard participation as an important means of empowering people, rather than as a goal in its own right (p. 9). People view participation as a way of achieving better services.
2. People require feedback on the effect their participation has on improving services. To deny them this may disempower them (p. 9).
3. Organisations, agencies and practitioners need to change their ways of working, so that changes can follow in the wake of people taking part (pp. 14–17) (see Chapters 7 and 54).
4. Attempts should be made to include the diversity of carers and people who use services – especially those such as older people, people from ethnic minorities, carers who are physically isolated and people in stigmatised groups such as those with HIV/AIDS and regarded as 'hard to reach' or 'seldom heard' – in initiatives to improve participation (pp. 18–22).

FURTHER
READING

Carr, S. (2004) *Has Service User Participation Made a Difference to Social Care Services?* Position Paper 3, London Social Care Institute for Excellence (SCIE)

Empowerment and Advocacy

40

ROBERT ADAMS

Learning outcomes

By the end of this chapter, you should be able to:

- UNDERSTAND what is meant by empowerment
- KNOW the meaning of the word 'advocacy'
- IDENTIFY some of the many uses of empowerment and advocacy in practice.

This chapter deals with two linked approaches to work with people, which present staff – managers and practitioners – in health and social care with one of the greatest challenges, namely, to achieve progress with the empowerment of carers and people who receive services. Empowerment has become a buzzword since the early 1990s, whereas advocacy is a somewhat overshadowed idea, which, in order to avoid being interpreted as taking over from someone and speaking for them, still needs developing in its own right.

What is Empowerment?

I have defined empowerment as:

> the capacity of individuals, groups and/or communities to take control of their circumstances and achieve their own goals, thereby being able to work towards helping themselves and others to maximise the quality of their lives. (Adams, 2003, p. 8)

In health and social care this means patients, carers and service users exercising choice and taking control of their lives. Empowerment is not an absolute, that is, when we say a person becomes empowered, it does not mean that he or she becomes all-powerful and other people – relatives and friends – have none. Even the most extreme dictator has to accept that some people will disobey when they feel they can get away with it. More commonly, it means the person feels able and feels powerful enough in certain situations to take part in decision-making. Steel (2004, p. 10), writing about empowerment, notes that taking control does not entail service users excluding professionals or 'undertaking every stage' of the work themselves. This has the added benefit of freeing them from the experience of being disempowered, stigmatised and excluded.

Research approaches that set out to empower the subject of the research (that is, the person 'researched') include 'collaborative' research, so called because it emphasises the researched person working with the researchers. In the social sciences and the humanities, notably history, 'oral history' has become a widely used approach, based on taking full, usually tape recorded, accounts of particular aspects of people's lives and experiences. In the social sciences, biographical research has developed the art of what health and social care practitioners might call 'history-taking' from a patient or service user into a research methodology (see Resource File: Life Experiences and Biographical Research, at the end of Chapter 35).

Emancipation is a commonly used word in other Western European countries to refer to what we in the UK mean by empowerment. The word emancipation is useful because it has overtones of the struggle for votes for women in Britain at the beginning of the twentieth century, so it reminds us that empowerment in the health and social services has a political aspect. When carers and people who use services experience being disempowered and excluded, this is a form of political disenfranchisement. In other words, it is as though they have no vote and are not treated as full members of society. In contrast, when people become empowered, they can exercise choices and have the possibility of maximising their potential and living full and active lives.

Partnership

Partnership is a popular word and it is often assumed that all partnerships must be beneficial for all the partners. But partnerships, of course, can be of many kinds. Not all partnerships involve two equal partners. There may be one dominant partner and one subordinate one. The dominant partner may force the subordinate one to agree to things. There may be different aspects of the partnership in a complex situation, where one partner dominates in one area and the other in a different area. This can happen where the two partners have different backgrounds and skills, for example where the disabled person is a retired, experienced doctor and the carer is young and in her first job. Or, there may be several partners, in which case the situation becomes even more complicated. So partnerships can be a form of empowerment, but if you are one of the junior partners, they can be disempowering. On the other hand, in a situation where there is 'user control', this means that the people who use services have the power rather than the professionals. The users have what we sometimes call the *balance of power*.

We should bear in mind that this is not abstracted from reality. Care managers have a duty under the NHS and Community Care Act 1990 to work in partnership with service users and carers to assess their needs and ensure that they are met through the care plan.

What is Advocacy?

Advocacy is a general term covering a range of activities to enable the views and feelings of carers and people who use services to be heard, particularly those who are seldom heard, including people with multiple impairments, substance misusers, people with HIV/AIDS, homeless people, ex-prisoners, young carers, asylum seekers and people from some ethnic groups whose particular circumstances are less recognised (Teasdale, 1998). Types of advocacy include advocacy, self-advocacy, peer advocacy and citizen advocacy. Advocacy is a double-edged practice. On one hand, vulnerable citizens may value an advocate to speak up for them. On the other hand, advocacy, like professionalism, can take power from people to speak up for themselves. This is a particular issue in work with vulnerable people and people with severe learning disabilities (Gray and Jackson, 2002). The difficulty for practitioners is to decide how to handle this tension.

There are policy initiatives that aim to maintain the fine balance between intervening too far in people's lives and not intervening enough, to maintain and safeguard their interests. Effective advocacy needs a code of practice to ensure that it does this (Coulan, 1997). For example, the Mental Capacity Act 2005 aims to protect people who are judged not to have the capacity to make their own decisions. As a safeguard, the Act introduces the independent mental capacity advocate (IMCA), intended to ensure that the person's interests and rights are protected. In any circumstances where the person needs to make a decision about accommodation or serious medical treatment, an IMCA is appointed to represent them, including challenging professional decisions where appropriate.

In some ways, of course, advocacy has much in common with that traditional idea – self-help.

Self-help and Self-care

The tradition of self-help – literally, doing it for yourself without professional help – is as old as society, although since Victorian times in Britain, alongside the values of hard work and respectability, it has been advocated as a particular virtue. There is what some people regard as an unacceptable opting out by the state in the Victorian principle of the Charity Organisation Society, founded in 1869, which only gave support to those families deemed capable of helping themselves. The true paupers, the 'residuum' as they called them, were left to their own devices. In the late twentieth century, self-help came into its own as governments encouraged voluntary and private organisations to develop health and welfare services in partnership with the state. This makes self-help sound a reactionary approach, but this is not the case. A broad spectrum of approaches can be found under the umbrella of self-help, some of which, like the self-build movement in community architecture, claim to empower the individual. In social work, many examples of self-help by individuals and groups can be found, not least in the plethora of treatment and therapy groups such as women's therapy and consciousness-raising groups and the more mainstream Depressives Anonymous and Alcoholics Anonymous. From the 1960s, the self-care model of healthcare was developed in nursing in the USA and spread to Britain. Direct payments are a form of self-care, which from a progressive viewpoint may seem to be linked with an empowering form of self-advocacy, or from a reactionary viewpoint may be regarded as the state handing back responsibility to the individual, to survive or not. Self-care should not be regarded as a reactionary force. In fact, the concept is complex, with social and political as well as individual ramifications, based on the two linked ideas that:

- the patient has the right to be viewed as an individual with unique needs
- the patient has the ability to meet his or her own needs (Pearson et al., 1996, p. 91).

Empowerment and Advocacy in Practice

There is a tension between enabling people to take control of their lives and recognising that workers may need to intervene and take control sometimes, in order to protect other people. This applies to both empowerment and advocacy.

Empowerment in Action

Health and social care workers need to recognise that it is difficult to avoid perpetuating tokenism in empowerment, without making major changes in the ways we practise. One of the key changes is for the worker to shift roles from *being in charge* of the intervention to *facilitating* what happens next. This sounds insignificant, but properly managed it can have a truly emancipatory effect on the person using services and, where appropriate, the carer.

The difference between being in charge and facilitating is straightforward to describe. The worker shifts sideways and tries to ensure that he or she is no longer in the powerful, privileged position. Instead, the facilitator works at the same level as the patient, client or service user. The facilitator steps aside so that the service user, with the carer where appropriate, has the freedom and power to make choices and decisions about the kind of service he or she wants. Another key change is that the relationship between the worker and the service user becomes reciprocal, that is, information and views are passed both ways between them. In this situation, their interpretations of what is happening are more likely to converge. We summarise below seven tasks or stages which need to be worked through in order to empower the service user or carer, although we emphasise there is no fixed sequence. They can be taken in the order that suggests itself as most suitable to those involved:

- analysing areas of disempowerment in the current situation
- ensuring that relationships with service users and carers are equal
- setting up reciprocal working relationships with service users and carers that lead to meaningful dialogue
- gathering the views of service users and carers so as to validate their experiences
- offering views and analauses to service users and carers about structural factors that disempower them, including information about areas that may be invisible to them
- maintaining the views of service users and carers in their own words rather than translating them into official reports, which might imply that somebody viewed the original statements as deficient in some way
- enabling service users and carers to empower themselves.

Perhaps empowerment may reach a point (see Chapter 39) where the person who uses services is called upon as a kind of consultant to advise on the details of the service being provided, as Raynes (2001) describes in her publication about involving service users in defining the specifications of home care services.

Practice study

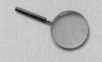

Mrs Ali

Mrs Ali lives on the first floor of a flat and looks after her bed-bound husband full time. She regards it as her duty, as a Moslem and an Arab, to serve her family. Jean is the care worker who visits and provides a basic level of domiciliary support. Mr Ali has a long-term condition which will not deteriorate in the immediate future, but will not improve.

Jean is concerned about the difference between her own view and that of Mrs Ali about how much Mrs Ali has to do. Jean regards Mrs Ali as disempowered. In contrast, Mrs Ali takes the view that she is very lucky. Allah has granted her a sick husband as an opportunity to pay for her past sins and, perhaps, to redeem herself. Whatever happens, her daily life is what is willed. It is her duty to accept it.

Jean wants to talk to Mrs Ali about having an assessment as a carer and developing a life outside the home, perhaps using a respite carer to enable her to leave him, to go to town shopping and even take a regular time every week to attend a further education class in flower arranging, which is Mrs Ali's particular delight.

Jean spends months getting to know how Mrs Ali experiences her life and what her deeply held religious beliefs allow her, and do not allow her, to do. Eventually, she makes it possible for Mrs Ali to justify leaving her husband early in the afternoon for an hour once a week, when he is having his after-lunch nap, and attend the flower arranging class. This does not conflict with Mrs Ali's beliefs because her husband is happily asleep. It is the first step towards further respite support that Jean puts in place over the following 12 months.

Part VI

Advocacy in Action

The service user and survivor movements in mental health are a testament to the power of people to act as self-advocates. Peter Campbell (1996, pp. 218–25) has written a useful, brief account of the history of these movements in the UK.

Advocacy requires a willingness to challenge other people. It is easier for the less experienced worker to back down in the face of a confident, experienced colleague, partly from a wish to avoid hurting other people's feelings. Also there is a tension between the desire to maintain positive working relationships and the need to be appropriately critical of one's own practice and that of colleagues.

Practice study

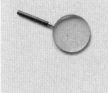

Michael

Michael is a 59-year-old man suffering from the terminal stages of prostate cancer, who wants to die at home. His wife is willing to care for him. The worker overcomes the resistance of some healthcare professionals, including his regular doctor at the local surgery, and recruits support from one of the other doctors in the primary care team. The worker establishes Michael's right to assessment for continuing care from the NHS without means-testing and the services are provided at home to support him and his wife until his death six weeks later.

Postscript on Social Security

We need to take note that poverty is an enduring problem for many vulnerable people and no amount of rhetoric about empowering them will remove it. The often unforeseen changes that affect people's lives – which may, in the case of carers and service users, be tragic – can add to the existing burden of limited budgets. On the whole, the social fund and other arrangements in the UK to provide financial help for people from state funding add to the complexity of managing their lives without ensuring a route out of hardship and poverty, as the helpful research brought together by Buck and Smith (2003) shows. Further information is obtainable from the Child Poverty Action Group (www.cpag.org.uk) and Age Concern (www.ageconcern.org.uk).

Conclusion

This chapter has explored the nature of ideas about empowerment and advocacy. It has examined some examples of empowerment and advocacy in action, indicating some of the tensions and difficulties that exist for professionals. In particular, it has highlighted the balance that needs striking between enabling people to take power and doing their empowering for them. Similarly, it has discussed the need for advocates to be sensitive to people's vulnerabilities, yet willing to step back and make space for them to act as self-advocates.

REVIEW QUESTIONS

1 What is empowerment in health and social care?

2 Can you describe what is meant by advocacy?

3 Can you identify some key tensions for the practitioner wanting to empower a person?

FURTHER READING

Adams, R. (2003) *Social Work and Empowerment*, Basingstoke, Palgrave Macmillan

Atkinson, D. (1999) *Advocacy: A Review*, Brighton, Pavilion Publishing

Barnes, M. and Bowl, R. (2001) *Taking over the Asylum: Empowerment and Mental Health*, Basingstoke, Palgrave – now Palgrave Macmillan

Barnes, M. and Warren, L. (eds) (1999) *Paths to Empowerment*, Bristol, Policy Press

Barnes, M., Harrison, S., Mort, M. and Shardlow, P. (1999) *Unequal Partners: User Groups and Community Care*, Bristol, Policy Press

Brandon, D. (1995) *Advocacy: Power to People with Disabilities*, Birmingham, Venture Press

Raynes, N.V. (2001) *Quality at Home for Older People: Involving Service Users in Defining Home Care Specifications*, Bristol, Policy Press

Sayce, L. (2000) *From Psychiatric Patient to Citizen: Overcoming Discrimination and Social Exclusion*, Basingstoke, Palgrave – now Palgrave Macmillan

Stein, J.S. (1997) *Empowerment and Women's Health: Theory, Methods and Practice*, London, Zed Books

RESOURCE FILE: Life Experiences and Biographical Research, at the end of Chapter 35, for approaches to research based on empowering principles – gathering the experiences of people as told by themselves.

41 Communicating Effectively

ROBERT ADAMS

Communication makes a crucial contribution to working relationships. Without the ability to communicate, the worker cannot be effective and will be unable to convey to people what he or she wants them to know and will not be able to gauge how they are responding.

What is Communication?

Communication is defined by Kadushin and Kadushin (1997) as 'the sharing of thoughts, feelings, attitudes and ideas through the exchange of verbal and nonverbal symbols'. Communication affects how we interact and is affected by many factors. Our prior learning and experiences influence how we engage with people and communicate with them. Our 'body language' – the way we sit, our facial expressions, the movements of our hands – all convey information about our mood and how we feel about the people near us.

Many years ago, I was attending a conference on family therapy at the Family Institute in Cardiff. We were given a dramatic illustration of how much people communicate through body language alone by one of the speakers. The volunteer family were invited onto the rostrum in the middle of the audience and the therapist put them at their ease while all the family members – grandparents, parents and children – took their seats, except one child, who flitted between the seats occupied by her grandparents and sister. For the next few minutes, without asking a question, the therapist talked about how the family members had chosen to sit, who sat next to whom, the husband whose legs were together, pointed away from his wife, and the child who avoided her parents and flitted between the others, apparently not finding a place in the family. It is not just in family therapy, but in all our work with people, that body language can give us crucial and detailed information about the dynamics of a person's interaction with her or his environment, as well as with other people, including colleagues, friends and other family members.

Models of Communication

The process model of communication was developed by Shannon (1949) and was basically mathematical. It can be understood by thinking about communication in terms of old-style war movies where wireless operators on ships and aeroplanes received messages on a secret channel (carrying the message) from the headquarters (the brain). The message was sent from the brain on a transmitter (initiating the message) to the wireless operator in code, which he or she had to translate from the secret code (decoding). Sometimes there was so much atmospheric disturbance that the crackling on the line (interference) distorted the message (changing the meaning). There are four main weaknesses of this model:

1. It uses a mechanical analogy and so is quite mechanistic.
2. It is based on the idea that communication is linear, with you sending me a message to which I respond and you respond to with a further message.
3. It follows the single signals from the sender to the recipient without allowing for the complexities of other factors, verbal and non-verbal, which provide crucial information.
4. It assumes that the essence of communication skills is the transmitting of information.

Subsequently, linguistic analysts pointed out the importance to communication of the structure and content of our statements and questions. We only have to watch an actor uttering a single word dramatically to realise how important the subtleties of expression can be. Additionally, social scientists (psychologists, social psychologists and sociologists) emphasised the significance of interaction and the interpretation of meanings to the communication process. It is significant who sends the message, what factors affect how it is said and how the person receiving it interprets it. To return to our comparison with wartime transmitters, in a typical conversation or meeting, there is a constant exchange between participants, with those who receive 'messages' decoding (interpreting) them, exchanging roles and becoming transmitters of the next message. The entire process becomes extremely complex. Additionally, face-to-face communication involves not just speech but also body language. How many ways can you find to say 'No'?

Language and Communication

While accepting that people communicate non-verbally, verbal communication is important and relies on the subtleties of language. Language is more than a means of communication and can be used, and abused, when people interact. Consider what happens when two lovers meet. They exchange soft words and these provide the basis for the following courtship. In contrast, consider the wife who arrives home to find her husband entertaining his secret mistress. The wife harangues him, using all the expressions she can think of to describe how despicable he is.

Theories of language and communication link language with the self, identity and the wider environment. These relate to theories about discourse. We can define a discourse as a way of speaking or writing about ideas and the beliefs associated with them.

The French social theorist Michel Foucault (1982) wrote at length about all the ways in which people, especially in penal institutions, mental hospitals and other institutions, keep information to themselves as a way of retaining power. Language and communication are weapons in such power struggles. The expression often used is 'information is power'.

We might say 'language is power' as well. I recall a visit to the hospital consultant at the audiology clinic. He called 'Come in' and sat with his back to me while I stood, waiting for several minutes in strained silence while he continued to read the notes. Finally he turned round and asked me to sit down. By this time I was in no doubt who was in charge of the encounter.

Just as we may describe good communication as dependent on more than speech, so it is necessary also to ensure that people are not disempowered by faulty communication, that is, using inaccessible language. After the examination, the consultant audiologist fed back to me the results of the tests, talking about frequencies and the response across the higher and lower registers in percentages of hearing loss. Fortunately, I had the presence of mind to ask him to translate this before I left his office. I should have given him some feedback about his techniques of communication.

Means of Communication

We might assume that good communication is speaking in a monotone slowly and, if the other person does not respond, simply repeating the same message louder and louder. But communication is more than a mechanical, largely one-way, process. At the heart of communication are two linked activities of engagement with people and interaction between people.

Engagement includes the skill of forming a professional, helping relationship or, in modern terms, 'making a connection'. *Interaction* involves the nature and quality of verbal and physical signals and responses, which pass between people and sustain, or break, their relationships. Interaction takes place when people chat together in a bar, or in the lounge of a residential home for older people. This may be successful conversation, but does it count towards purposeful, effective work? Ironically, while the skilled worker is able to hold relaxed conversations with people, it does not follow that every relaxed conversation between staff and patients, carers or service users is contributing to effective work.

Good communication goes far beyond words and depends on many ways of interacting. Speech, tone of voice, choice of formal or colloquial language, body language, gestures, facial expression and how we dress are all factors contributing to our interaction with each other.

A portrait artist will spend a long time painting the eyes of a person. The expression 'the eyes are the window to the soul' is perhaps an attempt to convey the expressiveness of people's gaze, if we know how to interpret it. Argyle (1969) discusses the complexities of body language, such as eye contact, which may be affected by factors such as social class and culture. In some circumstances, when two people meet and one asks the question 'Tell me honestly ...', avoiding eye contact when replying may be taken as an indication of a less than honest reply. Eye contact in this situation is interpreted as a sign of directness. In other circumstances, a child or a vulnerable person may find direct eye contact intimidating. Again, in some cultures, it is regarded as rude for a person to look at another. Looking may be culturally forbidden in some situations, especially where one person is much higher in status than the other.

I recall being invited by John Bazalgette in the 1960s to attend one of his group projects, which involved meetings with young, working-class men, totally unused to coming together, sitting around talking to a middle-class stranger. At an early stage in one meeting, there was almost a fight between two of the young men, after one accused another of staring at him. Apparently, to stare was to challenge.

Interviewing

Thompson (2002, p. 120) refers to an interview as any discussion – formal or semi-formal – between a practitioner and a person using services. Chapter 13 in his book *People Skills* has a number of useful tips on conducting interviews. There are four main stages in the interview: planning, engaging, responding and ending. *Planning* is the stage where the practitioner establishes the setting, so as to set the service user at ease, ensuring a non-stigmatising atmosphere, a balance between doing the task and enabling the service user to share thoughts and feelings. *Engaging* involves listening and, where necessary, adjusting the message to avoid misinterpretation. *Responding* involves giving feedback. Lack of opportunity for this implies a lack of respect for the carer or service user. Responding also includes, where appropriate, demonstrating warmth, empathy, active listening and being non-judgemental, as well as taking responsibility for clarifying the purpose of the encounter and expectations, giving information and advice as needed and dealing with the end of the encounter.

In interviews, effective communication involves making a constructive link or bridge between the interviewer and the person being interviewed. Lishman (1994) gives many tips in her practical book. Good interviewing depends on a variety of formal and informal modes of interaction. Interviews can, and probably should, be informal, when working with people who are intimidated by professionals or formality, or when working with children and young people. The carer who visits the lone widow in the morning does not do her job well if she interviews her formally about how she is feeling, but relies on informal conversation to update the existing assessment and attempts to motivate and empower her as she chats. This informal interview as part of ongoing work with the person is at one extreme. At the other extreme, there is the formal interview. In between, there are many interviews conducted with a mixture of formality and informality. This is not simply a matter of personal preference. People have varying concentration spans (the time over which a person can concentrate on an activity).

There are tensions between completing formal tasks and maintaining a relaxed, supportive setting. Sometimes information has to be gathered and time is limited. Ways have to be found of giving clear verbal and non-verbal indications to people that we are aware of, and in tune with, their anxieties and want to reassure them. Physical cues can be crucial. When I attended an interview at the Home Office, I knocked at the huge door, heard someone say something and assumed it was 'Come in', only to be faced by a line of people behind a table at the far end of the large room, one of whom called across the vast social distance separating us: 'Wait outside a moment, you're too soon.' During the next few minutes of waiting, I seriously considered walking away and not attending the interview.

There are sensitive ways of arranging office interviews. The desk does not have to be placed between the interviewer and the visitor. It could be in one corner so the interviewer can swivel round and speak away from the desk. The visitor's chair does not have to be an easy chair so he or she looks up at the interviewer, but can be at the same height.

Particular care should be taken when interviewing vulnerable people and children. Activities are sometimes used when talking with children. Art therapists use painting as a means of communication, chatting while drawing or painting. Other play techniques include the dolls used by practitioners when asking young children diagnostic questions about abuse. Music, drama and art therapies all have highly developed skills in working with people who have experienced major traumas. A growing area of concern is work with people who are seeking asylum and who are suffering the consequences (sometimes this is post-traumatic stress) of extreme situations before leaving their country.

It is important to practise techniques of asking questions and prompting for further information in ways that do not interrupt the person's flow and enhance rather than impair memories (Seager and Kebbell, 1999, pp. 99–103). Without such care, the entire basis of health and social care work is weakened.

Skills of Communicating

It is important to convey basic values in the ways we communicate. Even before sitting down to chat, the worker can signal in body language and general demeanour an attitude towards the person of respect and fair treatment (Argyle, 1988).

Using Words

The most common way of communicating with service users and carers is by speaking. Of course, there are occasions when sign language will be used in communication with a deaf person, but speech is the most commonly used means for communicating our ideas, views, decisions and emotions. Our *expressive use of words* and the intonation in our voice when we speak can convey as much to the listener as the words themselves. It may be necessary for us to *slow down our speech* so that the person has the chance to listen, take in what we are saying and respond to it. We may have to *choose clear words* to convey our meaning. Our language should be *not too casual* in case the person infers that we do not mean what we are saying, but on the other hand our speech should *not be too formal*. We should *match our words* to the developmental stage of the person listening. We need to gauge the pace and proceed slowly enough to build a trusting relationship, to enable the person to confide where necessary.

It is necessary to use an accessible style of speech, plain words, simple sentences, and, where possible at the start of the encounter, some open-ended questions to give the person an opportunity to say how she or he is feeling. The details associated with how to ask questions would fill this chapter. Sometimes a less experienced interviewer will become nervous and prompt the person being interviewed to try to speed up the process of gaining information. One obvious prompt is a 'leading question'. For example, you might say: 'I expect you're very upset at having to leave your home and go into residential care.' This comment is loaded towards one response rather than another.

Another common problem with some interviews is that the interviewer is too repetitive. There is too much 'noise', distracting the person from responding. This is particularly important with, say, children or adults with communication difficulties, such as sight and hearing impairments, autism or Asperger's syndrome, or those for whom English is their second language.

It is important to summarise from time to time and give feedback to the person for them to check out and confirm the appropriateness or otherwise of your responses to what they are saying. It is also reassuring and helps to let them know that you are listening and are sensitive to their feelings and thoughts.

Sometimes you will be aware early on in the encounter of the need to seek an interpreter. This may happen where a person is deaf, or English is not their first language and they are struggling to use it to express themselves.

Active Listening

When we are talking, we need to listen to what the other person is saying in response to us and on their own behalf. We need to listen actively, giving them clear verbal and physical messages that their views and feelings are important to us. We should not jump to conclusions about these, even if they seem predictable to us. We should wait for the person to express them. Often there are surprises in the messages. For instance, many people will hesitate near the end of the time limit, or by the door, and add as a seeming afterthought some important items, which may have been left until last because they were uncertain about whether to say them.

Skills in Assessing

Communication is at the heart of good assessment. The ability to assess the immediate situation is a crucial ingredient in the worker's effectiveness as a communicator. The range of items discussed in the chapter on assessment (Chapter 30) apply here. For instance, you can ask wider questions about the environment of a person, which enables him or her to bring the life course and cultural perspectives into play. You can gain a deeper understanding of the importance to the carer or service user of environmental, employment, housing, community, physiological, psychological and social factors in their personal, family and social life.

Using Non-verbal Communication

We saw a dramatic example of body language at the start of this chapter. Body language is a form of non-verbal communication. When it accompanies spoken words, it can be extremely powerful, either reinforcing the message or contradicting it. For example, if the worker is saying to the person 'I really am sorry, tell me all about it', but his eyes are darting around the room, he is drumming the fingers of one hand on his desk and with his other hand stabbing at the open diary with his pen, he is not conveying a very positive message about his attentiveness. Our words may contrast with our non-verbal behaviour. We may say 'I'm interested to hear this', but turn away frequently, doodle on a pad and look bored or disinterested.

There are *empathising* skills and skills of *empowering* people. People need encouraging, but not smothering. We should find ways, where possible, of recruiting the person as a partner in the interview, drawing on their experience, knowledge and skills. In terms of non-verbal behaviour, vulnerable children and adults, in particular, benefit from recognising the qualities of empathy and honesty when they interact with practitioners. Here, as elsewhere, the practitioner needs to strike a balance between too much warmth and sheer indifference; excessive warmth can be as claustrophobic and overpowering as indifference can be demotivating.

Written Communications

An important aspect of communication occurs alongside our interaction with the person, namely communication – in speech and writing – with our colleagues and in recording our practice. Chapter 2 in Prince's book on communication (1996, pp. 12–28) is very good on this subject and, although it is about childcare, has many important, and more general messages.

Conclusion

In this chapter we have introduced some of the complex responsibilities associated with communication. The skills of communicating have been touched on and some of the pitfalls as well as the opportunities. It is apparent that good communication is much more than applying a few simple techniques. It is an art and, like all art, it can be a creative achievement or a dismal failure.

REVIEW QUESTIONS

1 What are the main differences between communication and interaction?

2 What is active listening?

3 Can you list the main skills you would employ to maximise your chances of communicating with a service user who has a learning disability and no personal assistant?

FURTHER READING

Argyle, M. (1988) *Bodily Communication*, London, Methuen

Davies, H. and Fallowfield, L. (1991) *Counselling and Communication in Healthcare*, Chichester, John Wiley & Son

Hinde, R.A. (1972) *Non Verbal Communication*, Cambridge, Cambridge University Press

Lishman, J. (1994) *Communication in Social Work*, Basingstoke, BASW/Macmillan

Prince, K. (1996) *Boring Records? Communication, Speech and Writing in Social Work*, London, Jessica Kingsley

Seager, P. and Kebbell, M. (1999) 'Pitfalls in Interviewing: A Psychological Perspective', in D. Messer and F. Jones (eds) *Psychology and Social Care*, London, Jessica Kingsley

Thompson, N. (2003) *Communication and Language: A Handbook of Theory and Practice*, Basingstoke, Palgrave Macmillan

Part VI

Resource file

Doing a presentation

Doing an individual presentation

Preparation

■ Look carefully at the task and decide how to tackle it.

■ Remember a presentation is not the same as writing an essay.

■ Let your imagination come up with interesting ways of presenting material.

■ Use diagrams, photos, a poster collage of headlines and pictures cut from newspapers.

■ Don't prepare too much material. Reading 2,200 words takes 15 minutes, but explaining them can take an hour. One good diagram can take just as long to explain.

On the day

- Don't rely on your memory. Make detailed notes of everything you want to say.
- Print them in 18 point bold type or write in big capitals if you need to.
- Don't panic. It's never as bad as you feared.
- Don't be afraid to pause to read through the next bit before saying it. People will wait if they know you're being thoughtful and careful.

Doing a group presentation

Preparing

- Make sure you allow enough time to meet as a group.
- Agree together the task you've been set.
- Decide what outcome you want to achieve.
- Decide how you're going to set about it.
- Break the job down into tasks.
- Make individuals responsible for each task.
- Work in pairs, threes or fours where necessary.
- Meet regularly, phone, chat or email to check progress.
- Ask anyone who isn't coping to tell the others.
- Finish the work before the last day if possible.

On the day

- Don't panic.
- Use flip charts and other similar visual aids where they help to make your points.
- Stick to your agreed division of the presentation between you.
- Make one of you the timekeeper who can warn people who are going on too long.

Cognitive-behavioural Work

ROBERT ADAMS

> ## Learning outcomes
>
> By the end of this chapter, you should be able to:
>
> ■ SUMMARISE the main features of cognitive-behavioural work
>
> ■ OUTLINE the major theories inherent in cognitive-behavioural work
>
> ■ DESCRIBE the main stages of cognitive-behavioural work.

This chapter deals with a well-developed and popular approach in the health and social and penal services, namely cognitive-behavioural practice. The main assumptions inherent in this approach are reviewed using a practice example and its main strengths and weaknesses are summarised.

What is Cognitive-behavioural Work?

Cognitive-behavioural work sounds fearsome, but its use is simple and logical, and, provided the symptoms are not indicative of a more deep-seated problem, it can be very effective.

In the late 1970s, I spent a short period working in the psychiatric ward at Leeds General Infirmary, where I worked with a team led by a psychologist, who used a biofeedback machine to help a young woman to develop ways of controlling her impulse towards having a drink. The biofeedback device, which some call neurofeedback, showed the woman her brain activity on a screen, so that she could try to exercise control over her responses to the questions from the psychologist. Any responses she made in the desired direction were reinforced with praise, while others were given negative feedback or ignored. These two forms of feedback – negative or no feedback – form the basis of classical conditioning or operant conditioning respectively, which in turn form two of the three bases of cognitive-behavioural therapy (CBT). CBT draws its theoretical underpinning from psychological theories and research linked with learning theory. Cognitive-behavioural practice links behaviour therapy with cognitive work, both of which are equally important. *Cognition* refers to our consciousness and our feelings, thoughts, intentions and decisions. This amounts to that part of us which we can influence or even control. *Behaviour* refers to what we actually do. CBT concentrates on the link between people's conscious thoughts and their behaviour. It is assumed they can reason about, and control, what they do. By implication, the problem behaviour they seek to change is assumed to arise from some fault in their reasoning, leading to them doing the 'wrong' thing.

The strength of CBT is that it focuses on mobilising people's thoughts and powers to decide to change their behaviour (Marshall and Turnbull, 1996). Thus, it is useful in situations where a person, with support, can carry out practical plans to tackle her or his own problems. In work with children, CBT has been used to manage behaviour problems and curb young children's disorderly conduct. It works best when combined with training parents and family-based work.

Theory of CBT

The aim of CBT is to use individual meetings or groupwork, or both, to establish a collaborative relationship with the service user and develop a learning programme that modifies the thinking (cognition) and behaviour which need to change. Undesirable behaviour is not treated like a disease (as it is under the medical treatment model). All behaviour, from maladaptive to adaptive, is looked at the same way. Problem behaviour is not regarded as a symptom of underlying psychological disturbance, but is simply viewed as undesirable behaviour that needs to be unlearned. By regarding a person's behaviour in this way, it is the behaviour which is viewed as abnormal, rather than the whole person being regarded as in some way abnormal.

We can define learning as *changed behaviour resulting from experience*. The roots of CBT lie in three main behavioural approaches, which relate to psychological theories to do with learning: classical conditioning, operant conditioning and social learning. A good deal of subsequent work has made these distinctions much less clear-cut than previously. The main therapeutic technique used in CBT is conditioning. This provides a means by which desirable behaviour can be learned.

In *classical conditioning*, Pavlov ([1897]1982) rewarded or reinforced the desirable behaviour of dogs and they learned new behaviour. A bell rang when they were offered food and eventually they salivated when the bell rang, without the food being offered. They had learned a new behaviour.

Operant conditioning originated in the work of Thorndike (1898) and was elaborated by Skinner (1953, 1974). It focuses on the consequences of the behaviour, positively reinforcing the desirable consequence or negatively reinforcing the undesirable consequence of the behaviour.

Social learning includes approaches that encourage people to learn desirable behaviour through raising their expectations rather than creating a 'mechanical' stimulus–response effect (Sheldon, 1995, p. 94). The work of Bandura (1977, 1986) illustrates this trend towards therapists working for changes in people that are more cognitive than merely behavioural. For instance, this may be achieved by enabling the person to model (copy) the behaviour. Bandura proposed what he called 'social cognitivism', suggesting that children, for example copying aggression, can learn new behaviour by imitating others without the need for other stimuli or rewards. This is likely to work better if the person identifies some similarities with the situation of the model, if the opportunity to model the desirable behaviour comes soon after seeing it and if the consequent reinforcement of the behaviour helps to embed it.

Outline of CBT

1. The assessment of a person focuses on their suitability for CBT. The criteria for this includes answering the following questions, each scored 0 to 5, where 5 is the score for greatest suitability (Blackburn and Twaddle, 1996, pp. 69–70):

   - How far does the person spontaneously report key negative automatic thoughts?
   - To what extent does the person show awareness of emotions?
   - To what extent does the person accept personal responsibility for the problem?
   - To what extent does the person accept the validity of the cognitive approach?
   - To what extent is the person willing to ally with the therapist?
   - To what extent are the problems recent in nature?
   - To what extent would the person be unlikely to miss appointments or cancel the programme regardless of any feelings of shame or similar?
   - To what extent is the person able to remain focused on the problem without prompting being necessary?
   - To what extent is the person optimistic that CBT can work?

2. One or two assessment sessions followed by a similar number of treatment sessions generally lead to an initial formulation of the problem.

3. Later in the sequence of sessions, this is made more detailed, clarifying problems and working on them, focusing on changing behaviour by setting behavioural tasks, or homework, between sessions. Some sessions involved recording automatic thoughts when undesirable behaviour took place and then challenging them in the session and later the person challenging them alone.

4. Continued recording and challenging of negative thoughts continues. Various behavioural experiments are tried.

5. The initial formulation (2 above) is reviewed and where necessary modified. The person makes a written list of achievements.

6. The final formulation takes place.

7. Termination of the programme.

8. Outcomes of the programme include asking the person to score on the severity measures.

9. Relapse prevention. The final session tackles this, being reviewed at follow-up, three months and six months later. The person is asked to share with the cognitive behavioural therapist a written list of critical incidents related to the condition being tackled. A list is also made of hazards and risks in the future, related to past events, which relate to the person's condition. Questions about hazards and risks often follow the 'What if …' formula (Blackburn and Twaddle, 1996, pp. 77–84).

CBT in Action

We have adapted this programme of six–eight sessions of 90 minutes each that the cognitive-behavioural therapist Scott (1989, pp. 46–55) developed for anger control for parents in relation to their children. We shall illustrate CBT in action with reference to a programme of anger management with Mrs Jehu, who finds herself arguing constantly with her sister Beth, with whom she shares a large house that is too big for them to cope with. In this study, we are a health and social care practitioner who visits Mrs Jehu at home and later meets her at the office.

The programme has three interrelated components:

1. Teaching regarding physiological and other factors affecting how we are roused to anger.
2. Teaching how to use self-reinforcement, self-teaching, self-monitoring, deep breathing and relaxation to control angry feelings and situations that create anger.
3. Giving opportunities to practise in simulated conditions.

The aim of the programme is to reduce the aversive behaviour (Mrs Jehu's excessive anger) not to encourage positive behaviour.

Session 1

This begins by inviting Mrs Jehu to work with the practitioner to develop ways of coping with a high-risk situation where she shows signs of being aroused to anger. The practitioner asks Mrs Jehu to enact the situation in slow motion. Afterwards she asks Mrs Jehu to repeat the situation and stop at the first sign of anger arousal. At this point, Mrs Jehu wants to set off in the car for their drive, but is being kept waiting by her sister and is pacing up and down in a state of high anxiety, making self-statements under her breath such as 'She does this deliberately.' The practitioner gives her three alternative self-statements that she has noted from their conversation earlier in the session. She can use one of these as she chooses, depending on whether her anger is high, medium or low:

■ *High:* 'Beth is so tired from staying up late last night that she has no energy to get ready.'

- *Medium:* 'Beth was probably late having lunch and is still getting ready.'
- *Low:* 'Beth doesn't remember as well as she used to and has probably forgotten.'

Giving Mrs Jehu these choices between her own statements increases her sense of being in control of the therapy. The practitioner does a simulation with Mrs Jehu, asking her to be moderately angry, then very angry and select an appropriate self-statement to stave off her anger. It takes a little while to simulate the situation between them and get used to practising the alternative self-management statements.

Session 2

This begins by listening to Mrs Jehu telling stories about her attempts to use the techniques learned so far. Even tiny reductions in her irritability with her sister are praised by the practitioner, who then gives Mrs Jehu the invitation to select another situation she finds anger-provoking. The aim is to move Mrs Jehu from being aggressive to being assertive. So, instead of her saying to her sister 'You know how much that annoys me …', the therapist gives her the statement to say: 'I don't like it when you …'. Or when her sister delays getting ready until Mr and Mrs Jehu are ready and the car is on the drive: 'we waited another 10 minutes before you came out.'

Mrs Jehu selects the situation where she is speaking and her sister interrupts her. This normally makes Mrs Jehu extremely irritated and after a few such incidents she normally explodes with anger. The practitioner encourages Mrs Jehu to give her sister space to think and cope with her interruptions, which normally irritate her. Instead of concluding that her sister is insensitive or wants to annoy her, the practitioner offers her the task of thinking of a more neutral reason. For instance, Mrs Jehu is to say to herself 'My sister is excited today, which makes her interrupt me.'

Sessions 3 and 4

The practitioner asks Mrs Jehu to express her feelings and thoughts. At first the practitioner focuses on the last 'homework'. The practitioner develops more self-coping statements and negotiates them with Mrs Jehu. They cover a minimum of two problematic situations already written by Mrs Jehu in her 'Angry Thoughts' diary.

Session 5

This begins with a review of the last homework. It moves on from the previous sessions, focusing on anger-producing cognition and developing rational responses to the dysfunctional (problematic) cognitions. The practitioner drafts a list of self-statements to be used, in order to keep Mrs Jehu motivated to complete the programme.

Session 6

The programme is completed by teaching Mrs Jehu her own framework for developing her own list of coping self-statements.

Part VI

Sessions 7 and 8

Each of these last two sessions starts by the practitioner checking Mrs Jehu's homework from the previous session. The aim of these last sessions is to consolidate what Mrs Jehu has learned during the programme.

Practice study

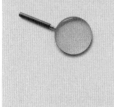

Biva

Biva, 25, has been mildly depressed for a few weeks, crying at home repeatedly and unable to face colleagues in the department store where she works. She has been to the doctor and is taking medication, but lately her feelings of inadequacy have become worse. She goes to see her GP who refers her to a therapist based at the surgery, who offers to try a course of CBT with her.

Let us consider how the therapist proceeds with Biva. To begin with, the therapist points out that CBT will not be devised *for* her and imposed on her, but will be carried out *with* her, with the aim of giving her the confidence to curb her depression independently. The therapist gives her homework, to keep a careful diary during the week of the events and situations that make her feel worse.

The first areas identified are Biva's tendencies towards self-blame and self-pity. She is also hard on herself and does not allow herself to make mistakes. The therapist points out that when we feel that we are inadequate and cannot measure up to the standards of the world around us, we should bear in mind that none of us are perfect and neither is the world around us perfect. We are little different to everybody else. She helps Biva to plan ways to allow herself to make mistakes and give herself small rewards when she finds alternatives to self-blame and self-pity.

Biva plans and achieves small ways to make mistakes, forgive herself and reward herself. For instance, she learns how to give herself permission to take a lunch break and reward herself with her favourite healthy snacks when she has done particularly well at work in the morning. Over a period, her confidence grows, her depression disappears and she flushes the medication down the sink.

Strengths and Weaknesses of Cognitive-behavioural Therapy

There are many applications of CBT, but in particular it is used where a change in immediate behaviour is sought, such as parent 'training', reducing violent and angry behaviour (through an anger management programme), communication, direct work with children such as curbing difficult teenage behaviour, or dealing with mental health problems such as depression, anxiety disorder, panic disorder, obsessive-compulsive disorder, agoraphobia and bulimia nervosa.

Strengths of CBT include the following:

- It has a positive emphasis on the present.
- It offers power to the person to change behaviour, so can have an immediate impact on their future life.
- It offers a short-term technique for changing problem behaviour; it can achieve change when it targets a specific behaviour in a focused way.
- It works best when the person's problem behaviour is not rigidly established over a long period and is still amenable to therapy to change it.

Weaknesses of CBT include the following:

- It may be unable to deal with deep-rooted problems requiring a person to do more than use reason to make decisions about their next actions. Not all behaviour can be changed through reasoning and logical argument.
- It may only be superficially effective, since it deals only with those aspects of a person's life and behaviour under conscious control, whereas people may not have access to their thoughts and feelings and the problems may not be visible in identifiable 'workable' problems.
- People may not be motivated to 'do homework' and help themselves.
- It may be unethical to use CBT to change behaviour, since CBT involves manipulation of the problem behaviour by the practitioner rather than leaving it under the control of the 'client'. Sheldon notes that this is a particular concern in a residential setting where staff may take short cuts with a programme of treatment and people may be manipulated in a programme of treatment (Sheldon, 1995, pp. 244–5).

Practice study

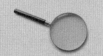

Ada

The therapist is working with Ada, 49, who, since her husband died three years ago, has developed a drink problem. Last month she was disqualified from driving for 12 months, after being found drunk in her car late at night outside the local pub. Ada agreed in court to a course of cognitive-behavioural work.

The therapist works in the following way:

- she encourages Ada to talk about ways in which she wants to change her behaviour
- she helps Ada to identify the circumstances in which she turns to problem drinking
- when Ada says she drinks when she feels fed up, the therapist sets Ada a series of small-scale objectives that she needs to achieve in order to change her problem drinking pattern
- she works on the first objective with Ada, breaking it down into a series of even smaller tasks and tackling them one by one, successively
- each time Ada succeeds in achieving her goal, the therapist moves on to the next one and plans with her how to achieve it

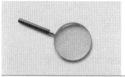

■ whenever Ada fails to achieve her goal, the therapist helps her to identify where it did not succeed and tries, flexibly, to rework the goal and other related goals, before suggesting to Ada that she tries again.

Activity 42.1

Having read this practice study, spend 10 minutes making notes on the features of cognitive-behavioural work likely to help Ada.

Here are notes on the study.
Cognitive-behavioural work with Ada:

■ focuses on achieving practical outcomes
■ involves action rather than talk
■ is about doing rather than thinking
■ is based in the present rather than dwelling on the past or the future
■ gives the person the tools to change their behaviour rather than sticking with existing patterns of behaviour.

The therapist talks to Ada about a recurrence of her drinking. Ada says she feels depressed and cannot control her reactions. The therapist suggests to Ada that her depression *can* be controlled by her and sets up a number of small experiments for Ada to attempt to achieve changes in her behaviour.

This gives us important information about two sets of assumptions underlying cognitive-behavioural therapy:

■ It is assumed that although Ada's repeated depressions may on occasions be triggered by external events, she has lost control of her moods, primarily because of what are called 'cognitive deficits', or faults in her attitudes.
■ It is assumed that the therapy can apply the approach of experimental psychology to problems such as mental health difficulties (Klosko and Sanderson, 1999) and addictions (Grant et al., 2004).

Wider Uses of CBT beyond Therapy

Cognitive behavioural therapy is widely used in psychiatric work. One group of psychiatrists have written about its benefits in work with phobic disorders, depression, obsessive disorders, eating disorders and anxiety states (Hawton et al., 1991). Applications are by no means restricted to therapeutic settings and mental health problems in particular. One use is in treating chronic medical problems (White,

2001) and another widespread use is in social skills training, which may be linked with therapeutic aims, but may be an end in itself. Typically, there are five stages, in the following example of enabling a person to feel better about handling arriving at work in the morning, which may not be sequential, but may overlap:

1. Teaching the person to say good morning and look people in the face when doing so
2. Giving feedback indicating where improvements can be made, for example looking pleased next time
3. Offering practice through mimicking, on the principle that giving feedback is not always sufficient to embed the desired behaviour
4. Offering therapeutic models, then ensuring that the person tries the behaviour, then offering feedback and, perhaps, repeating the sequence
5. Giving praise for any improvement, no matter how small, such as making an additional positive remark (adapted from Scott, 1989, pp. 119–23).

Conclusion

This chapter has described the main features of cognitive-behavioural work and illustrated how it works. It has discussed some of the main applications of cognitive-behavioural therapies. Finally, it has evaluated cognitive-behavioural work, high-lighting the fact that it is by no means a suitable treatment for all circumstances.

REVIEW QUESTIONS

1 What is cognitive-behavioural therapy?

2 What are the main similarities and differences between classical conditioning, operant conditioning and social learning approaches?

3 Can you think of three health and social care applications for CBT?

FURTHER READING

Curwen, B., Palmer, S., Ruddell, P. and Houston, G. (2000) *Brief Cognitive Behaviour Therapy*, London, Sage

Grant, A., Mills, G., Mulhern, R. and Short, N. (2004) *Cognitive Behavioural Therapy in Mental Health Care*, London, Sage
A series of detailed studies of different mental health problems and treatments.

Klosko, J.S. and Sanderson, W.S. (1999) *Cognitive-Behavioural Treatment of Depression*, Northvale, NJ, Jason Aronson
A detailed analysis of sessions of CBT treatment.

Marshall, S. and Turnbull, J. (ed.) (1996) *Cognitive Behaviour Therapy: An Introduction to Theory and Practice*, London, Ballière Tindall
A practical guide to principles and practice of CBT.

Scott, M.J., Stradling, S.G. and Dryden, W. (1995) *Developing Cognitive-Behavioural Counselling*, London, Sage
An easy-to-read guide to aspects of practice.

Part VI

Sheldon, B. (1995) *Cognitive-Behavioural Therapy; Research, Practice and Philosophy*, London, Routledge
A detailed work of reference on theories and practice.

White, C.A. (2001) *Cognitive Behaviour Therapy for Chronic Medical Problems: A Guide to Assessment and Treatment in Practice*, Chichester, John Wiley & Son
Deals with the assessment and formulation of plans in CBT dealing with problems such as cancer, chronic pain, diabetes and cardiac conditions.

Therapeutic Work

ROBERT ADAMS

Learning outcomes

By the end of this chapter, you should be able to:

- IDENTIFY some of the most widely known therapeutic approaches to working with people
- DISCUSS some of the main features of these therapeutic approaches
- SUGGEST some of the most appropriate uses of the main therapeutic approaches.

It would be impossible in a book of this size, let alone one chapter, to summarise the hundreds of different therapies that exist. In this chapter, we shall select several important ones and focus on them in turn.

Psychoanalysis and Psychotherapy

There are many approaches to psychotherapy, but most can be traced back to the psychoanalytic practice of Sigmund Freud and his later followers and critics. Freud, renowned both as the populariser of the idea of delving into our unconscious for explanations of the feelings and thoughts that underlie our behaviour and as the originator of psychoanalysis, was born in Moravia in 1856, studied medicine and practised in Vienna for many years and died in London in 1939. His writings were based partly on his self-analysis and psychoanalysis of others, including the interpretation of their dreams as a clue to their unconsciousness. His writings dealt with the nature and development of the personality – the ego (the I), the id (the instincts and drives) and the superego (the conscience) – emphasising the way people's early experiences from infancy shaped their later lives, building on basic drives such as sex and aggression. His views became more pessimistic in the light of the traumatic consequences of violence that he saw in soldiers returning from the First World War.

In 1909, Freud met and befriended Carl Jung (1875–1961), who created new and distinctive dynasties of psychotherapists. Jung developed a more optimistic view of human development (the ego, the individual unconscious and the collective unconscious), not entirely rooted in sexuality nor infant and childhood traumas, but based in psychic energy, drawing on mythology, art and patterns of thinking and action that he thought of as lying in the collective unconscious of different peoples.

We can distinguish between psychodynamic and psychoanalytic perspectives on therapy. The former make more general links between people's thoughts and feelings and how they act (see Chapter 45). The latter owe more to the psychoanalytic theories of Freud and his successors (see Chapter 7).

Therapeutic Communities

Therapeutic communities are one form of environmental therapeutic approach in which care is taken to design the regime (or daily programme of activities for staff and people using services) so that every part of it contributes to the therapy (Kennard, 1998). Mental hospitals (see Maxwell Jones's 1968 work in psychiatric hospitals such as the Henderson hospital), community homes with education on the premises, young offenders' institutions and prisons (Morris, 2004) are settings where therapeutic approaches have been taken. Many so-called 'total institutions' have been described by Erving Goffman (1961) as having a number of features: a tightly regimented regime; block treatment requiring every patient, resident or inmate to carry out basic activities – such as getting up, washing and going to bed – at the same time; and a social gulf between the staff and the patients, residents or inmates (see Chapter 15). One aim of the therapeutic community is to substitute for these negative and dehumanising characteristics a more positive atmosphere, values and goals. The heyday of the therapeutic community idea in Britain was the 1960s and early 1970s. I recall attending some regular small meetings of psychiatrists in the late 1960s, all of whom were involved in therapeutic community work at the large mental hospitals in Middlesex, Surrey and surrounding districts. The discussion tended to focus on how to engineer systemic change in these rather rigid and depressing institutions.

Therapeutic communities share a number of common features, among which are:

- Managing the hospital democratically and giving patients more power relative to staff
- Using group meetings as a key method of day-to-day management of the hospital
- Using group meetings as a way of tackling day-to-day problems between people
- Nurturing an atmosphere of openness and sharing between staff and patients
- Focusing on understanding the dynamics and processes of life and work in the hospital.

Therapeutic Groupwork

Therapeutic groupwork is the general term used to describe a great range of group-work approaches that can take place in residential care in particular (see Chapter 54 on group living and group care). From the 1960s, group counselling and encounter groups, widely described as forms of group therapy, were increasingly popular in the UK. Bizarrely, there were group counselling programmes run by staff in several prisons, including Pentonville. In one institution, Pollington, East York-shire, where I acted as governor in the early 1970s, for two full evenings every week every young person and many staff met in counselling groups, lending the entire institution the temporary atmosphere of a therapeutic community. The traditional staff–inmate relations were loosened in group meetings and the use of first names and the passing of 'confidential' information from inmates to staff were not uncommon. More recently, social and cognitive-behavioural groups that lack the dimension of institutional change have become more popular. Some commentators and practitioners, notably Mullender and Ward (1991), have promoted a view of groupwork as empowering for its members, who share much of the power traditionally vested in the leader or the therapist. Ward (2005, p. 152) points out that groupwork can be intrinsically anti-oppressive and democratic in the way it is run. There is a close link between this form of groupwork and mutual aid or self-help groups (Adams, 2003).

Family Therapy

Family therapy involves treatment of the whole family together, even though one person may be presented or referred to the agency as 'the problem'. The assumption of family therapy is that family situations contribute to the circumstances of individual family members and therefore have a part to play in creating the problem and generating ways forward. Health and social care workers may encounter family therapists, although they are unlikely to practise family therapy themselves.

Solution-focused Brief Therapy

Solution-focused brief therapy describes a particular form of practice in which the client is encouraged to focus on changes that she or he can envisage making now or in the immediate future. The brief therapist encourages the client to identify these, by asking the client what he or she wants from the therapy, how his or her life would look if these wants were achieved and details of anything he or she has already done which could contribute to achieving this. The role of the therapist is to ask the questions so as to enable the client to find the responses. Solution-focused work is a quite straightforward approach to intervention, with the problem identified and agreed between the practitioner and the service user and an explicit agreement made about building, from the present into the future, on the strengths identified during the assessment process and avoiding referring back to the past deficits of the person. Of course, we should emphasise that not every problem is amenable to this approach (see Chapter 45).

Expressive Arts Therapies

There is a vast range of approaches to therapy that rely for their character and effectiveness on their creative and expressive nature, and here we focus on drama, music, poetry, art and photography.

Drama Therapy

Drama therapy has been used for many years as a therapeutic tool. Drama therapy originated in drama and the theatre, but is uniquely inclusive in the expressive therapies in incoporating music, movement, storytelling, performance and design (Chesner, 1995, p. 5). Drama therapists may work closely with other therapists, for example using drama therapy in anger management (Thompson, 1999) or to contribute to family sculpting in family therapy. Sculpting is a technique which takes many forms. In one of these, family sculpting may involve asking family members to group themselves in what for them is a typical attitude or stance and then, when everybody is in position, encouraging each person in turn to talk about why they have chosen this stance and how they feel about it. As therapy progresses, people can be asked to sculpt their ideal for themselves and this can have a great impact on them and on other people also in the same sculpt.

Work with disabled people proceeds from a careful, open-minded 'tuning in' to the person's mood during assessment (Chesner, 1995, p. 19). Following assessment, a short – six or twelve – structured sequence of sessions may be agreed in a contractual arrangement. In the case of people with a profound learning disability, Chesner (p. 15) suggests a long period of time is needed over which change may take place. Drama therapy is a group as well as an individual therapy and group therapy offers wide therapeutic possibilities (Chesner, 1995, pp. 128–90).

Music Therapy

Pauline Etkin (1999, p. 155) illustrates how musical improvisation can be used to gain insights into the world of an abused child, through the three-stage process of:

1. Establishing a relationship with the child
2. Offering a way of communicating and self-expression
3. Bringing about change and enabling the child's potential to be realised.

Poetry Therapy

Poetry therapy is often overlooked, but has the potential to make a major contribution to therapy, for four reasons:

1. Poems selected can be short.
2. They tend to appeal to the emotions.
3. They tend to be focused sharply on particular aspects.
4. They often possess the power of expression to make a unique contribution to the therapeutic process.

Art Therapy

Art therapy is often carried out in settings where people have difficulty expressing in words the emotions they are experiencing. For example, children who have been abused may be encouraged to use drawing and painting as ways of expressing themselves, while the therapist accompanies them and enables them to talk about their painting if they wish. The use of art in this way dates at least from the early years of psychoanalysis, if not earlier. Klein (1997) used people's, including children's, paintings as diagnostic clues to their thoughts and feelings.

Art and music therapy are also used in rehabilitative work with people with mental health problems or people who have suffered traumas (Carey, 2006). Sometimes art therapists will work with offenders (Liebmann, 1994) or NHS Trusts will employ art therapists in hospitals.

Photography

Photography can be used therapeutically, either as a technique in its own right or in conjunction with other treatment. Jackson and Jackson (1999) have written a fascinating and easy-to-read little book giving important insights into how photography can be used in work with people with a learning disability. They maintain that photography can help a person to gain new skills, reach emotional stability or reduce uncertainties (pp. 7–8). Photography can give a sense of achievement, help a person to grieve, provide instant feedback and a trigger for memories after a special event or outing and reinforce learning (Jackson and Jackson, 1999, pp. 9–10).

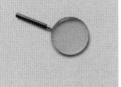

Practice study

Bill

Jackson and Jackson illustrate the use of photography in the work done with one man, Bill, who has limited speech and uses Makaton to communicate. The aim is to use photography to help him travel independently by bus to the day centre from the staffed group home he shares with two other people.

There are four stages to the process, which are outlined below.

Stage 1

The community nurse begins by using a holistic approach to *assessing* what Bill already can understand and do. A photographic record of his life helps at this stage. One photograph shows him at the day centre and helps to remind him of his destination when going there by bus. Another shows him enjoying himself with friends at the day centre and reinforces how important it is to him to go there independently each day.

Stage 2

The *training programme* is developed, building the photographs used at the assessment stage into a larger selection used to compare the advantages of Bill travelling by bus, over other forms of transport where he is not independent. There are photographs of Bill at each stage in the journey, clearly visible in the photograph, showing how the bus is quicker than the minibus.

Stage 3

During the *action* phase, the carer takes Bill on the bus to the day centre, using photographs of him on the journey to reinforce key landmarks and at the centre to reinforce where they are going. He is provided with a little wallet containing the photographs. The carer gradually withdraws from accompanying him by getting off at the last but one stop, then getting off at successive stops earlier each time. At intervals, she talks through with Bill the landmarks on the journey to ensure that he has learned the journey well.

Stage 4

At the *evaluation* meeting, six questions were asked:

1. Has the programme met its *main aim*?
2. Has the programme met any *subsidiary aims*?
3. Have any *further issues* arisen that need tackling?
4. Is Bill now travelling to work independently and safely?
5. What are the *benefits* from the programme and what are its *costs*?
6. Are there any other concerns about Bill's travel?

The carer reported that within eight weeks Bill succeeded in travelling to the day centre independently. On one occasion, he had got off at the wrong stop, but later he talked this through with the carer and community nurse. Bill attended the meeting and expressed his pleasure at his achievement. His parents also were pleased.

General Comments

We can generalise from the important point Jackson and Jackson make about photography used as a cathartic tool needing the support of a therapist. It must be emphasised that professional supervision and support are needed where the expressive arts are used therapeutically to enable people to release feelings. The expressive therapies are not suitable for all problems or all carers, service users or patients. Careful assessment is needed to ensure that unsuitable arrangements are not made with people who will not benefit.

Conclusion

This chapter has surveyed a various and rapidly expanding field of therapies. It is ironic that this is expanding as many adult care services departments have damped down any public commitment to therapeutic work as such. They tend to commission private and voluntary organisations to carry this out. We have surveyed the main strands of therapy and have illustrated some of the main ones from practice.

REVIEW QUESTIONS

1   How would you describe and distinguish between psychoanalytic and psychodynamic approaches to therapy?

2   What is family therapy?

3   What contribution can the expressive therapies make to helping people?

FURTHER READING

Appendix 3 for information about complementary therapies

Burck, C. and Daniel, G. (1995) *Gender and Family Therapy*, London, Karnac

Houston, G. (2003) *Brief Gestalt Therapy*, London, Sage

Mander, G. (2002) *A Psychodynamic Approach to Brief Therapy*, London, Sage

Nichols, M.P. and Schwartz, R.C. (2006) *Family Therapy: Concepts and Methods*, Boston, MA, Pearson/Allyn & Bacon
Considers different models of family therapy and their applications.

O'Connell, B. (1998) *Solution-focused Therapy*, London, Sage

O'Connell, B. and Palmer, S. (2003) *Handbook of Solution-focused Therapy*, London, Sage

Stratton, P., Preston-Shoot, M. and Hanks, H. (1990) *Family Therapy: Training and Practice*, Birmingham, Venture

Tudor, K. (2002) *Transactional Analysis Approaches to Brief Therapy, or, What Do you Say between Saying Hello and Goodbye?*, London, Sage

Wilkins, P. (2003) *Person-centred Therapy in Focus*, London, Sage

Part VI

Writing an essay

Preparing for the essay

- Check that you understand the title or question set.
- Confirm the deadline and what you have to hand in.

Collecting the information for the essay

- Set a timetable for yourself with a deadline well before the hand-in date.
- Decide what kind of information you need.
- Gather the information, avoiding being diverted from your topic.
- Modify the topic and your information if necessary:
  - Don't stick with a topic you become convinced is unworkable.
  - Renegotiate an unworkable topic or change it if you can.
  - Don't collect too much information.
  - Don't gather information you feel is irrelevant but interesting.

Planning the essay

Plan the main headings of the essay. Most essays have three sections – Introduction, main body of the essay and Conclusion – plus, at the very end, a list of the work referred to (for how to refer to other people's work, see Resource File: References and Bibliography, at the end of Chapter 44).

Introduction

The most important first job is to try to come up with a sentence in the introduction, summarising your approach – which we call here the argument – in your essay. Here are some common ways of starting your essay as an argument:

- 'This essay discusses the pros and cons of ...'
- 'In this essay, we examine the evidence for the statement that ...'
- 'This essay critically reviews the statement that ...'

- 'I have chosen to study ... for my special topic and I am tackling the question of whether ... or ...'.

Main body of the essay

Jot down the topic for each paragraph. Try to map out the whole essay in paragraphs or sections, based on the chunks of information you've collected.

Put your plan on one side for a while and come back to it after a gap of several hours or preferably a day or two.

Conclusion or Conclusions

The Conclusion or Conclusions (whichever you prefer) is a few sentences bringing your essay to an end, perhaps by rounding off the argument or saying what you've found or shown. Your conclusion should not introduce any new ideas, particularly those quoted as references from things you've read.

Writing the essay

- Now have another look at your essay plan. Alter anything which looks wrong.
- Confirm the sequence of your main paragraphs. Say, for example, your word limit is 2,000 words. Have no more than 10 long paragraphs or 20 short ones.
- Write a simple sentence summarising the main point of each paragraph. Each single sentence should be no more than 30 words long (three lines). Any longer and you should try to split it into two sentences.
- Each single sentence now becomes the first sentence in each paragraph. Add four or five more sentences to it explaining its key point in that paragraph. Repeat for every paragraph in the essay. Your essay should be near its final length.
- You may be able to add a paragraph at the end under the heading 'Conclusions'. This brings together all the points you've made in a few sentences summarising your argument.

Systemic Work

ROBERT ADAMS

Learning outcomes

By the end of this chapter, you should be able to:

- DEFINE systemic work
- IDENTIFY the key features of systemic work
- DISCUSS the strengths and limitations of systemic practice.

This chapter deals with a group of perspectives on health and social care work which have become increasingly important, now that more agencies and professionals are working together in various forms of teamwork, collaboration and partnership to deliver community care, mental health and childcare and other similar services.

What is Systemic Work?

Systemic or systems working relates to systems theories, which have had a significant impact on consultancy management and practice in commercial organisations (Campbell et al., 1991). Teamwork and collaborative work between professionals and agencies owe much to the ideas about systemic work (see Chapters 47–50). Systemic practice owes much to systems theory as well and you should read the following account without becoming too hypnotised by all the times the word 'system' appears. You should think of the system simply as an individual, group or organisation, depending on the circumstances. If the basic system is a group, then we might refer to the individuals in the group as subsystems, because they are in the next layer, composing the group. The organisation would be called the supersystem, in the next layer above, made up of lots of other systems (groups). The idea of the system is really a way of arranging lots of clumps of supersystems and breaking them down into systems and subsystems, rather than saying here we have lots of organisations, composed of groups, each group containing these individual people.

Theory

Systems theory has become valuable in industry as a means of exploring the links between individuals, groups, organisations and the wider environment. The general concept of the system, composed of subsystems that contribute to supersystems and relate to other supersystems, has been present in philosophy and the social sciences for many generations. A familiar theme in the late nineteenth and early twentieth century was to liken people in the city to corpuscles in the subsystem of the blood, circulating through the arteries, as though human communities were composite animals. The city, like the body in this analogy, is a system. To examine the system of the body for a few moments, without *input* (food), the system would not maintain *entropy* (the energy to keep it going) and produce *outputs* (energy spent on other things like relationships) and would not sustain *equilibrium* (a balanced state).

In health and social care, systems approaches enable us to analyse how we can tackle the problems of individual people by distinguishing the different systems involved in people's lives, working to restore equilibrium and keep the systems going.

Theory into Practice

Systemic practice depends on the practitioner being able to achieve two things:

1. Analyse people's problems so as to produce statements of aims that are not abstract but involve changing people.
2. Analyse and use the different systems involved in a person's situation.

The following sentence summarises what is involved, highlighting in italic the four systems contributing to the practice. Effectiveness rests on the practitioner as a member of the *change agent system* being able to focus on the *target system* and work with the *action system* to enable the *client system* to work with the change agent system to achieve change. For the sake of completeness, we should add that alongside the action system there is the *social system*, these two systems being concerned with meeting aims and maintaining functions. Only one system is a permanent feature of this wider system of practice, namely the change agent system. The change agent system includes the practitioner and colleagues in the change agent's employing organisation. The other three systems are temporary members of the broader system including the entire system of practice. Within this, these are the client system, which includes the family of the person using services, the target system, which includes those whom the change agent needs to change or influence so as to achieve the aims, and the action system, which includes those whom the practitioner works with to achieve the change (Pincus and Minahan, 1973, pp. 56–8).

This pattern of systems provides a general framework that helps the practitioner to identify tasks which need to be carried out in order to progress the treatment. The purpose of the *professional* relationship between the practitioner and the service user, carer or patient is to enable this to happen, to achieve the planned change. This is different from a *personal* relationship, which would not need aims attached to it, but would be satisfying in itself.

We shall now take the practice one stage at a time. First, we shall take aim 1 above, with an example from practice.

Practice study

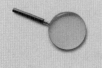

Mr and Mrs Hakim

Let us briefly check what might happen in a community care situation, where older couple Mr and Mrs Hakim cannot make up their minds whether to go along with Mr Hakim's wish to stay independent, or to go along with Mrs Hakim's and their grown-up children's wish to move from their flat into sheltered housing. The action system includes the family and the sheltered housing.

The practitioner converts the goals agreed with Mr and Mrs Hakim into tasks, draws on background insights into social inequalities and discrimination, as well as psychological knowledge about how the life course affects older people (Part II of this book), knowledge for practice (Part III) and practice skills (Parts IV and VI), and develops a programme as the basis for the contract. The specific skills drawn on in work with people include assessing problems, collecting information, making initial contact with people in the different systems, negotiating contracts, forming action systems, sustaining and coordinating systems (including influencing people) and ending the action (hopefully, at the point where, whatever the outcome of the decision, planned change can be assured).

Now let us take the entire process through from start to finish, spelling out more of the detail with another example from practice.

Practice study

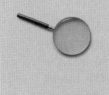

Mr and Mrs Nor

Mr and Mrs Nor, who migrated to London from a Jewish community in Russia 50 years ago, are in their seventies and occupy a rented flat in a downtown district. Mr Nor has a heart condition and is finding it difficult to walk distances. Mrs Nor has an anxiety-related condition which means going out is an ordeal. Their prime languages remain Yiddish, Hebrew and Russian. They are not in touch with any agencies, as their culture and faith puts self-reliance and family values as the top priority. They have children and grandchildren living in the surrounding suburbs and villages, but do not see much of

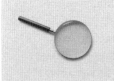

them. One day, a neighbour notes that the curtains are closed and, not having seen Mrs Nor for several days, rings social services. An assessment is made by the local community care team, working in partnership with Mr and Mrs Nor.

As the assessment proceeds, it becomes clear that Mrs Nor has not been coping with the housework and shopping for some time. The flat is dirty and the bedding has not been washed for months. From a systems perspective, workers in the agency identify themselves as the *change agent system*. They identify the isolation of Mr and Mrs Nor as individual 'systems' and as a couple in the *client system*, their isolation from their family members, and their lack of connection with the wider *target system* of local neighbourhood and community support and health and social services. Using a systems approach to working with Mr and Mrs Nor, we are aware of three levels of support within the target system that can be used to help them. These are informal, formal and societal.

Informal supports include family members and neighbours who can support Mr and Mrs Nor on a day-to-day basis. *Formal* supports include local neighbourhood groups in the Jewish community and organisations such as Age Concern, who run a local centre with many activities for people from a diversity of ethnic backgrounds. *Societal* supports include local health and social services agencies with their range of services, from the Primary Care Trusts with GPs and community nursing services to hospitals and day and residential services.

Gradually, these systems are mobilised and over a period of six months sufficient support and resources are provided to enable Mr and Mrs Nor to receive the services they need. Their resistance to being helped is overcome and their lives open up, as they meet other people from similar backgrounds, at a similar point in their life course and with similar problems.

Strengths and Limitations of Systemic Work

Mr and Mrs Nor may be happier and more fulfilled through a systems approach to working with them. The strengths of systemic approaches are that they enable us to look beyond the boundaries of the individual and the isolated couple and make connections with the wider systems, resources and services from which they may benefit.

The limitations of systems thinking are less apparent but no less real. Some of the limitations arise from the history and location of systems theories alongside other functionalist theories in sociology. These tend to emphasise equilibrium and the status quo as the norm and departures from these as problem-ridden. This means that any aspect involving conflict is perceived as a state of disequilibrium and disharmony which is abnormal and needs resolution. However, in the real world of human relations at individual, group and organisational levels, we cannot assume that all the different layers of systems work in harmony with each other. There may be tensions and conflicts in many areas and at different levels. Mr and Mrs Nor may be isolated from their children and grandchildren because they do not agree and have had conflicts in the past. They may continue to reject assessment and intervention by health and social care agencies. The services provided by the agencies, while supportive, in the long run may undermine their motivation to remain independent.

At a more basic level, Mr and Mrs Nor may not have any 'systems' to support them in their lives. They may have no relatives and no desire to link up with neighbourhood and community resources. In such circumstances, it makes little sense to use a systems approach, which works best where there is a richness of resources and systems on which to draw.

Conclusion

This chapter has examined the main features of a systemic approach to work with people. It is clear that while there is a certain level of jargon associated with systemic work, if we can move beyond this, in situations where there are different kinds of resources on which to draw, people may benefit from adopting this approach. The chapter concludes by acknowledging some of the main limitations of the approach.

REVIEW QUESTIONS

1 What are the main systems involved in health and social care practice?

2 What are inputs, entropy and equilibrium?

3 What are the main strengths and limitations of a systemic approach to health and social care practice?

FURTHER READING

Boscolo, L. and Bertrando, P. (1996) *Systemic Work with Individuals*, London, Karnac

Campbell, D., Draper, R. and Huffington, C. (1991) *A Systemic Approach to Consultation*, London, Karnac

Farmer, C. (1995) *Psychodrama and Systemic Therapy*, London, Karnac

Healy, K. (2005) *Social Work Theories in Context: Frameworks for Practice*, Basingstoke, Palgrave Macmillan

Jones, E. and Asen, E. (2000) *Systemic Couple Therapy and Depression*, London, Karnac

Payne, M. (2005) *Modern Social Work Theory* (3rd edn) Basingstoke, Palgrave Macmillan

Part VI

Resource file

References and bibliography

Note: If you copy or paraphrase (that is, summarise) the words or ideas of an author or web-based source and do not acknowledge this in your writing, you will be guilty of plagiarism. Plagiarism is a serious offence and is treated as dishonesty. Plagiarism can be direct – quoting other people's words without putting quotation marks round your extract – and also summarising their ideas without acknowledging the source, so always make written acknowledgement of other people's work, as indicated below.

Two approaches to references

Sometimes we need to quote or refer to other people's writing in our own work. There are two common ways to do this:

1. Listing references: You can go through your written work putting a number in brackets after each item you refer to or quote from. Then, at the end of the written work, you list the numbers and after each give a full statement of the source of the reference: author or editor, initials or forenames, date, title, edition (if later than the first) place of publisher, name of publisher.
2. Bibliography (Harvard system used below): This is an easier system for you to use. You put a main name, date and, if necessary, page number in brackets at the point where you refer to a person's work. Then, you list in alphabetical order at the end of your written work all the items you have referred to.

We shall use the Harvard system below and throughout this book.

Quoting or referring to extracts from books

In the main part of your written work, put a bracket like this (Webb and Jones, 2003: 94). Or, if you mention Webb and Jones: As Webb and Jones (2003: 94) say 'blackberries are sweet'. At the end of your written work, list all the books and articles you've quoted or referred to, like this: Webb, J.H. and Jones K.D. (eds) (2003) *Fruits of the Forest* (3rd edn) London, Best Books. So the formula is author(s)' or editor(s)' surname, initials of forenames, (ed.) if edited, date using all four numbers (2003), title in italics and edition, if later than the first edition, place of publication and name of publisher.

Quoting or referring to extracts from journal articles

Journal articles are similar. In your written work, put a bracket as for books (Brown, 2004: 274). At the end, in the bibliography, put the author(s)' surname, initials, date in brackets, the title of the article inside single quotation marks, the title of the journal in italics, the volume number, issue number in brackets and finally the page numbers of the entire article. For example: Brown, L. (2006) 'Health and Safety in England', *Journal of Fire Prevention*, **88**(2): 40–9.

Quoting from or referring to websites

Follow the same sequence as above for authors and their works. Then put the website followed by the date you referred to it. For example: http://www.west.ac.uk/central (accessed 4 May 2006).

Counselling and Advice-giving

45

ROBERT ADAMS

Learning outcomes

By the end of this chapter, you should be able to:

- UNDERSTAND the nature of counselling and advice-giving
- DISTINGUISH the three main approaches to counselling – psychodynamic, humanistic person-centred and cognitive-behavioural
- IDENTIFY the qualities and skills needed in a counsellor
- BE AWARE OF some major issues affecting the decision as to whether to counsel a person.

Just as some people view jobs with 'care' or 'caring' in the title as everyday helping that anyone can do, so some people regard counselling as simply talking. Others maintain that counselling is no more than giving advice. This chapter demonstrates that neither of these are the case. Counselling requires a high level of knowledge and expertise, ethical commitment, sensitivity and self-awareness.

What are Counselling and Advice-giving?

Counselling is

> an approach to human interaction that enables people to reflect on their situation and empowers them to deal with it themselves.

The aim of counselling is not to change people but to enable them to acquire the means to understand and do what they wish, for themselves.

Advice-giving is the activity of giving guidance. It is often allied to counselling and may be confused with it. Linking counselling and advice-giving in this chapter enables us to sharpen up the differences between them and emphasise what each has to offer.

Who can Counsel?

You would be unwise to advertise yourself as a counsellor without training and accreditation by the British Association for Counselling and Psychotherapy (BACP) or its equivalent. Counselling is a skilled activity that requires practising with due regard for the ethical guidelines laid down by the BACP (Burnard, 2005, p. 8). However, counselling is not something mysterious and rarefied that no ordinary person can understand or do. Whatever our roles, we can learn from the values and techniques of counselling and, through this knowledge, improve our health and social care practice. Counselling should not just be viewed as the territory of the practitioner. It is equally open to friends, relatives, carers and service users themselves to acquire and use counselling techniques to improve the quality of their relationships and their everyday lives.

Approaches to Counselling

There are three main approaches to counselling: psychodynamic, humanistic person-centred and cognitive-behavioural.

Psychodynamic Counselling

Psychodynamic counselling is a general term covering a huge variety of approaches that share their origins in ideas which, broadly, come from psychoanalysis. They include many Freudian concepts that have been built on, adapted and altered by many other practitioners over the past century, including Jung, Klein, Bion and Winnicott (see Chapters 7 and 43).

Humanistic Person-centred Counselling

Humanistic person-centred counselling is based on theories and ideas that presume all issues and problems in human existence revolve around what we experience at this second, in what we call 'the here and now'. The movements in philosophy to which these ideas relate are called 'existentialism' and 'phenomenology', both of which emphasise the primary significance of people's experience. This element is prominent in person-centred counselling, which regards the client as the expert in her or his own problems and the counsellor as the reflector, interpreter and supporter. Carl Rogers was a leading practitioner of person-centred counselling and has written many bestselling books on the subject (Rogers, 1942, 1961, 1980).

Egan (1998) identifies four main stages of counselling – defining the problem, clarifying the problem, developing goals, and linking goals to actions. Velleman (1992, p. 27) expands these to six stages: 'developing trust, exploring problem areas, helping to set goals, empowering into action, helping to maintain change, agreeing when to end'. The advantage of this expanded list is that it emphasises the way the major stages are negotiated with the person and it highlights that, as far as possible, the person is put in charge of the process.

Brown (2005, p. 146) notes that Egan's model of counselling has lent itself to adaptation to the fields of community care assessment and care management. This is not surprising when we consider that both person-centred counselling and community care emphasise working in partnership *with* the people who receive services, rather than providing services *for* them.

Cognitive-behavioural Counselling

Cognitive-behavioural counselling brings together ideas and research from the fields of behavioural psychology and cognitive learning (see Chapter 42 for a lengthier discussion). It is important to recognise that cognitive-behavioural counselling can be a powerful therapeutic tool, when used in specialised circumstances where the problem is simply the behaviour and the aim is to effect a change within a restricted area. For example, Rose was enuretic (a bed-wetter) until the age of 11, when she was referred to a cognitive-behavioural therapist for counselling. She persuaded Rose of the benefits of trying a number of cognitive-behavioural techniques and after a few weeks of trial and error Rose was rewarded with success and the end of her bed-wetting. The key to this approach with Rose reflects a general principle of cognitive-behavioural counselling, in that it focuses on the behaviour that needs to change, without paying any attention to questions about causes or underlying problems.

Behavioural counselling may also be used where the goal is the elimination of a single behaviour, such as smoking. This form of counselling can be directive and may involve setting strict behavioural targets with the person and keeping in intensive contact immediately following ceasing taking the last 'smoke'. It may be linked with supportive measures such as nicotine replacement therapy (see Resource File: Health Promotion (2) Stopping Smoking, at the end of Chapter 19).

Counselling Qualities, Knowledge and Skills

Activity 45.1

Make a list of the qualities and skills you feel would make a good counsellor.

Here is a typical extract from a brainstorming session with students. A good counsellor would be:

- a good listener
- sympathetic
- able to draw on life experience
- able to advise me.

You can look at your list and, perhaps, make similar comments. There is a mixture of items on the list, some more to do with qualities and others closer to skills. By a quality, I mean something inherent in you as a person. By a skill, I mean a technique you can acquire. For example, 'sympathetic' is more of a quality than a skill. On the other hand, 'able to advise' is a reference to the skill of advice-giving. Interestingly, as we noted above, this is distinct from counselling, although this is an example of a person who would like their counsellor to do this for them. The note about 'able to draw on life experience' implies something to do with wanting to feel confident that the counsellor can understand, on the basis of life experience rather than knowledge and understanding gained through reading books or training.

Let us try to clarify the kinds of qualities that might give a person a head start in becoming a counsellor and what skills he or she is likely to need.

If you are a caring, sensitive, warm, sympathetic person, you have many of the qualities that would make you a good counsellor.

If you are able to listen without interrupting, recollect what the other person has said, reflect on it and interpret what they mean, feed back constructively this interpretation to the person, you are well on the way to acquiring skills you would find useful as a counsellor.

As a skilled counsellor, you would be able:

- To listen, but this is not sufficient
- To care, but care for other people is not enough
- To communicate, but communication is not sufficient
- To influence another person's behaviour, but not this alone.

The skilled counsellor sets out to be more than a caring, listening, friendly presence. Perhaps the counsellor is able to view the person in their situation from an independent vantage point and is in a position to do more than nod in an understanding way. The counsellor can act as a support and helper, but again is in a position to do more than this. The counsellor may be able to enable the person to probe into their own motives and reasons for acting and thinking the way they do and examine possible ways they may wish to change. For the counsellor to facilitate this process requires confidence, skills and resources, perhaps to carry out a planned series of meetings with the person, with scope to review and evaluate at their conclusion.

Particular Areas of Counselling Practice

Dealing with Loss and Change

Many aspects of loss occur throughout our lives and are not restricted to old age.

Activity 45.2

Write down all the different kinds of losses that affect people throughout life.

Here is my list of losses I have experienced:

- Death of a much-loved pet
- Moving house and losing touch with former friends
- Death of a school friend in a motorcycle accident
- Loss of job when changed careers and went on a year-long training course
- Death of my mother and sister
- Loss of mobility when suffering infections, accidents and conditions accompanied by physical impairment of asthma.

This activity highlights the reality that contrary to the narrower view that loss only means bereavement through death of a relative or friend, we experience a variety of losses as we move through the life course, sometimes accompanied by a change that masks the loss by bringing a gain. For example, in my list was the loss of a job when I chose to train in a new career. The loss is no less real, although its impact is no doubt masked by the change. Accidents and illnesses involve losses of mobility and access to friends and activities, so can have major consequences.

In my case, the losses through deaths were mostly in my younger days, although inevitably as people grow older, the friends of their generation grow more prone to illness and are more likely to die. Often, when older people suffer losses, they withdraw and do not move on. In part, this is related to other people's expectations of old age, as much as with the older people's attitudes themselves (see Resource File: Attachment and Loss: Death and Bereavement, at the end of Chapter 28).

Activity 45.3

Think of the particular losses an older person might experience.

An older person might experience some of the following losses:

- Death of older relatives, such as brothers and sisters
- Death of a partner

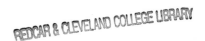

Part VI

- Children leaving home
- Losing contact with grandchildren when children leave their partners
- Retirement: loss of job, status and income associated with it
- Impairment: loss of physical mobility, sensory impairment
- Chronic illness: restricted contact with friends, loss of leisure activities.

Brief Counselling

This approach to counselling involves a focused series of steps, of which the following are typical, say, for a situation in which Ada, a waitress, has developed a fear of going to work (Dryden and Feltham, 1992, pp. 62–80):

- Agree with Ada which are her main concerns
- Prioritise one of them as the target goal – she has lost confidence
- Identify previous occasions when she has felt confident at work
- Identify when she has failed to be confident at work
- Identify the obstacles to being confident – it emerges she thinks people are talking about her appearance, because she has put on weight
- Discuss specific interventions to help Ada tackle her view about her weight (see also Chapter 43).

Practice Issues in Counselling Work with People in Health and Social care

Visiting People in their Own Homes

Some therapists advise against visiting clients at home, yet health and social care workers based in the community have no choice, as home visits are an essential part of their jobs. Does this mean they cannot use counselling skills? The answer, fortunately, is that there is no consensus among 'experts' about this matter, so advocates can be found on both sides of the argument (Nicholas, 1992, pp. 23–4). The gifted paediatrician Dr Winnicott states that, in the home visit, the therapist faces the reality of all the distress and muddle of the mind of the client.

> He [Winnicott] continues by saying how one should not be frightened by the client going mad, or feel guilty because of this or the client's disintegration, extreme behaviour, or attempts at suicide, successful or otherwise. All these are signs of despair because of loss of hope for help. (Nicholas, 1992, p. 24)

Counselling People who are Vulnerable

Counselling people with physical impairments, older people and people with mental health problems raises particular issues and it is not the case that counselling skills simply can be applied, irrespective of the circumstances of these people. For example, a person may have restricted sight and hearing and this will make it necessary to communicate with care, so as to ensure that particular points are not missed.

Also, people with mental health problems and disabilities may feel excluded and undervalued. This may lead them to understate their views and feelings, in the light of previous experiences where their expectations have not been recognised, appreciated and endorsed by agencies or practitioners.

It is important to recognise that while counselling (leaving group counselling on one side) is basically a one-to-one activity, it requires the ability to put the person's situation in its wider social context. Below are two examples, the first challenging discrimination and the second challenging ageism.

Challenging Discrimination

Practice study

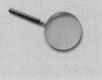

John

John may put forward the view that his inability to succeed in obtaining work is due to his lack of relevant skills and abilities, but the counsellor may know that young, black, male applicants from his housing estate have been discriminated against in the past. The counsellor may be able to use this wider knowledge to enable John to move from being excluded by changing his address, buying a suit, shirt and tie and practising his interview skills.

Challenging Ageism

Practice study

Maude

Maude is an 80-year-old woman who is extremely physically and mentally active and healthy. She still lives independently in a house by a park, which she struggles to clean but has lived in for 50 years and wants to stay in, because of happy memories of her husband, who died five years ago. Her two daughters are pressurising her to give up the house, because she is 80 and old, and move into a private residential home. While she does not want to sell up, she has reached the stage where she is inclined to go along with them, 'for the sake of a quiet life' as she puts it.

Maude has the means to continue to pay for various domiciliary care services. One of the care workers talks regularly with her and Maude shares her concerns. The worker gives her the support to say 'no' to her daughters and carry on living in the house, which she does for another 10 years before dying peacefully in her sleep.

We can see that the daughters are following their assumptions about the so-called natural and inevitable process of ageing, linked with various ages. They apparently have a threshold in their minds about people over 80 not having the capacity to

Part VI

remain independent. While many of the widespread views about ageing and growing incapacity have a basis in fact, they are *socially constructed*, that is, they are part of what many people believe, but are not universally true. The care worker does well in this case to use counselling techniques not only to resist the pressure from Maude's daughters, but also to resist the dominant assumption that growing old necessarily means growing more infirm. The care worker achieves the difficult task of empowering Maude to convince her daughters that her situation is in contrast with the way age and dependence are socially constructed and the way her daughters have applied it to her circumstances.

We can draw a general message from this as well. The care worker has been able to challenge the consequences of ageing in Maude's case and enable her to find the strength to combat her daughters' ageism.

Conclusion

This chapter has surveyed the main approaches to counselling and highlighted their distinctive features. It has explored the qualities and skills needed in order to practise counselling. It has illustrated some of the main ways in which counselling is used to help people.

REVIEW QUESTIONS

1   What are the three main approaches to counselling?

2   What are the main qualities you would expect to find in a counsellor?

3   What skills would you expect in a trained counsellor?

4   In what areas of practice is counselling particularly relevant?

FURTHER READING

Burnard, P. (1992) *Counselling: A Guide to Practice in Nursing*, Oxford, Butterworth Heinemann

Burnard, P. (2005) *Counselling Skills for Health Professionals* (4th edn) Cheltenham, Nelson Thornes

Dryden, W. (2006) *Counselling in a Nutshell*, London, Sage

Dryden, W. and Feltham, C. (1992) *Brief Counselling: A Practical Guide for Beginning Practitioners*, Buckingham, Open University Press
A useful handbook containing many examples.

McLeod, E. (1993) *An Introduction to Counselling*, Buckingham, Open University Press
A good introduction to counselling practice.

Palmer, S. and Dryden, W. (1995) *Counselling for Stress Problems*, London, Sage

Scrutton, S. (1989) *Counselling Older People*, London, Edward Arnold
Although quite an old book, it is full of practical wisdom.

Street, E. (1994) *Counselling for Family Problems*, London, Sage

Tudor, K. (1998) *Counselling in Groups*, London, Sage

Emergency, Crisis and Task-centred Work

ROBERT ADAMS

Learning outcomes

By the end of this chapter, you should be able to:

■ IDENTIFY the key features of emergency work, crisis intervention and task-centred practice

■ SPECIFY the circumstances in which emergency, short-term, problem-focused work is appropriate.

This chapter deals with three quite distinct but related ways of working with people which we can put under the general heading of problem-solving: crisis intervention, emergency and task-centred work. We are blurring some boundaries in doing this. The idea of crisis is not the same as that of emergency. A crisis is located in a person's life, whereas medical emergencies have implications for the speed of response of the service. So medical and social care cultures construct these events differently and, as a few minutes watching a television dramatisation of an A&E ward in a hospital illustrates, respond to them very differently. A crisis can develop slowly in a person's life and for a long time may not even be acknowledged, while in general we expect an emergency to present a major threat to health or life. However, even while writing this, I am aware that, perhaps with the exception of public traffic accidents, emergency hospital admissions may be preceded by a period during which the person may deny the problem until it reaches crisis point.

Emergency Work

An emergency is an event or other change in circumstances which interrupts and threatens normal functioning so as to require immediate action to restore this.

In health and social care services, emergencies may threaten serious injury or loss of life. In the public view, emergency work begins with ambulance services and the practice of paramedical staff, although associated with these staff is the massive infrastructure of A&E departments in hospitals. The huge range of specialist medical support services provided by these staff is not our concern here. What we focus on is the process of the work. It is clear that emergency care in the streets (Caroline, 1995), in the ambulance (Browner et al., 2002) and in the hospital (Saunders, 2000) shares many features of acute services, or what social workers know as short-term work. We link them because they are concerned with responding immediately to problems presented in the here and now.

Crisis Intervention

Crisis intervention came to prominence through the formative work of Gerald Caplan in the 1960s (Caplan, 1961, 1964), although the work of Naomi Golan (1978) offers a clear exposition of its theory and practice. Basically, she describes crises as a range of happenings which disturb the equilibrium of an individual, group or organisation and create tensions and stresses if we fail to surmount the problems created by this. This leads to an active crisis, with the potential for the person to be open to learning new ways of coping during this uncertain period. A crisis can be defined as:

> an unplanned, event or problem, which may or may not be anticipated, and which disrupts a person's life and functioning.

Crisis intervention may be defined as:

> a range of actions and treatments aiming to interrupt the crisis and minimise or prevent its harmful consequences.

However, it can be argued that since all people approaching an agency do so because of a crisis they perceive in one way or another, there is a sense in which the idea of crisis applies to all users of services. Another argument is that a crisis is a situation dealt with by an A&E duty person or team. Often, for practical reasons to do with regular services closing down after hours, crises tend to arise in the evenings, late in the night or at weekends. Furthermore, crisis work often is perceived as taking place in the field of health or mental health, since these are where many emergencies arise.

Strengths and Limitations of Crisis Intervention

The strengths of crisis intervention include the positive techniques it offers for dealing with situations that have generated stress and tension in people's lives. It is not restricted, as is task-centred work, to tackling visible problems of which the person is aware, but because of its links with psychodynamic ideas, it offers ways of responding to emotions and behaviour that are beyond the person's conscious awareness.

Crisis intervention has two main limitations:

1. It may aim and claim to be democratic, but can be criticised for offering people a false sense of empowerment. In fact, people undergoing a crisis are likely to be vulnerable and in that vulnerable state are prone to agreeing to whatever the practitioner suggests. In such circumstances, it is false to pretend that the relations between the practitioner and the service user are equal in power terms.
2. Crisis intervention is suitable for use only in a restricted range of situations and problems. For example, it is not appropriate to use it in situations where long-term work is anticipated. Crisis intervention is likely to be effective only where there is an identifiable crisis that can be tackled within a few weeks.

Practice study

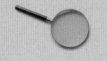

Anna

In actual work with people, it will soon become apparent that the crisis they present often is a manifestation or 'symptom' (to use a word from the individual or 'medical' rather than the 'social' model – see Chapter 14) of a preceding event or crisis that precipitated it. In work with Anna, this soon became apparent. She rang the office in tears to say she had returned home to find a dead rat in the kitchen. There seemed to be more in her hysteria, so two workers visited. They found Anna, 68, sitting in the parlour of her small terraced home opposite the body of her mother who had died some days ago. The entire room was full of rubbish that had piled up and was creating a major health hazard, but the earlier crisis had been Anna's inability to face the reality and cope with the illness and death of her mother.

Task-centred Work

Task-centred work originated in the work of Reid and colleagues in the USA from the late 1960s (Reid, 1963; Reid and Shyne, 1969; Reid and Epstein, 1972) and has been carried forward in Britain by Doel and Marsh (1992). Task-centred work typically concentrates on offering short-term solutions, or at least ways forward, for immediately and clearly apparent problems. The programme needs to be based on goals determined and agreed by the service user. There is no attempt to set up a long-term arrangement between the worker and the client, patient or service user. The agreement or 'contract' is more likely to be for up to half a dozen sessions, or in the longer term programmes, 10–12 sessions. During these, the worker will agree with the person what will be worked on and each session will be clearly driven by its own task. The work done with the person can feel very businesslike and is different from the kind of delving into people's backgrounds and history that tends to take place in psychotherapy, for example. Task-centred work steers away from asking questions about the deep-seated causes and long-lasting character of a person's problems and instead concentrates on tackling the difficulties that are immediately visible.

The practical nature of task-centred work makes it particularly useful where a person can benefit from carrying out certain practical tasks, as a means of helping them with emotional problems. The most useful way of viewing task-centred work is as a structured plan worked out with a person to enable them to accomplish certain goals, which they have agreed in advance with the worker. In this sense, it can be an empowering way of working and, where the person makes progress, it can be rewarding, because the agreed aims are practicable, tangible and realisable. The application of the approach depends on whether the problem can be broken down into tasks that can be accomplished within a limited period of time.

Work done with people may be individually based or in groups, including work with couples. For example, work may be done with a couple, under some stress because of various health and mobility problems, who cannot make up their minds about whether to continue living independently or to move into a residential home.

Practice study

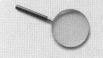

Khalid

Khalid, aged 67, was living alone in his flat and was taken to the A&E department of the local hospital in the early hours of the morning when the milkman found him crawling about on the hall floor in his underwear.

After a thorough check-up and a spring-clean of the flat, to which Khalid readily agreed, a task-centred approach was used to move from agreed problems to agreed goals, planning and programming.

Khalid wanted to move from his second-floor flat, but did not know where to go. He had become mildly depressed and was lonely. An agreement negotiated with him was based around the problems he identified: lack of motivation since retiring as a teacher, two years ago, depression at his declining physical condition through chronic problems with continence and loneliness through moving from his home area to this seaside town on retirement.

Work with Khalid went through the following stages: exploring the problem, negotiating goals, planning, implementing and evaluating, as follows.

Over a period, Khalid explored how to find and apply for sheltered accommodation, deal with his incontinence by continence treatment (see Chapter 24), and visit a coffee bar in the local Age Concern centre and join an evening class meeting two evenings a week to counteract his loneliness. He had to spend occasional periods in hospital overnight and had reached the stage of hating this, feeling his incontinence put him back in the position of childish dependence on adults, a feeling he hated. He learned to reframe this when he used various continence techniques and took control of his life by using the pads and commode when he spent short periods in hospital, rather than perceiving himself as infantilised.

Strengths and Limitations of Task-centred Work

Task-centred work has the advantage of enabling complicated situations to be analysed and broken down into simpler, achievable tasks. By the same token, the limitations of task-centred work include the risk that applying it too rigidly can lead to oversimplification of the many facets of a situation, with all their uncertainties and tensions, and thereby distort complex reality.

Crisis Intervention and Task-centred Work Compared

Theoretical Aspects of Crisis Intervention and Task-centred Work

Crisis intervention and task-centred work share a focus on identifying and solving problems. Problems are the origins of crises and therefore are the focus of crisis intervention; they also are the targets of problem-solving contracts in task-centred work. The problem-solving approach inherent in task-centred work is similar to that adopted in crisis intervention. The main aim is to alleviate the problems of individuals and families (Reid, 1978, p. 13). Problems and problem-solving were given detailed attention a generation earlier in Helen Perlman's pioneering work (Perlman, 1957). Reid (1978, pp. 35–6) listed the types of problem that could be tackled by a problem-solving approach:

- interpersonal conflict
- dissatisfaction with relationships
- difficulties in formal organisations such as hospitals or schools
- difficulties in performing roles, such as being able to curb children's problem behaviour
- difficulties with decision-making, such as whether to have another baby
- reactive emotional stress, such as health concerns or job loss
- psychological problems, such as addiction.

Problem-solving approaches in general are not manipulative, in the sense that an outsider to the problems, the practitioner, 'fixes' it. Instead, the practitioner works to empower the service user, the patient, to do the fixing, by being in the driving seat of decision-making and finding a way forward.

The roots of problem-oriented theory are claimed by advocates of task-centred work to lie in psychoanalytic theory and problem-solving theories, social roles, small group theory, social systems and learning theories (Reid, 1978, p. 123). Indeed, the reality, as Payne (2005b, pp. 103, 116) acknowledges, is that the range of problems dealt with is far too wide to be encompassed by one specific psychologically or sociologically based theory. There are five stages in task-centred work, specified originally by Reid and Epstein (1972) and spelled out more flexibly by Marsh and Doel (2005, pp. 15–17):

1. Exploring and specifying the problem
2. Reaching agreement and negotiating the contract

3. Discussing and agreeing the task most appropriate for alleviating the problem
4. Use of basic techniques and strategies involving the practitioner
5. Termination and review of the work.

Crisis theory does have links with systems theory and O'Hagan (1986, p. 61) tries to reformulate this to give it both a functional (maintenance) basis and a progressive (change) orientation, calling these *morphostasis* and *morphogenesis* respectively. O'Hagan (1986, pp. 62–3) calls for practitioners to be realistic and pragmatic and limit the system which is the focus of the work, to enable the work to remain manageable. This does not mean that we as practitioners will not respond with a degree of flexibility to the wants of people. We may be called upon to use our counselling knowledge and skills on occasions, for example in a medical emergency (East, 1995).

General Similarities and Differences

The most obvious areas where crisis intervention is practised are in abuse and protection work, in mental health and healthcare work. Task-centred work is likely to be used in situations such as difficulties making key decisions, less entrenched and fundamental relationship problems, interpersonal disagreements and stressses brought about by 'acute' situations.

Crisis intervention and task-centred work share several features:

■ The priority given to short-term, structured work, such as a series of meetings or hospital treatment, to tackle problems.
■ An agreement or 'contract' with the client, patient or service user or close relatives, specifying which problems are being tackled.
■ A tendency to give immediate advice and treatment to deal with pressing difficulties.
■ A focus on preventing the continuance of the problems.

They differ in the following ways:

■ Crisis intervention aims to interrupt events that disrupt people's lives, whereas task-centred work is a structured programme of problem-solving.
■ Task-centred work targets practical problems in people's lives, whereas crisis intervention relates to psychological theories about how people cope with emergencies.

Conclusion

This chapter has examined the main features of crisis intervention and task-centred work. Whereas crisis intervention is capable of responding to major emergencies and disruptions to people's lives, the task-centred approach is geared to more minor problems, which they can tackle consciously, rationally and purposefully.

REVIEW QUESTIONS

1 Can you give details of the main features of emergency, crisis and task-centred work?

2 Can you outline the key stages of task-centred work?

3 Can you summarise the main characteristics shared by crisis intervention and task-centred approaches to work with people?

FURTHER READING

Browner, B.D., Pottack, A.N. and Gupton, C. (eds) (2002) *Emergency Care and Transportation of the Sick and Injured*, Sudbury, MA, Jones & Bartlett

Caroline, N.L. (1995) *Emergency Care in the Streets* (5th edn) Boston, MA, Little, Brown

Greaves, I., Porter, K., Hodgetts, T. and Wollard, M. (eds) (1997) *Emergency Care: A Textbook for Paramedics* (2nd edn) London, W.B. Saunders

Healy, K. (2005) *Social Work Theories in Context: Frameworks for Practice*, Basingstoke, Palgrave Macmillan

Marsh, P. and Doel, M. (2005) *The Task-Centred Book*, London, Routledge/Community Care

Payne, M. (2005) *Modern Social Work Theory* (3rd edn) Basingstoke, Palgrave Macmillan

WEBSITES: http://www.doh.gov.uk/consent/ (Department of Health website concerning consent by patients)
http@www.emedicine.com/emerg.index.shtml
http://www.jrcalc.org.uk (Joint Royal Colleges Ambulance Service)

Resource file

Writing a review

Writing a review may be of anything, but most commonly, it will be of a book or article.

Essentials

- You need peace and quiet and space and time around you to think properly.
- Switch off your mobile.
- Tell people to go away.
- You are thinking. Thinking is as much work as digging the garden or cleaning the bathroom. Without space and time, your mind is like a muscle that can't expand.
- Exercise your mind by thinking critically and it will grow stronger every time you use it. Again, think of your mind as a muscle. The more you exercise your mind, the more confident you will become.

Preparation

- Read the item through and take notes of the major points.
- Make particular note of anything you strongly agree or disagree with.
- Spend time afterwards thinking about how the item relates to anything else you have come across or read.
- Write down a list of the strengths and a list of the weaknesses of the item.
- Spend time writing down points of interest that either agree or differ in the two items.
- If you have time, look up any other similar items and check whether they agree or disagree.

Writing

- Put yourself in a creative mood.

- Become confident.
- You are about to give your opinion. Your opinion is as valuable as anybody's.
- Don't hold your views back. Don't be afraid to commit yourself.
- Spend a few minutes jotting down the main points you want to make, in note form, not in full sentences.
- Look at the points you've made and try numbering them in a logical sequence.
- Try different sequences. You may want to go through the strengths first and the weaknesses second. Or, it may work better with your strongest criticisms first.
- Write a simple sentence summarising each point.
- Make each sentence the first sentence in a short paragraph. Write two or three more sentences explaining each key point.
- Try to round off at the end with a paragraph summing up whether, on balance, you like or dislike the item, whether its strengths impress you more than its weaknesses and whether you think the author could have tackled it another way. Don't be afraid to suggest this.

Roles and Tasks in Practice

Part VII
Roles and Tasks in Practice

Introduction

Part VII of the book deals with examples of key roles and tasks in contemporary health and social care. There are two main trends, which create additional work and responsibilities for staff:

- An increasing tendency towards a variety of agencies and professionals contributing to services for one person and towards increasing joint working between them.

- The growing complexity of working relationships between those involved in working together.

It is necessary to find ways to work together, within the same organisation, between disciplines and across boundaries between different organisations and agencies. There are degrees of working together, from the least to the most 'togetherness'. Sometimes when people mention working together, they simply mean liaising, keeping in touch. A more demanding situation is where cooperation between partners is required. At a higher level still, collaboration involves the sharing of tasks and redistribution of responsibilities across boundaries.

Working together in teams and joint working between agencies make it even more necessary to be clear about what information can be shared and what needs protecting (see the Resource File below).

Freedom of Information and Data Protection Acts

More than 100,000 public bodies are covered under the Freedom of Information Act 2000, including government departments and local authorities, voluntary and private organisations. People have the right to ask for information about themselves and their treatment. A person's right to this information continues to be governed by the Data Protection Act 1998. This can only be refused on certain, strictly governed, grounds, such as if it is 'vexatious' or likely to cause serious physical or mental harm to the person asking. A request is submitted in writing and the public authority normally has 20 working days to respond.

The Data Protection Act 1998 introduces strict guidelines on how data (information) on people is stored. This is particularly important for health and social care practitioners in agencies where there are many items of personal information about people who use services and carers, some of which refer to intimate aspects of people's health and lives. Under the Act,

there are eight principles governing the proper handling of data. Data must be:

- lawfully and fairly processed
- processed for limited reasons
- relevant and adequate but not excessive for its purpose
- accurate
- kept only as long as is necessary
- processed so as not to undermine the person's rights
- secure
- only transferred to another country with adequate protection.

There are tensions for practitioners in health and social care between satisfying the legal requirement for disclosure and meeting their professional responsibilities to protect the confidentiality of matters to do with the treatment of carers and service users, including patients. This is particularly the case when practitioners share information in the course of their daily work.

FURTHER READING   Wadham, J. (2001) *Blackstone's Guide to the Freedom of Information Act 2000*, Oxford, Blackstone Press

47 Working in Teams and Partnerships

ROBERT ADAMS

Learning outcomes

By the end of this chapter, you should be able to:

■ DEFINE what is meant by partnerships and teams

■ UNDERSTAND the implications of different styles of team leadership

■ KNOW the ingredients for effective work in teams.

This chapter deals with a continuously expanding area of health and social care work, namely the work practitioners do with other paid staff and volunteers in a wide range of roles. Some of these arrangements are called *partnerships* – an increasingly popular idea since the 1980s (see Chapter 48).

There is a great diversity of situations where we could describe practitioners as being 'in a team', but if the word 'team' was applied strictly, we would reserve it for cases where there was a measure of shared agreement among them about their values, aims, objectives and methods of achieving them. Many so-called teams are teams in name only and work on linked tasks or in the same office or department because their functions are described by management as dependent on each other. They are carrying out common tasks together, rather than working as a team.

Partnerships

In legal terms, a partnership is an arrangement between two or more business managers which enables them to run the business together. In the health and social services, a great diversity of partnership arrangements have come into existence.

Some are basically liaison committees, while others are fully fledged organisations in which each partner takes some legal responsibilities for some aspect of the organisation's role. Since the 1990s, partnerships have become increasingly important in the organisation and running of health and social care services. The number of partnerships involving carers and people using services working alongside agencies and professionals is growing all the time.

Partnerships have a number of strengths:

- They reassure people that cooperation and collaboration between diverse groups and organisations are possible.
- They enable people as individuals and in groups to join forces to achieve shared goals.
- They are a means by which agencies can work together to solve problems they could not tackle alone, for example through enhanced, shared training and by widening access to a broader range of staff resources and skills.

Partnerships may suffer from problems:

- Where there are lots of groups and partnerships, this may lead to muddle and confusion about the allocation of tasks and responsibilities within and between them.
- When ineffective, they may be short-lived and leave weak groups and vulnerable individuals in a worse position than before.
- It is more difficult for organisations with diverse cultures and ways of working to work together. Thus, social services are likely to have inclusion of the unruly person as their main goal, while health services will prioritise treating patients. Thus, the unruly patient is likely to be viewed differently by a partnership of health and social services agencies. Similarly, head teachers in schools are more likely to exclude the unruly pupil, while social workers may be committed to working against excluding them.
- The expectations and commitment of different partners may vary widely and disagreements and conflicts may arise between them.
- Because they may be poorly resourced, they may not tackle the more fundamental causes of social problems and may focus on more easily attainable, short-term gains.

Working in partnership is not just about attending meetings and being a member of multiprofessional and multiagency conferences and working groups. To be effective, partners must be able to work openly, share power and make decisions jointly. There are often tensions, such as:

- Competitor agencies, for example education and social services, striving for the same sources of limited funding for their work.
- Overconfidentiality and sharing information within and between agencies.

Spend a few minutes jotting down half dozen or so key points that you believe underlie successful partnerships.

Here is our list of what comprises successful partnerships:

- They display agreement over goals.
- Each partner has clearly agreed expectations of the others.
- The partners have pooled resources and avoided duplication.
- All the partners have the chance of shared learning from experience.
- All the partners may gain from the higher profile of the partnership than they enjoyed individually before, offering them enhanced opportunities to bid for additional funding.
- Workers in each partner group or organisation are committed to making the partnership work, by building on its strengths rather than undermining it.

Teams

A team is a group of staff members sharing tasks and working together for common goals. Teamworking has attracted positive views since the 1960s when the 'human relations' movement in industry and management made the study of how group members work together popular (Burns and Stalker, 1961). From the 1970s, the popular study of the social psychology of groups and group relations had a great impact on health and social care organisations. Many staff training courses in the public services were influenced. In the 1990s, the Department of Health funded the Open University to provide the Management Education Scheme by Open Learning (MESOL) under the title of Managing Personal and Team Effectiveness, with the aim of improving joint working between NHS organisations and social services departments (Salaman et al., 1994). Such joint working arrangements have become increasingly common, even a necessity since the 1980s, especially in areas of work such as child and adult protection and mental health (HM Government, 2006). The fact that the Department of Health funded the MESOL programme managers and an Advanced MESOL for senior managers is a clue to the existence of widespread concern that joint working between health and social services was experiencing problems.

Managers and Leadership

Managing care occurs at many levels. If managing care is about taking decisions on a moment-by-moment basis in the light of known circumstances, having regard to all possible relevant sources of information first, then it can happen to anybody in the spectrum of care workers. Any health and social care practitioners, from health-care assistants to home care visitors, community nurses, occupational therapists to night-sitting care workers, can find themselves in the position of managing care.

Management takes place in small, tactical areas of work as well as large, strategic ones. Practitioners deal routinely not just with difficult decisions but with ethical and practical issues, often involving tensions between competing demands and possible outcomes.

Styles of team leadership create different types of team

Ideas about the desirable approach to team leadership vary according to the many different conditions in which health and social care services are delivered. In a formal work organisation, a more traditional managerial style may be appropriate. However, this approach may not be effective in the 'third sector' (voluntary, private, 'not for profit' and informal groups and organisations) and where networks of people are working together in the community.

We can distinguish the job of managing a group of staff from that of leading a team. Broadly speaking, the manager often works to a prescription, a series of responsibilities, laid down by the organisation. In contrast, the leader of a team – which may be composed of staff from a range of different organisations – is more like a community organiser than a commander in a single hierarchy. The team leader in this situation is likely to be most effective when seeking people's views and attempting to reach decisions democratically. Leadership styles range from authoritarian and directive to consultative. The extreme of being consultative is the laid-back or 'laissez-faire' leader who can contribute to anarchy in the team. Out of the limitless possible combinations of leaders with different styles interacting with other team members, Payne (2000, pp. 202–3) highlights in his comprehensive study of teamworking the five styles of team leadership identified by Vroom and Yetton (1983), which I have illustrated with imaginary monologues:

1. *Autocratic 1* – 'I decide on my own'
2. *Autocratic 2* – 'I direct subordinates to find information, then I decide'
3. *Consultative 1* – 'I gather ideas from subordinates individually, then I decide
4. *Consultative 2* – 'I meet with subordinates, share problems, then I decide'
5. *Group* – 'I share the problems, we discuss them and try to find a consensus that I accept.'

Activity 47.2

With these five styles in mind, consider the following questions:

1. In your present, or most recent, job, which style most accurately describes you?
2. In your ideal world, which style would you most like to cultivate?
3. Share this exercise with a colleague. Discuss your responses, including any differences between your answers to questions 1 and 2.

Group dynamics affect teamworking

Of course, teams vary and their responsibilities as well as their membership will differ. There are different types of teamwork, largely because teams are groups of people, small or large, and once we set up a group of people working together, group dynamics come into play. If you have ever sat in a newly formed group of people and tried to reach a collective decision, you will know how chaotic and energy-consuming this can be. You may recognise a number of stages that many new groups typically go through, as described by an observer (Bion, 1968) – forming, norming, storming and performing; establishing norms and ways of working; working through the stage of group members sparring and sometimes arguing as roles are clarified; and finally arriving at the stage of performing, that is, carrying out the task.

Teamwork Settings

Payne (2000, p. 74) identifies four kinds of settings where teamworking happens:

1. *Organisations* from which practitioners mutually support each other as they set off from their workbase.
2. *Multiprofessional* contexts where practitioners from different disciplines work together.
3. *Community settings* where people network to bring different groups and organisations together.
4. *Institutional settings* where service users, for example, are living and all the disciplines contributing to the quality of their lives converge to do their work.

Working across Boundaries in Joint and Collaborative Work

Boundary crossing is increasingly a feature of health and social care work. The boundaries can exist between disciplines, different professions, different organisations, cultures and geographical locations. The situation is more complicated than this, because sometimes the boundaries are lowered and at other times they may be blurred or abolished altogether. Some staff will perceive the boundaries as a barrier, while others see their existence as a focus for their efforts to reach out and work collaboratively. To some practitioners, this is a threat, while others may see it as a challenge or an opportunity.

There are also many variants of team approaches where the participant practitioners are employed by different agencies (multiagency), or share work from their different disciplinary (multidisciplinary) or professional backgrounds (multiprofessional) within the same agency. Multiprofessional work is often held up as the ideal, yet working together is also the focus of much criticism when practised badly.

Reasons for non-effective work include:

- practitioners not communicating adequately
- lack of opportunities between meetings for workers to make collective decisions

- lack of mechanisms to enable information to be shared between agencies
- lack of a culture of joint working in partner organisations and agencies.

Working across different professions can, however, be necessary, desirable and more effective than working alone as a professional. Thus there are several advantages of multiprofessional work:

- It improves coordination between different workers from different professions who in any case are involved in a situation with a service user and carer.
- It enhances the skills that individual workers bring to bear on the situation.
- It enables workers to share information and distribute responsibility for carrying out tasks.
- It enables workers to clarify their different accountabilities.
- It improves the chance that in complex situations the service user and carer will benefit.

Conditions for Effective Teamwork

In working for the best outcomes for service users and carers, effective teamwork should meet the following conditions:

- Clearly stated goals are shared and understood by all partner agencies.
- All the partner agencies subscribe to accepted working methods.
- Work by all members of partner agencies is valued by other partners.
- Open communication between partners, enabling roles, activities and authority to be challenged and critically examined.

Practice study

Cezar

Cezar, aged 16, was admitted to a residential childcare unit after a considerable period of support from the child and family psychiatry team. His withdrawn character and obsessive patterns of behaviour – cleaning and arranging household items – alternated with short periods of aggressive behaviour. He hadn't attended school for some time, after brief periods of attendance were followed by exclusion after violent outbursts in the classroom. The worker is a residential childcare worker.

A planning meeting was organised, which representatives from social services, health, education and the youth offending team attended.

At the planning meeting, the different professionals came with very different ideas about the reasons for Cezar's present difficulties. The perceptions respectively of the social worker, youth worker, teachers and clinical psychologist were that school was not engaging him, he was awkward and difficult, and suffering from psychosis and attention deficit hyperactivity disorder (ADHD).

Conflicts in the meeting were exposed, explored and real communication began as

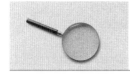

open dialogue took place. This represented a real move forward. Cezar took part at later stages, with his parents. Negotiation occurred, the worker managing the tension between submissiveness and non-assertion and assertiveness.

Conclusion

This chapter has introduced teamwork as a concept and put teamworking in the health and social services in the wider context of its growing popularity in industry in the second half of the twentieth century. The chapter has explored the nature of teams and partnerships and discussed the kinds of circumstances in which teamworking can be most effective.

REVIEW QUESTIONS

1 What is a team?

2 What is a partnership?

3 What style of leadership is best suited to teamworking?

4 What kinds of conditions are best suited to teamwork?

FURTHER READING

Atkinson, M., Wilkin, A., Stott, A., Doherty, P. and Kinder, K. (2002) *Multi-Agency Working: A Detailed Study*, LGA Research Report 26, Slough, NFER

Henderson, J. and Atkinson, D. (eds) (2003) *Managing Care in Context*, London, Routledge/Open University

HM Government (2006) *Working Together to Safeguard Children: A Guide to Inter-agency Working to Safeguard and Promote the Welfare of Children*, London, TSO

Keen, J. (2001) *Clients with Complex Needs: Interprofessional Practice*, Oxford, Blackwell

Payne, M. (2000) *Teamwork in Multiprofessional Care*, Basingstoke, Palgrave – now Palgrave Macmillan

Weinstein, J., Whittington, C. and Leiba, T. (2003) *Collaboration in Social Work Practice*, London, Jessica Kingsley

White, V. and Harris, J. (2001) *Developing Good Practice in Community Care: Partnership and Participation*, London, Jessica Kingsley

Multiprofessional Work with Adults

ROBERT ADAMS

Learning outcomes

By the end of this chapter, you should be able to:

■ SPECIFY the main stages of work with adults

■ WORK THROUGH the sequence of work with adults

■ IDENTIFY some of the main issues arising in the work.

Multiprofessional work with adults is a necessity where their needs and problems are complex and demand responses and resources from more than one agency or organisation. This chapter is entirely devoted to a detailed examination of one case where this occurs, so as to highlight some of the main issues in practice. First, let us put the idea of multiagency and multiprofessional work in context.

Effective Joint Working

There have been problems in England for people wanting to obtain funding for continuing care, often related to a lack of seamless collaboration between health and social services, a problem we have referred to in Chapter 47. Ann Abraham, the health ombudsman, highlighted the lack of health and social services working together. She reported on numerous problems for individuals trying to secure funding for their long-term care and found confusion about whether it was continuing care, free nursing care only covering the costs of the nursing, or a care package to meet health needs funded in full by the NHS. She recommended clarifying national, minimum eligibility criteria for continuing care, with a clear set of assessment tools and practice guidance to support them (Abraham, 2005).

Effective joint work between different agencies and professionals depends on a number of conditions being fulfilled:

■ A high level of understanding of overlapping and common areas of responsibility
■ A willingness to share tasks
■ High trust between different professionals
■ Openness and good communications.

Partnership Arrangements and Partnership in Practice

In the first place, the agencies have to set up the partnership and make it work. Let us follow this through from the general, policy level to the actual working arrangements between health and social care staff, day by day, hour by hour. We begin with some general points, but you will soon see how necessary it is to clarify them in order for the practice of joint working to be smooth running, well coordinated and effective:

■ The arrangements have to be consistent with the legal framework. That is, the partnership must comply with, and ensure it implements, laws such as the NHS and Community Care Act 1990, Carers (Recognition and Services) Act 1995, Carers and Disabled Children Act 2000, Carers (Equal Opportunities) Act 2004, Disability Discrimination Act 1995 and the Human Rights Act 1998, and it must ensure that the services are delivered to the standards of the relevant NSF. For instance, the mental health NSF (DoH, 1999a) requires specialist health and social care teams of staff to be integrated and the partnership is responsible for ensuring this happens.
■ The policy has to be agreed.
■ The agencies must build in flexibility, which enables services to be supplied that meet the emerging needs of people, rather than trying to fit the needs to the existing services.
■ There have to be working agreements between the agencies about who does what. This will affect the details at every stage. For example, if a person is receiving domiciliary care and a carer is supplied at night to give the spouse some respite from full-time caring, is the carer empowered to give the medication, through the night? Similarly, on emergency admission to the hospital, accompanied by the spouse, is the nurse in A&E empowered to put a plaster on the spouse's arm for an injury unrelated to the admission? Actual working practice in these aspects may vary from area to area according to local protocols.
■ There needs to be agreement between agencies – health and social services – about where the resources are to be shared and how they should be made available. For example, the local PCT has agreed to resource full-time home care for a terminally ill man being cared for at home by his sister. Should the changes of bedding be supplied by health or adult care services?
■ There should be agreement on who takes the lead and makes decisions about treatment in particular situations. For example, where a terminally ill woman is

living alone with no relatives, and is suffering from mood swings and therefore not capable of making a consistent decision, who should decide whether the last weeks of her life are spent at home, in hospital or at the local hospice?

■ There is a need to develop and maintain effective working relationships between the different health and social care staff.

We can see that it takes preparation, time, resources and hard work to set up, build and maintain the partnership. The partnership is more likely to work if it is developed with staff rather than imposed on them and if attention is paid not just to the structure but to the way it is actually organised and operates. At the point where the health and social care workers interact with carers and service users (sometimes called 'the interface'), there is a need to make sure that all the different staff are working consistently together. This sounds straightforward and logical, but in practice may be difficult to achieve.

We shall take an example to illustrate some of the practical issues that arise. We shall go straight into the detail, as though we are a community nurse and care worker jointly visiting from the local PCT and Adult Care Resource Centre to acquaint ourselves with the case.

Practice study

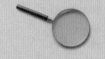

Mr and Mrs H

Home care for terminally ill Mrs H has been arranged and during a 24-hour period, half a dozen different staff are coming and going. Here is the diary of a typical day:

6.45: emergency doctor arrives in response to a phone call by Mr H, who heard Mrs H moaning when he went to the toilet, and wants pain relief for her
7.00: night sitter from Marie Curie (supplied by PCT) leaves
7.15: two carers arrive to wash Mrs H
7.30: Mr H gets up
7.45: the two carers leave
8.00: Mr H puts out the soiled bed linen for the laundry service to collect
9.15: community nurse visits from PCT and meets Macmillan nurse
10.00: doctor visits from PCT
13.00: carer visits to allow Mr H respite to get a haircut and go to the shops
14.00: pharmacist visits with medication for Mr H, who has his own sleep problems
15.00: emergency admission of Mrs H to hospital with acute pains
14.00: Mrs H admitted to ward, accompanied by Mr H
18.00: Mrs H cleared for discharge after medication and evening meal
19.00: Mr and Mrs H arrive home in hospital transport with two paramedical staff to carry Mrs H into the house and ensure she is safely in bed
21.30: night sitter arrives.

We examine this routine and discuss it with staff at the next opportunity. It is clear that the different staff need a protocol (working arrangement) that enables them to coordinate their work. At the interface with the carer and service user, they need to have a single point of access to shared information, for instance. One way of achieving this is through the maintenance of running notes at the home, which each staff member reads, checks and adds to through the day and night. These notes must be written clearly and observations need to be distinct from decisions.

Also, it needs to be clear who is empowered to make the decisions, for example, about medication. The emergency doctor visited and prescribed liquid morphine for pain relief because the patch on Mrs H's arm apparently was not curbing the pain sufficiently to allow her to sleep. However, when the community nurses arrived, they regarded this as not helpful in the medium term because the morphine was tried a couple of days ago and caused stomach upsets and discomfort. They ask Mr H for his view and remind him of what happened a couple of days ago, which he had forgotten. He agrees to them telephoning Mrs H's regular GP to ask her to visit and consider prescribing a stronger patch.

This implies that the agencies must take care:

- to develop joint ownership of the partnership
- to involve carers and service users – in this case, Mr and Mrs H – in the decisions made
- to make sure that there are no gaps between agreeing the assessment of Mr H's needs for respite as part of his carer's assessment and Mrs H's need for home care, and the joint arrangements between health and social care agencies for the implementation, monitoring, reviewing and evaluation of the agencies' performance throughout the process.

Have you noticed how we have been plunged into the heart of this situation without time or space to think? Think back to Chapter 34 on reflective and critical practice. If we are to maintain our reflectiveness and criticality as well as our capacity to make good decisions, we need to create space. We shall do this artificially by choosing an item to reflect on, which will enable us to put the work with Mr and Mrs H into its wider context. I have chosen some writing on counselling at different stages of the life course to do this. You may choose something different.

Léonie Sugarman (2004) writes about how people's expectations of their relationships with others vary at different stages of the life course:

- 0–1:   *trust* is the priority to the infant
- 1–6:   the young child seeks more *autonomy* as he or she grows
- 10–14: *competence* is the priority as the child learns
- 14–20: *identity* is the priority as the young person seeks to establish him or herself
- 21–35: the adult seeks *intimacy* through relationships with others
- 35–65: the adult prioritises a sense of *relating to other generations*
- 65+ : the adult attaches particular importance to *integrity*, that is, trust and reliability in others and in the services provided.

This exercise has given us space to put Mr and Mrs H's priorities in the context of their position in the life course. Mr and Mrs H have chosen to receive home care, which meets their needs for a trustworthy, reliable service. At the point of delivery of services, they simply want to ensure that Mrs H is cared for as well at home as she would be in hospital or in a hospice. To achieve this, there needs to be a high level of communication and coordination between the different agencies and practitioners, namely:

- social services: carer, laundry service, pharmacist
- PCT: GP, district nurses
- Macmillan nurses
- emergency duty service: doctor
- carer/night sitter from Marie Curie Cancer Care
- staff in acute hospital: A&E, acute ward, discharge planning staff.

Here is a checklist of the kinds of issues that have been considered to date, in the primary assessment of Mrs H's needs.

Anti-discriminatory practice

It is necessary to focus primarily on Mrs H's needs as a person first rather than on her medical condition.

Moving through the process of the work

- *What do we know about Mr and Mrs H at the start?*
  From previous contact with health and social services, we have information about Mrs H's progressive condition, which has now become terminal.
- *Are there any particular factors?*
  Yes, they have chosen to receive home care.
- *What is the level of concern about risks to individual family members?*
  Mrs H is vulnerable. Mr H seems able to cope.
- *What is Mr H's view?*
  He seems a typical caring husband and clearly wants to support his wife.
- *What is Mrs H's view?*
  She will accept what is prescribed.
- *What other information do we need?*
  We haven't identified any other significant relatives or neighbours who can offer information, help or support.
- *What other sources of information are there?*
  None that we are aware of.
- *What is our assessment, with family members, about what they need?*
  Mrs H needs constant monitoring to ensure that her condition is stabilised as far as possible, bearing in mind no cure is possible, to minimise pain and inconvenience to her.
- *What existing interventions or orders are currently in force?*
  None.

■ *What level of concern do we have about this couple, in terms of how pressing their need is and how much risk is presented, either to them or by them?*
Not applicable in this case.

Practice study

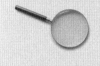

Mr and Mrs H (cont'd)

Three days later, we find ourselves back at the house, following a confused message left on the office voicemail by Mr H after the night sitter has left. It sounds as though Mr H is crying. He then says it doesn't matter and rings off.

When we visit, at first Mr H blocks our attempts to find out what lay behind the phone call. We persuade him to sit down and have a cup of tea. Mrs H starts to moan in the other room and he shouts something, muttering about her being unreasonable. He is clearly stressed. Five minutes later, he starts to cry and stops himself, as he did on the phone.

It takes a while, but over the next half-hour, Mr H reveals symptoms of chronic depression, which nobody has identified, because of the other emotions expected of a carer of a terminally ill spouse in this situation. This visit leads to a proper assessment of Mr H's depression, relating this to his needs as a carer.

Questions are asked back at the office about how Mr H's situation could have been taken for granted and his needs as a carer ignored. The response by staff involved at the time is that he seemed to be coping and refused an assessment.

We are committed to evidence-based practice. Even in a busy office, our line managers and supervisors maintain a shelf of up-to-date books and articles. We go to the section on depression. First we revisit some important and influential research about the social origins of depression by George Brown, first published in 1978 and now available in a book published in 1996 (Brown, 1996). The importance to us of the earlier book by Brown is that he shows a hidden side of depression experienced by women who may be quite isolated at home, doing the housework. He shows that there may be social factors contributing to their depression. The second publication we find useful is the brief and clearly written research study by Jill Manthorpe and Steve Iliff (2005) on depression among older people, a must-read for all those who work with older people. We are thinking about Mr H's state of mind, his attempts to keep going and support his wife and what we now know, that he has been depressed for a long time, but felt it wrong to reveal this, believing that he would seem weak and unable to cope, thereby risking his wife being taken away into a nursing home, hospital or hospice.

So, we have some additional questions on our checklist:

■ *What existing supports exist for Mr and Mrs H?*
We haven't taken into proper account so far the support needed for Mr H and are now ensuring that he has a carer's assessment under relevant legislation

(Carers (Recognition and Services) Act 1995, strengthened by the Carers and Disabled Children Act 2000).

- *What additional supports would be desirable?*
  Mr H's depression needs assessment. He needs carer support.
- *What are we trying to achieve by intervening?*
  We are trying to stabilise the situation for Mr and Mrs H, as a couple and as two people, each of whom has needs.
- *What kinds of services and what levels of resources are required?*
  Before responding to these questions, we need to take into account our discussions with colleagues and our reading above of relevant research and related writing. The books and journal articles we read have relevance, but we need to link their generalised messages with this particular situation faced by these service users and carers. There is little doubt that Mr H is lonely, but to establish his condition more definitely, he would need to attend either a doctor's surgery or one of the weekly mobile surgeries.

Given his special circumstances, the doctor visits at home with a nurse and care practitioner and his assessment is completed on this flexible basis. The result of the assessment is that Mr H needs treatment for his depression and support as a carer.

Networks are important to family members as a source of support. Seed (1990, p. 72), in his useful book on the use of networks and network analysis in social work, notes that analysis of a person's networks enables us to put the assessment of the individual factors affecting a person's situation in the wider context of family and environmental factors.

Intervention

- We put the plan into action
- Mr H's needs as carer begin to be tackled and Mrs H receives the flexible regime of support.

Reviewing effectiveness

Several weeks later, we review how Mr and Mrs H are getting on. Here is a checklist of the questions we ask at that stage:

- *What were our goals?*
- *Which practitioners were involved?*
- *What did we do?*
- *What outcomes did we perceive?*
- *What outcomes did Mrs H as the service user and Mr H as the carer perceive?*
- *What, if anything, would we do differently if we could?*
- *What are we happy with?*
- *What, if anything, would Mrs and Mr H have us do differently?*
- *What are Mrs and Mr H happy with?*

Part VII

Conclusion

This chapter has been unusual, because of its focus on a practice example. It highlights the difference between actually doing the work and writing and talking about it at one remove. This chapter has attempted to pitch you, the reader, into the middle of the practice and show you how what we have covered in this book begins to translate into our work with people, both service users and carers. It particularly shows how it is necessary for primary healthcare teams and social care partners, together with colleagues in hospitals and communities, to move closer together, becoming more than two agencies doing joint work and actually integrating their services so they become shared work together.

REVIEW
QUESTIONS

1 What conditions do you regard as necessary for effective joint working?

2 What are the main laws that have to be complied with in joint working?

3 What contribution does an understanding of networks make to the assessment of people's needs?

FURTHER
READING

Anstey, K. (1999) *Patient Assessment in Continuing Care*, London, NT Books

DoH (2001) *Domiciliary Care: National Minimum Standards: Regulations: Consultation Document*, London, DoH

DoH (2002) *NSF for Older People: Supporting Implementation: Intermediate Care: Moving Forward*, London, DoH

DoH (2003) *Domiciliary Care: National Minimum Standards Regulations*, London, DoH

Manthorpe, J. and Iliffe, S. (2005) *Depression in Later Life*, London, Jessica Kingsley

Marshal, M. (1997) *The State of the Art in Dementia Care*, London, Centre for Policy on Ageing (CPA), www.cpa.org.uk

Steiner, A., Vaughan, B. and Hanford, L. (1998) *Intermediate Care: Approaches to Evaluation*, London, King's Fund

Terry, P. (1997) *Counselling the Elderly and their Carers*, Basingstoke, Macmillan – now Palgrave Macmillan

Wade, S. (ed.) (2004) *Intermediate Care of Older People*, London, Whurr Books

Multiprofessional Work with Children and Families ROBERT ADAMS

Learning outcomes

By the end of this chapter, you should be able to:

■ SPECIFY what is involved in the main stages of work with children and families

■ WORK THROUGH the sequence of work with children and families

■ IDENTIFY some of the main areas of difficulty in the work.

The Children Act 1989 states that the welfare of the child is the paramount principle governing practice. The inquiry report into the tragic circumstances of the death of Victoria Climbié highlights the need for improved coordination of children's services (Laming, 2003). The Children Act 2004 emphasises the importance of local agencies developing stronger partnerships to deliver better services for children.

Children's services (see Chapter 17), including children's trusts, are expected to be formed from newly joined-up children's education and social services. They should be organised so that the network of agencies and public, private and informal (family-based) supports and services radiate like the spokes of a wheel or, rather, converge on the child at their hub. A seamless web of services should be created to meet the needs of the child.

We follow the pattern established in the previous chapter and devote this entire chapter to one detailed example. It is important to take space to examine a single situation in detail, as this enables us to highlight the key issues involved, when practitioners from different agencies bring together theory, experience of practice, research evidence and practice.

The Structure for Joined-up Children's Education and Social Services

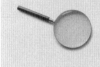

The Davis family

This is the case of a family who have been in contact with health and social services agencies. There have been child protection issues in the past, involving one of the mother's previous partners, but there has been no evidence of child protection issues since they moved to this present house two years ago. A local voluntary agency which supports families had been involved in supporting them, until six months ago when the situation apparently stabilised. It is called Families and Children First (FCF – a fictitious name) and this morning it was alerted by phone calls from neighbours that late night shouting and door slamming have been heard in a house in a rundown locality. Tracy, the mother, is 35 and Harry, the ex-partner, is 40. There are five children: twins Tina and Mick, aged 17, and Lisa, 4, Mary, 7 and Ben 11.

We are a health and a social care worker for FCF. We are following a checklist of questions, which you may like to note for your own use, since they provide a useful framework for noting what happens in this case, and can be used for any other case. These questions follow five headings: the preliminary stage at the start of the work, and then the four stages we have examined in detail in Chapters 30–33: assessment, planning, implementation/intervention and review/evaluation.

Preliminary Stage: Start of the Work

- *How does the work start?*
  As soon as FCF workers hear about the phone calls, we anticipate that this is another troublesome episode and, although it will need intervention and probably support, FCF does not have the lead role in work with this family, in the sense that it is not the statutory agency, but has been the organisation most involved over the past year and is probably best placed to assess what is going on. The question of who does what is sorted out first thing in the morning in a phone call between the manager of FCF and the local manager of children's services in the local authority. This is part of a protocol (arrangement) about how shared responsibilities work locally, to which different involved professionals and agencies contribute.
- *Which laws and procedures govern work with this family?*
  The workers in FCF need to be familiar with the legal context and ensure that we obey the law constantly throughout the work. The main laws to take account of include the Children Act 1989, NHS and Community Care Act 1990, Carers

(Recognition and Services) Act 1995, Sex Offenders Act 1997 (information about the implications of being a Schedule 1 offender), Human Rights Act 1998, Carers and Disabled Children Act 2000, Freedom of Information Act 2000 and Carers (Equal Opportunities) Act 2004.

Assessment

■ *What approach to assessment shall we use?*
The Department of Health *Framework for the Assessment of Children in Need and their Families* (DoH, 2000a) is the basis for all who have responsibility for the care and education of babies and children, for assessing and planning the work.

■ *Is there any information about previous agency contacts with the family?*
The family is known from previous contact with health and social services.

■ *Are any particular factors known?*
Yes, they lived on a travellers' site, but two years ago Tracy split up from her partner and left, taking the children with her. At that stage, allegations that her former partner Harry had sexually abused the older daughter were investigated and insufficient evidence was found to support a prosecution. Harry is on the sex offenders' register for another offence, not connected to this family.

■ *What is the level of concern about risks to individual family members?*
The question is whether any of the children are being harmed or are at risk of being harmed. The view is that the immediate risks are low. Two workers from FCF visit the home and confirm that inside it is surprisingly clean. Tracy appears to be prone to drinking too much alcohol, but the children seem to be very organised, well dressed and well fed.

■ *What is the mother's view?*
When the two FCF workers visit at about 11 in the morning, even though the visit was planned and agreed by her, Tracy is still in bed. She gets up and speaks briefly to them. She says she relies on the twins a lot to keep the house in order.

■ *What is each of the children's view?*
A male and a female worker visit the home, with the intention of talking to Tracy together and then chatting to the children individually. One of us can stay chatting to the others, while the other does the individual assessment. *As a basic principle, all family members, including every child, are seen on their own, at least for part of the visit.* No particular cause for concern is noted. The two younger children are not talkative, but their silence is not the 'frozen watchfulness' of the abused child. The practitioner sits down near Lisa and talks about the crayoning she is doing. When asked where she got the crayons and paper, she says Tina brought them home. The practitioner has in mind advice that it may be more productive simply to spend time with a child rather than asking questions and that joining in with the child's activity may be a good way of communicating (Thomas, 2002, pp. 94–5). We check out with every family member that Harry has not visited. We know he is on the sex offenders' register.

■ *How can we ensure that we remember what the family members tell us?*

We need to make sure that we record what each family member says, and especially what each child says, in their own words. Each child's views and assessment should be given a separate, easily identifiable section in the file.

■ *How can we make sure that all family members, including the children, participate actively throughout the work done with them?*

We need to empower family members, giving them confidence to make their views known in interviews, group discussions and review meetings. This requires preparation in the form of reassuring individuals that no sanctions will follow if they speak their minds. From experience, we know that once some family members have tried speaking out, the problem will be damping down their enthusiasm for saying what they think so as to allow the business of the meeting to proceed. However, it is possible to have tokenism in this area and this is a risk to guard against.

■ *What other information do we need?*

There are gaps in our knowledge about this family. We are used to using the Department of Health framework for assessment as our standard tool for assessing children and families.

■ *How shall we use the framework?*

The framework for assessment gives us three main headings, or domains of the child's world, in which to gather information: the child's developmental needs; the parenting capacity of the adults; and family and environmental factors (DoH, 2000a, p. 17). Because this is such an essential tool for all assessments of children, we describe it in some detail now.

The Child's Developmental Needs

It is necessary for the practitioners to use the assessment to identify the areas of the child's development to deal with and record, to plan how to measure progress, to ensure that this is matched to the child's age and stage of development, and to know how to analyse the information (DoH, 2000a, p. 18).

The dimensions of the child's developmental needs are as follows:

■ The health of the child
■ The child's education
■ Emotional and behavioural development
■ Identity: 'the child's growing sense of self' (D0H, 2000a, p. 19)
■ Family and social relationships: the growth of empathy
■ Social presentation: the child's growing sense of appropriateness of appearance and behaviour, including appropriateness of dress for gender, age, culture and religion and cleanliness
■ Self-care skills: the child's ability to demonstrate practical emotions and demonstrate effective communication.

The Parenting Capacity of the Adults

It is necessary to assess the parental capacity in terms of how the family functions and which adults play the main parenting roles. The more cause for concern about a child, the more important parenting is. It will be necessary to assess Tracy and her partner, and the partners of her children, in terms of the potential contribution they can make. The dimensions of parenting capacity include:

- Extent to which basic food, drink, shelter and care is provided
- Safety
- Emotional warmth
- Stimulation
- Guidance and boundaries
- Stability.

Family and Environmental Factors

The assessment needs to take account of the wider context of individual circumstances and family life. Its dimensions include:

- Family history and functioning, including any medical conditions or mental health problems
- The wider family, which in the example given includes the relationships of the fathers of Tracy's children to their own offspring
- Housing conditions, that is, whether it is free of damp and other problems
- Employment and unemployment in the household, including its impact on the children
- Income levels in the household, including whether it is adequate to keep the children
- Social integration of the family, including whether they are isolated and excluded in the wider community
- Community resources, including whether there are potential supports for family members.

Important Extra Item

Are there any specific concerns about discrimination or anti-discriminatory practice?

We do not feel the framework emphasises this sufficiently. It is one of our criticisms. We are committed to remaining critical in our practice and this is an example of our questioning approach. We have attracted some queries and comments from colleagues about this in the past, but challenge them as complacent.

The issue is that we have been aware in the past that other children at school have victimised the younger children, making fun of them because they were 'gippoes' and complaining that they smelt. Since they moved from the travellers' site, this appears not to have happened.

Planning

We return to the office. When we return we shall have completed our draft thoughts about the assessment, bearing in mind that this is an ongoing situation and not the first assessment to have been carried out on this family.

Quite quickly, we assemble a plan. We believe Tracy is only coping because the older twins are doing a lot of the parenting, possibly to the detriment of their schooling. We need to ensure enough support is given to the family, particularly the twins. Our plan is to develop this support, working with them and with Tracy. The plan will be negotiated with them, based on the following checklist of questions:

- *What are we trying to achieve in the plan?*
- *What do family members think and feel about this?*
- *What are the views of different agencies?*
- *What kinds of supports and interventions are available and appropriate?*
- *What supports can be expected from family members themselves?*
- *What supports might come from the local community and from agencies, such as Families and Children First?*
- *What kinds of services and what levels of resources does all this imply?*
- *What evidence do we have to back up our plan?*

This is one of the most difficult areas for us as workers. We need to gather our knowledge and check out relevant research and practice experience, to confirm that the skills we are going to use in this case are likely to lead to a productive and positive outcome for the family. One part of this is searching for relevant literature. A lot of the work we have done in earlier parts of this book are relevant. We should bear in mind that the articles, chapters and books we read, the commentaries and research are of general relevance. Before they can inform our practice, we still need to make the link between that generality and the particular circumstances of Tracy and her children.

From the information already gathered, we have formed the view that the two older children, the twins, are providing a lot of the care, compensating in part for the absent father and in part for Tracy's inability to keep sober all the time.

We search for information about the assessment of families and young carers. The edited book by Horwath (2001) is useful, as it contains a wealth of insights from the wide range of contributors to the different chapters. We also find the chapter by Deardon and Becker (2000) on the needs of young carers particularly useful.

Implementation/Intervention

- *How do we reassure ourselves that the children are safe?*
  As far as we can tell, the children are not at any more significant risk than they have been for two years. The ex-partner has not been in touch and their main vulnerability arises from Tracy's inability to cope without support from the twins.

- *What should we do to support family members?*
  We are working, with volunteer support and using our nearby family centre and meals service, to implement a plan to give extra support to Tracy and the children.
- *Does the planned intervention have legal support?*
  What we are doing falls within the legislation but does not require any specific legal action.

Reviewing and Evaluating

At the conclusion of this process, we meet again with Tracy and the children to review and evaluate what has gone on. We are keen to know what they feel has been achieved. At the meeting, we cover the following questions:

- *What were our aims?*
- *Which workers were involved?*
- *What did we carry out in the plan?*
- *What outcomes did we and family members notice?*
- *What, if anything, would we do differently if we could?*
- *What are we happy with?*
- *What, if anything would family members have us do differently?*
- *What are family members pleased with?*

Conclusion

Most of this chapter has been taken up with one detailed example. It has given you a general list of questions you can use to guide you through any case. It also ensures that you do not leave this book feeling you only have a superficial grasp of how values, knowledge, research evidence, policy guidance and skills come together in childcare practice. At whatever level we learn about health and social care, it is important that we appreciate the complexity of the task we undertake, in conjunction with other practitioners. In the case of work with children and families, almost every responsibility is shared between more than one agency. This makes the task of interagency liaison and joint working more complicated even than dealing with people's lives, which are complicated enough in themselves.

We hope you have found this brief journey through this case and the one in the previous chapter interesting and productive and will soon be ready to consider some general messages about teamwork and multiprofessional working. Before we do this, we have one more chapter that illustrates the complexity of different disciplines, professions and agencies sharing work, chosen from what may be viewed as one of the closest healthcare neighbours to social care – occupational therapy.

Acknowledgement

I should like to acknowledge the help given to me in using the checklist of questions for this and the preceding chapter, by the work I did when developing three case studies (older people, mental health, disability) for Research Mindedness, a virtual learning resource funded by the Social Care Institute for Excellence (SCIE) at www.sws.soton.ac.uk/rminded. I have adapted the questions from this checklist.

REVIEW
QUESTIONS

1   What three domains of the child's world are covered in the assessment of needs?

2   When visiting the home to assess the child, why does it matter if we visit alone and only have time to interview the child?

3   What do we mean by parenting capacity?

FURTHER
READING

Children First (2000) *Working Together to Safeguard Children: A Guide to Interagency Working to Safeguard and Promote the Welfare of Children*, Cardiff, National Assembly for Wales

DoH (2000) *Framework for the Assessment of Children in Need and their Families*, London, TSO

DoH/Social Services Inspectorate (1995) *The Challenge of Partnership in Child Protection: Practice Guide*, London, HMSO

Frost, N. (2005) *Professionalism, Partnership and Joined-up Thinking: A Research Review of Front-line Working with Children and Families*, Totnes, Devon, Research in Practice

Percy-Smith, J. (2005) *What Works in Strategic Partnerships for Children?*, Ilford, Barnardo's

Sure Start (undated) *Birth to 3 Matters: A Framework to Support Children in their Earliest Years*, London, Sure Start
This is a brief, but informative and well-illustrated pamphlet.

Resource file

Suspicion or disclosure of child abuse

Who counts as a 'child'?

A child is anybody under 18 years (Children Act 1989).

Responding to the child

- Do not overreact. The child disclosing invariably is not in immediate danger.
- Listen to the child and be positive, not disbelieving.
- Reassure the child that talking about it is best.
- Don't make the child unnecessarily repeat.
- Refuse to agree to listen 'in confidence'. State that you may have to pass on the information, but that it will go only to the professionals who need to know.
- Follow the policy and locally agreed procedure.
- As soon as you can, write down what the child has said as fully as possible.

Reporting the suspicion, allegation or incident

- Remember the welfare of the child is paramount.
- Carry out your duty to report the suspicion, allegation or incident
- Contact one of the following: local childcare team; out of hours duty team; or the police.

FURTHER READING

Children Act 1989

DfES (2006) *Working Together to Safeguard Children. A Guide for Inter-agency Working to Safeguard and Promote the Welfare of Children*, London, TSO

DfES (2006) *The Common Assessment Framework for Children and Young People: Practitioners' Guide*, London, DfES

Education Act 2002 (Part 11, S. 175)

National Council of Voluntary Child Care Organisations (2005) *Local Safeguarding Children Boards*, London, NCVCCO

Walker, S. and Thurston, C. (2006) *Safeguarding Children and Young People: A Guide to Integrated Practice*, Lyme Regis, Russell House

50 Occupational Therapy in Multiprofessional Practice JON ADAMS and RUTH GILI

This chapter is intended to be a brief introduction and overview of occupational therapy and the role of the occupational therapist within the multidisciplinary team. It will provide a context in which to develop the reader's understanding of occupational therapy by using a number of case studies.

What is Occupational Therapy?

As individuals, we have an inbuilt desire to engage in occupations (purposeful and meaningful activities). This desire or motivation is influenced by our beliefs and values, the physical and social environments in which we live, work and play, and our spiritual and emotional needs.

As these 'influences' interact and change, we make choices and decisions about what occupations we engage in and why in order to maintain and enhance our own health and wellbeing. However, if due to the impact of illness or disability or a change in our occupational circumstances, we are unable to make satisfactory occupational choices, this can have a negative effect on our wellbeing.

Occupational therapy focuses on enabling people to maintain and improve their ability to engage in purposeful and meaningful activity. The aim of occupational therapy is to enable individuals to maintain and restore optimum performance of purposeful and meaningful activities.

The purpose and meaning that an individual associates with a particular activity and the degree to which they can perform this activity are central to maintaining health and wellbeing. The notion of optimising an individual's performance within work, social, leisure and personal activities to create a sense of personal wellbeing and social integration is central to occupational therapy practice.

What Occupational Therapists Do

'Occupational therapy personnel work with people of all ages, with physical, mental and social impairments and learning disabilities' (Creek, 2003. p. 7). Occupational therapists work within a variety of health and social care settings in both the public and private sector. They work with people who have multiple and complex problems, people with minor coping difficulties and those who are functioning well and wish to maintain and promote their wellbeing. There is an increasing opportunity within the health promotion arena and the primary care setting for occupational therapists to work at a consultation level, providing support to other health and social care professionals.

As occupational therapy focuses on enabling people to maintain or improve their ability to perform purposeful and meaningful activities, the occupational therapist first needs to identify those activities an individual is finding difficult. The occupational therapist then analyses the individual's occupational performance through observing them carrying out activities, identifying which of the individual's skills are impacting on the performance and what environmental factors are causing the activity to be difficult.

Once the strengths and deficits of the skill have been identified, the occupational therapist works with the individual to develop a plan identifying treatment goals. This plan may include relearning old strategies and skills and/or developing new strategies and skills to overcome difficulties with occupational performance. The occupational therapist will also consider if any adaptations to the environment would enhance occupational performance. Throughout this process, the occupational therapist is aware of the balance between the individual's skills, the complexity of their occupations and the demands of the environment.

The activities performed by individuals themselves can be grouped into three main areas:

1. *Activities of daily living*, defined as 'self maintenance tasks' (AOTA, 1994, p. 1051), which include brushing hair, cleaning teeth, dressing and undressing and managing medication.
2. *Work and productive activities*, which are 'purposeful activities for self development, social contribution and livelihood' (AOTA, 1994, p. 1052), including maintaining

the home environment, looking after others and engaging in educational or vocational related activities.

3. *Play and/or leisure activities*, which can be defined as 'intrinsically motivating activities for amusement, relaxation, spontaneous enjoyment, or self-expression' (AOTA, 1994, p. 1052). It involves identifying skills and interests and participating in leisure and play activities.

The following three Practice studies give brief illustrations of how each of the three performance areas can be applied in practice.

Practice study

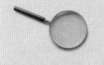

Joan

Joan is a 60-year-old female who, when asked about her activities of daily living, said: 'I cannot reach down to put my shoes and socks on any more so my husband has to do it, I would prefer to be able to do this by myself. This is particularly difficult in the mornings when my hips are much more stiff and painful.'

Through assessment, the occupational therapist identified that Joan's reaching skills were impacting on her ability to put her shoes on, and her manipulation skills and strength of grasp were impacting on her ability to pull her socks over her heal and tie up her laces.

The occupational therapist worked with Joan to explore alternative ways of putting her shoes and socks on without any assistance from her husband. By using a combination of providing some equipment, including a sock aid and long-handled shoe horn, changing her shoe laces to ones made of elastic and teaching her alternative ways of reaching her foot, she can now put her shoes and socks on independently.

Practice study

Davina

Davina is a 23-year-old female who, when asked questions about her work and productivity activities, said, 'I can't get to the school gates to pick up my children without having a panic attack, so now I have to rely on friends to pick the children up.'

The occupational therapist initially taught Davina about anxiety and ways in which to manage it, and then together they devised a graded programme for Davina to follow which gradually built up her exposure to school. By following this programme and using her techniques, she has learned to manage her anxiety and is now able to pick her children up from school.

Practice study

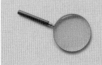

John

John is a 73-year-old male who, when asked about his leisure activities, said: 'I used to play bridge three times a week with a group of friends down at the local social club, but recently I have found it difficult to remember when we were supposed to be meeting up. I always seemed to be late and have even missed a couple of games by accident. I felt really embarrassed and decided not to go any more.'

Following assessment, the occupational therapist and John explored strategies to enable him to attend his bridge club. One strategy John and the occupational therapist identified was for him to talk to his friends about his difficulty remembering when they were supposed to meet and to ask if one of them could ring him up to remind him on the day of the bridge game. He had previously not wanted to do this in case they did not understand, but after speaking to them about his difficulties, he realised they were willing to support him as they had missed his company. John now regularly meets up with his friends to play cards and feels supported.

Multidisciplinary Teamwork

The multidisciplinary team includes team members from a multitude of professional backgrounds and clinical and administrative support staff. The multidisciplinary team takes on the responsibility for jointly assessing and reviewing the client's progress and making joint decisions about treatment plans. Consequently, the team's understanding of the client's problems is multifaceted, reflecting the multiple components of care (see Figure 50.1).

Each member of the team brings to the review process aspects that are unique to themselves and their specific training. For example, a medical doctor would diagnose an illness and inform the team and client about the physiological impact of illness and possible drug therapies available to enhance wellness. An occupational therapist, on the other hand, would provide advice and treatment to enhance the performance of activities of daily living. As well as profession-specific skills, team members bring with them shared skills, attitudes and personal qualities such as effective communication skills. The following is a list of the team members and their particular skills:

- *Psychologist:* Clinical psychologists work with people of all ages with mental or physical health problems. Their primary focus of treatment is to reduce psychological distress and enhance psychological wellbeing. Psychology assessments may include psychometric tests, interviews and direct observation of behaviour. After the assessment process, the client may receive therapy, counselling or advice.
- *Support worker:* Support workers are non-registered healthcare workers who bring to the team a wealth of practical, life and often work experience. They are

essential in supporting members of the team with the implementation of treatment plans and strategies.

■ *Physiotherapist:* Physiotherapists help and treat people of all ages recovering from physical and mental health problems. Physiotherapists identify and maximise an individual's movement potential through physical methods, including manipulation, massage, therapeutic exercise and the application of electrophysical modalities.

■ *Nurse:* Nurses work across a wide spectrum of healthcare services, focusing on obtaining and maintaining physical and mental health, and wellness. As well as assessing patient needs in order to monitor symptoms and progress, nurses administer medications and assist in the recovery process.

■ *Clerical officer:* The clerical officer supports the whole team with administrative tasks such as sending out appointment letters, typing assessment reports and inputting patient information onto the organisation's database.

■ *Social worker:* The social worker within the team aims to address the social impact of illness and disability. The social worker offers a broad range of services for both the client and carer. These services include the assessment of social circumstances and community care needs and providing advice and support with issues such as housing and benefits.

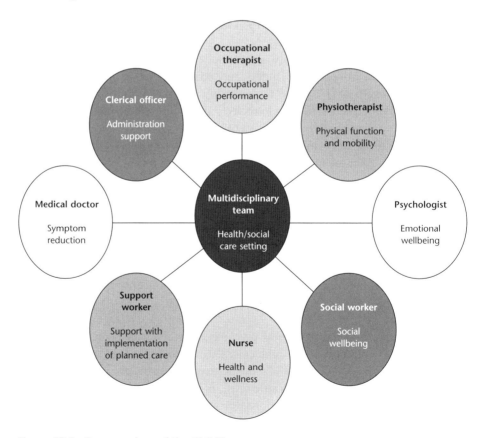

Figure 50.1 Core members of the CMHT

Practice study

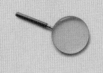

Mary

Mary is 75 years old; she lives alone and has been seen frequently by her GP following concerns from her daughter that Mary is finding it increasingly difficult to manage at home. Mary has been referred by her GP to the community mental health team (CMHT) for older aged adults.

The CMHT manager took the referral to the weekly team meeting, where a qualified member of the team was allocated to meet Mary and her daughter to carry out an initial assessment.

The initial assessment was brought back to the team and the following key points were identified:

- Mary has lived alone since her husband died five years ago. She lives in a rural area with limited public services. The GP surgery and local shop are within walking distance from her house. Mary's daughter lives in the same village and visits Mary on a daily basis, usually after work.
- Mary worked as a clerk in the local post office for 20 years before retiring at 60. Since her retirement, her daughter reports that she had been active in the local Women's Institute (WI) group but her participation in this has declined steadily over the last six months. She has been an active member of the local Methodist church in the past, and is a keen gardener and cook.
- She owns her own house which is a three-bedroom semi-detached property. Mary receives a pension from the post office and doesn't have any outstanding debts. She receives council tax reduction and pension credit.
- Mary has lost interest in the way she looks and finds it difficult to keep on top of household chores. Mary's daughter identified that Mary has needed more support from her over the last six months with shopping and household chores: 'She is becoming more forgetful, she forgets to meet up with her friends at the planned time.'

Following the presentation of the initial assessment, the team discussed Mary's needs. It was identified that a full risk assessment needed to be carried out, with particular attention to the impact of Mary's forgetfulness on her safety, but also considering her environment (stairs and steps and other items and obstacles that might increase Mary's risk of falling).

Clear roles were identified and established in the team discussion through individual professional expertise and skill identity (see Figure 50.2). The plan was for Mary and the team to have a formal review of her care in six months.

Part VII

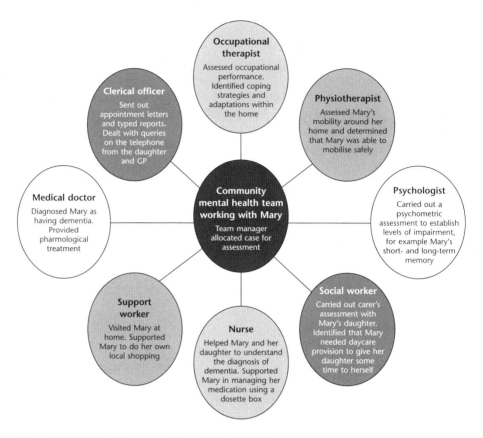

Figure 50.2 Tasks of core members of the CMHT

Occupational Therapy Assessment

The occupational therapist visited Mary initially with the member of the team already familiar to Mary in order to maintain a level of continuity with Mary's care. This initial contact was the opportunity to begin to establish a therapeutic relationship with Mary. Over a period of a few weeks, the occupational therapist visited Mary, sometimes when she was alone and sometimes when her daughter was present. These visits gave the occupational therapist the opportunity to assess Mary's level of occupational performance.

It became clear that getting to church on a Sunday morning was important but, although she was getting up early enough, getting dressed in time had become an obstacle to Mary achieving this. She stated: 'I am finding it difficult to get dressed in the morning because I can't find my clothes.'

Mary also identified that she used to have a lot of friends with whom she would meet on a regular basis. Mary said: 'I feel that I have to come to terms with spending more time on my own. I can't organise myself to get out of the house in time to go to WI meetings with my friends and I often forget the dates and times of the meetings.'

When exploring Mary's daily routine, it became apparent that large proportions of her day were unstructured. When this was highlighted to Mary, she stated that she found this dissatisfying but because she forgot her appointments with her friends and relied on her daughter to do her shopping and gardening, she was left with very little to do during the day.

As well as interviewing Mary and her daughter, the occupational therapist carried out an observational assessment to observe Mary engaged in a meaningful activity. This assessment provided the occupational therapist with information on which skills and environmental factors were impacting on Mary's performance of the activity. It also provided information on her safety when performing tasks. Mary was unable to complete the agreed task and was unable to initiate parts of the task. She also experienced difficulty locating items in the kitchen when they were inside cupboards. Mary was aware of safety issues during the task, such as turning the cooker off.

Occupational Therapy Intervention

Mary was very motivated to make changes to her life: 'I want to be able to take control of my life again.' Following discussions with Mary, it was identified that she would benefit from a more defined daily and weekly routine.

By addressing this using the following strategies, Mary was able to occupy herself in a more meaningful way:

- To help Mary to get dressed in the morning, the occupational therapist encouraged Mary and her daughter to sort out Mary's clothes and put small piles of each type of garment out on the top of the chest of drawers, making them clearly visible.
- Mary was keen to start doing her shopping again, so it was arranged that the support worker within the team would visit her once a week, to help Mary write her shopping list and walk with her to the local shops.
- Mary was happy for her daughter to continue to help with the gardening, as it meant that they had time together every Saturday. The daughter was also happy to continue to visit daily in the evenings.
- Mary was supplied with a calendar with large spaces in which to write appointments. The occupational therapist asked the daughter to make sure that the calendar was up to date, crossing off the day with Mary at the end of her daily evening visit. This enabled Mary to remain oriented to the day and date. The calendar was put up in Mary's kitchen on her fridge so that she regularly saw it throughout the day.
- The occupational therapist encouraged Mary to talk to her friends about her difficulties to see if they had any suggestions on how she could see them more often. Mary's friends agreed that they would take it in turns to pick Mary up on their way to the twice-weekly WI meetings. Mary asked them to provide her with a list of the dates of the WI meetings so that she could put them on her calendar.

Another friend said that she would be happy to pick Mary up on the way to church.

■ Mary's routine now had five days with identified activities. Mary and her daughter were worried about what she was going to do on the other two days. Following a carer's assessment by the social worker, it was identified that Mary could attend the local day centre on the remaining days.

Conclusion

This chapter has been a brief introduction to occupational therapy and the role of the occupational therapist. The chapter identified through case studies how occupational therapy can be applied within health and social care in a multidisciplinary team, and also explored the roles of other members of the team.

REVIEW
QUESTIONS

1 Can you describe briefly the practice of the occupational therapist within a health and social care setting?

2 What are the main elements of the role of the occupational therapist within the multidisciplinary team?

3 What are the main strengths and weaknesses of a multidisciplinary approach to clinical working?

FURTHER
READING

Christiansen, C. and Baum, C. (eds) (1997) *Occupational Therapy; Enabling Function and Well-being*, Thorofare, NJ, SLACK

Crepeau, E.B., Cohn, E.S. and Boyt Schell, B.A. (2003) *Willard and Spackman's Occupational Therapy* (10th edn) Philadelphia, Lippincott, Williams & Wilkins

Hagedorn, R. (1997) *Foundations for Practice in Occupational Therapy* (2nd edn) Edinburgh, Churchill Livingstone

Hagedorn, R. (2005) *Tools for Practice in Occupational Therapy: A Structured Approach to Core Skills and Processes*, Edinburgh, Churchill Livingstone

Wilcock, A.A. (1998) *An Occupational Perspective of Health*, Thorofare, NJ, SLACK

Making Good Decisions

TERENCE O'SULLIVAN

Learning outcomes

By the end of this chapter, you should be able to:

■ UNDERSTAND what is involved in making a good decision

■ APPRECIATE how good decisions are made.

This chapter is about making good decisions and uses actual practice situations to explain decision-making processes and the achievement of good outcomes. Decision-making is an important generic skill for all professional workers. It is involved in all the major practice stages of assessment, planning, implementation and review. Government practice guidance recognises the importance of good decision-making for providing effective services and interventions (for example see, DoH, 2000a, pp. 53–62). As such, decision-making skills are one of the foundations of good practice at the heart of professional work with both children and adults in health and social care. The making of a good decision is the result of a number of things being done well and the chapter will begin by explaining what is meant by a 'good decision'.

Activity 51.1

Think for a couple of moments about how you would explain what a 'good decision' is.

What is a Good Decision?

A good decision can be defined as having two elements, first, that it is well made and, second, that it has a good outcome after it is implemented. *Well-made decisions* are based on accurate information, have been carefully thought about, and all appropriate people have been included. A *good outcome* is one that achieves the decision-makers' goals. Well-made decisions and good outcomes do not always go together. When workers do not have time to think carefully about what to do, they still can achieve good outcomes. For example, on occasions, experienced workers may need to react quickly and make rapid decisions using their intuition. Also health and social care workers can make carefully thought through decisions that have bad outcomes, as when an at risk older person enters residential care to be safe, only to die soon after admission. No matter how well made a decision is, uncertainty about what will actually happen means that there still can be bad outcomes. Nobody can fully control how things turn out and life inevitably entails taking risks. Nevertheless, there is much that workers and services users can do to increase the chances of a good outcome.

Practice study

Freda

One Tuesday morning, Freda, an 84-year-old woman, was taken to A&E after having been found lying on the floor of her living room by the police. They had made a forced entry after being alerted by the milkman that she had not taken her milk in the previous day. The doctor found Freda had a painful hip but, as there were no bone injuries, decided there was no acute medical reason for her to be admitted to hospital. The hospital social worker and the A&E discharge coordinator were concerned about Freda's home situation, the circumstances surrounding her fall and her not being able to call for help. They were thinking of a brief admission to a ward or intermediate care to allow for a full multidisciplinary assessment. Freda was having none of this and demanded to be returned home immediately and for no interfering busybodies to be sent to check up on her. An ambulance returned Freda home and unfortunately she was brought back to hospital two weeks later with a fractured hip that necessitated hospital admission and then intermediate care.

This example shows that health and social care situations typically involve many decisions made at different points in time. Sometimes, when analysing how decisions are made, it is useful to select one or two decision points for closer examination. This chapter will use the examples of Freda discharging herself from A&E on the first occasion and her planned discharge on the second occasion.

Activity 51.2

Did Freda make a good decision that Tuesday morning?

What Makes a Good Decision?

In order to answer the question, What makes a good decision?, you would need to have some criteria by which to judge whether a decision was a good one. In this case, the criteria are that a good decision is one that:

- the service user has been fully involved in making
- stakeholders have been fully consulted and have worked together
- is based on accurate and full information
- has been given sufficient thought
- can be explained in a coherent and credible manner
- can be implemented in a sustainable way
- has a good outcome.

Briefly we will examine Freda's decision in relation to these criteria so as to be in a better position to judge whether she made a good decision. It may be unusual to you that Freda, the service user, is being regarded as the decision-maker and that we will be applying the 'good decision criteria' to her decision-making. The example reflects the importance of facilitating service users to make their own informed decisions.

Is Freda Fully Involved?

Freda was fully involved in the decision-making, having had the highest level of service user involvement in taking the decision for herself. Although we do not have much detail of what actually happened, it is worth considering whether the decision-makers worked together to engage with Freda. It is important that workers go out of their way to engage the service user in a positive way. To be fair to the workers, Freda may not have given them much chance; on the other hand, how much skill did the workers use in order to connect with Freda to check out whether she was making an informed decision or acting out of fear?

Did Freda Consult Stakeholders and Did the Stakeholders Work Together?

In this decision situation, the stakeholders include Freda, the hospital social worker, the discharge coordinator and the A&E doctor. Any relatives may also be stakeholders and Freda may have benefited from consulting them. It is unclear whether Freda fully consulted the doctor, hospital social worker and A&E discharge coordinator before making her decision. She certainly knew the doctor's opinion that she was well enough to be discharged and that the hospital social worker and A&E discharge coordinator felt she should not return home until a multidisciplinary assessment was carried out. We do not know how closely the three workers worked together. It is important that the different professional workers work together in a cooperative way, rather than in isolation from each other. There is a suggestion that the hospital social worker and discharge coordinator worked together but that once the A&E doctor had decided that there was no medical reason for keeping Freda in hospital, she left the other two workers to resolve the situation.

Is Freda Basing her Decision on Accurate and Full Information?

The workers are concerned about her home circumstances and the reason why she couldn't summon help. Freda knows her home circumstances better than anybody and she knows the circumstances of the fall and not being able to get up. There may be things she does not know about, for example the services, advice and equipment that might be available to her or what the workers' attitude would be towards her. Importantly, Freda may not have had full knowledge of the possible consequences of her decision.

Has Freda Given Sufficient Thought to the Decision?

We do not know how much thought Freda gave to the decision and whether she acted on intuition. It is often appropriate that particular decisions are based on intuition but others may need to be carefully thought about. It is likely to be an emotional time for Freda and emotions are an important factor to take into account; however, there are times when they can unduly influence decisions. For example, Freda's decision may have been ruled by her fear of what might happen if she allowed the workers to carry out their assessment.

Can Freda Explain her Decision in a Clear and Credible Manner?

When the workers asked Freda why she needed to return home immediately, she just replied because she wanted to. This does not necessarily mean she did not have a good explanation, she just might not have wanted to share it with the workers. However, not being able to explain why you believe a particular course of action is the best can indicate that the decision has not been sufficiently thought through or made on a sound basis.

Could Freda's Decision be Implemented in a Sustainable Way?

The fact that Freda was returned home meant that the decision was capable of being implemented but her readmission a fortnight later showed that it was not sustainable. The workers, believing that Freda had clearly stated that a home visit would not be welcomed, did not follow up her situation. There may have been a case for Freda being visited by someone who would take a sensitive approach, but it was important to achieve a balance between Freda's right to privacy and self-determination and giving her the opportunity to talk about her situation to somebody who would listen.

Was the Outcome a Good One?

The different stakeholders' views may have differed on whether the outcome of this decision was a good one. Freda's goals were to remain in her own home and not to have people interfering in her life, and for two weeks these goals were achieved but the situation proved not to be sustainable. Three weeks after her decision, she may have changed her mind and regarded her decision as having had a bad outcome, having experienced a serious fall and admission to hospital with a fractured hip.

Was Freda's Decision a Good One?

As you have seen, there is not always a straightforward answer to the question, Was the decision a good one? From the information we have it is not possible to give a clear opinion as to whether Freda made a good decision. Health and social care workers would tend to agree that she had the right to take the decision as she had the mental capacity to do so and was entitled to take risks in relation to her own life. They would also tend to say that they would have liked to be more reassured that Freda was in fact taking an informed decision and was not acting solely out of fear. More evidence of the workers effectively working together would also be needed, particularly in relation to positively engaging with Freda and alleviating her fears.

Activity 51.3

When Freda has sufficiently recovered from her broken hip, how will she and the workers make good discharge planning decisions?

▌How Good Decisions are Made

You may have correctly thought that the workers and Freda would need to work together to meet the criteria for what makes a good decision. After reading Efraimsson et al. (2004), the workers had become very aware of how lip service is often paid to service users participating in discharge planning and were determined to effectively involve Freda throughout. Each criterion for a good decision suggests things that need to happen if the discharge planning decisions are to be good ones. For example, what would giving sufficient thought to the decision mean in this particular situation? There are models that can guide decision-makers through a process that ensures they give sufficient thought to the situation. Most models of the decision-making process are similar in broad terms to the following:

- defining the problem or aim
- collecting information
- organising and analysing the information
- identifying the options
- coming to a conclusion.

Identifying the Aim

The workers are very careful that they and Freda are clear about her aim. As we know, she wants to stay in her own home and live independently without receiving services. Sometimes it is helpful to write the aim down in a way that does not suggest a particular course of action but instead concentrates on the life outcomes that a person wants to achieve. This enables different options to be considered to see which gives the best chance of achieving these outcomes. After a lot of discussion, Freda settles on the aim of retaining as much control as possible in the way she lives her life.

Collecting Information

The workers and Freda think about the information they need in order to plan her discharge in a way that achieves her aim and how they are going to get this information. For example, the current main threat to her retaining control over her own lifestyle is her falling. The workers, particularly those for whom this is a specialist area, need to assess her home environment for hazards to falling and other aspects such as Freda's balance. Information needs to be collected in a sensitive manner, with what Freda says being valued and listened to, and with respect shown for Freda's way of life and sense of identity.

Analysing the Information

The collected information is sifted, organised and analysed to produce an assessment. This process is often done with the aid of a form that has headings for the workers to use. For example, adult services workers use a single assessment form to help them build up a holistic picture. The workers and Freda organise and analyse the information. For example, they list the things that could be changed in the home environment.

Identifying the Options

The workers and Freda identify the options available and come up with two plans. The first involves returning home, with a few changes to the physical layout of her home environment, the installation of an emergency alarm and the inclusion of balance exercises in her daily routine. Freda rejected many of the changes to her home suggested by the workers and the use of various walking and transfer aids. Being aware of the research carried out for Help the Aged (undated), the workers were not too concerned about this as they didn't want to push these matters, knowing that to do so ran the danger of undermining Freda's confidence and self-esteem, two factors that were very important in preventing falls and her continuing to live a happy life. The other option was to move to a supported housing scheme where all the aspects of the first option were already in place along with some additional benefits.

Coming to a Conclusion

The workers and Freda compared the pros and cons of each option and assessed how likely each were to achieve Freda's aim of remaining in control of her life. After looking at the two options in this way, the workers and Freda came to the conclusion as to which was the best option. In fact, they did not agree. The workers felt that the supported housing was the best option. Freda could see that sheltered housing would be a safer place for her but was prepared to accept a higher level of risk in order to stay in her own home. The workers are clear that it is Freda's decision to take, that she is fully informed and start to think about how to formulate and implement a discharge plan for her return home.

Activity 51.4

Note down some points about how Freda and the workers can implement the decision in a way that achieves Freda's aim of retaining control over her own life.

What Happens after a Decision is Made

The detail of Freda's discharge will need to be carefully planned if she is to achieve her aim of retaining control over her own life. Three aspects of what should happen after the decision has been made are:

- organising the implementation
- monitoring progress
- achieving a good outcome.

Organising the Implementation

Freda's return home takes a bit of organising. For example, her house hasn't been lived in for some time and there are practical preparatory tasks to complete before she can happily live there. Freda will still need to take things easy at first and is happy for these practical tasks to be completed prior to her return home.

Monitoring Progress

Freda and the workers plan how her return home will be monitored during the first weeks in relation to how things go and how well she settles down again. Freda agrees to a number of visits to see if changes and adjustments are needed. For example, having returned home, Freda changes her mind and accepts some of the changes to the layout of her home that she previously rejected.

Part VII

Achieving a Good Outcome

In situations like Freda's, it is difficult to know at what point in time it is possible to say that the decision has had an outcome. Three months after her discharge, Freda is living independently in her own home and has not experienced another fall. At this point in time, both the workers and Freda believe that the discharge planning decisions have had a good outcome. If, however, Freda has a serious fall tomorrow that results in her losing her confidence and ending up in residential care, the workers may feel that their work has in fact had a bad outcome. Nevertheless, Freda may continue to value the three months she has spent in her own home without, as she sees it, interference (see Chapter 13).

Conclusion

This chapter has explained that good decisions have two elements – they are well made and have good outcomes. Criteria for making a good decision were presented and applied to an actual situation. We found that it is not always straightforward to judge whether a decision is a good one or not. The chapter went on to illustrate a process of making and implementing a good decision so there was the best chance of achieving a good outcome. The chapter has stressed the importance of successfully engaging and involving service users in decision-making, decisions being made on an informed basis and workers effectively working together.

REVIEW QUESTIONS

Think about a decision that you or your family made in the past and answer the questions below. For the first question, think of service users as the person or persons whose life will be most affected and stakeholders as those who have an interest, but the decision will not impinge upon them directly.

1   Which of the good decision criteria were met?

2   How far was anything like the process of decision-making explained in this chapter followed?

3   What was done during the decision's implementation, if anything, to increase the chances of a good outcome?

FURTHER READING

Adair, J. (1999) *Decision Making and Problem Solving*, London, Institute of Personnel and Development
Chapter 2 is a readable and useful introduction to 'the art of effective decision making'.

O'Sullivan, T. (1999) *Decision Making in Social Work*, Basingstoke, Macmillan – now Palgrave Macmillan
Fully explains the subject matter of this chapter. For example, Chapter 3 explains in a clear and accessible way what is involved in engaging service users in decision-making.

Thompson, N. (2002) *People Skills* (2nd edn) Basingstoke, Palgrave Macmillan
Chapter 21 gives a good basic introduction to making decisions when working with people.

Illustrating Practice in Different Settings

Part VIII
Illustrating Practice in Different Settings

Introduction

We have taken a considerable journey in this book to reach this point. In Part VIII we can afford to test out some of what we have gained in previous parts. In the light of the Health and Social Care (Community Health and Standards) Act 2003, the government set out the standards for planning, commissioning and delivering local services (DoH, 2004g) through local authorities and NHS organisations:

- focusing on health and wellbeing across the entire health and social care system
- empowering patients, service users and the public to choose and improve their health and self-care
- improving the quality and equality of services
- tackling the needs of children as well as adults
- reviewing and changing working practices to improve service delivery.

Four-fifths of the health budget is spent by PCTs, working in partnership with adult care and children's services, the quality of their work being based on National Service Frameworks (NSFs) and the work of the National Institute for Clinical Excellence (NICE) and the Social Care Institute for Excellence (SCIE). The 2003 Act prescribed outcomes against which the work should be judged in the following seven domains: safety, clinical and cost-effectiveness, governance, patient focus, accessible and responsive care, care environment and amenities and public health. Against this context, we spend the next two chapters dealing in some detail with practice examples from community care, one from health and social care work with children and the other with adults. Chapter 54, with its accompanying Resource File, tackles theories and practices in day and residential services, which arguably are two of those areas most in need of improvement under the government's modernisation agenda.

FURTHER READING	RESOURCE FILE: Writing a Case Study/Integrative Study, at the end of Chapter 37

Health and Social Care 52
Work with Children

JACQUIE HORNER

Learning outcomes

By the end of this chapter, you should be able to:

■ CONSIDER the issues arising in health and social care work with children and young people

■ WORK through the stages of practice

■ TAKE INTO ACCOUNT the tensions and dilemmas of practice.

This chapter examines some of the similarities and differences between health and social care. It uses illustrations to show how issues arise in different settings for health and social care practice with children and young people. Healthcare uses all the personal features required to help a patient remain as independent as possible and enables them to use the choices they are offered to improve their health status and individual requirements. Social care, on the other hand, is care that enhances a patient's health and wellbeing in order that they remain independent and can include such things as meal provision, daycare facilities to enhance their social activity and interaction with other like-minded people.

Working Together in Diverse Settings Delivering Health and Social Care

Patients, carers and service users may receive health and social care in a number of settings and from a variety of professionals, non-professionals and voluntary organisations. This involves joint working arrangements between different agencies and practitioners, who come from different professional backgrounds where they are trained to focus very differently on how they apply their knowledge and skills. Depending on the kinds of problems faced by patients, service users and carers, the task of coordinating this health and social care may become extremely complex. Health and social care can be delivered, in theory, almost anywhere. Care may take place in the person's home, doctor's surgery, hospital, the workplace, day centre, school, residential home, mental hospital or penal custody. Many experienced nurses may suggest that they offer advice in a variety of places, such as the local supermarket, library or post office, but they always ensure that the individual follows up that advice in an appropriate designated place such as the doctor's surgery or hospital clinic. In order that people receive the appropriate care, they will be referred to the practitioner who can best help that situation.

A wide range of health and social care services may be required in a particular situation. In this chapter, we focus on services for children.

Activity 52.1

Think about an instance where a child has required health or social care. Identify the practitioners who provided that care and describe what they did and what that care consisted of. Spend a few minutes considering whether that care was or was not beneficial.

Now make some brief notes on whether or not you feel that care promoted the child's independence.

Keep your notes by you and add to them as you read through this chapter.

The range of professionals who deliver health and social care includes health visitors, domiciliary care workers, nurses, care assistants, doctors, healthcare assistants, physiotherapists, occupational therapists, radiographers, midwives, social workers and volunteers.

Practice Issues in Health and Social Care: Children

The following example enables us to explore practice issues, including the tensions that can arise in complex cases, where there is no simple, single solution to problems.

Practice study

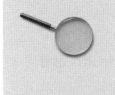

Susan

Susan, a young girl who says she is 15, calls at the office and asks for a confidential chat with somebody. She has spoken to the school nurse, with whom she has developed a trusting relationship over recent months.

She lives at home with her mother who is a lone parent. Susan reveals that she has had a sexual relationship with an older man. In the more relaxed setting of the interview, Susan admits that this relationship began when she was 12 and now she is only 14 and is scared of having become pregnant. She mentions that she fears she may

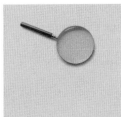

have contracted a sexually transmitted disease. She claims that she has not seen the man recently and is entering a relationship with a boy she has met aged 15. She wants the worker to make her an appointment to see a doctor other than her own, before the relationship with the boy becomes sexual, so that her mother, a devout Roman Catholic, will not find out about her situation. She says that if she becomes pregnant, she really wants to have the baby. Susan says that her mother and her mother's family would never speak to her again if she had an abortion.

There are four main areas of concern for professionals:

- Susan's comment that she may be pregnant. There are mixed messages here from Susan. Her relationship may already be sexual, hence her fears about pregnancy and disease. Suspecting or finding out that you are pregnant can create a number of emotions regardless of what age you are. Susan may be finding it difficult to come to terms with her possible pregnancy and may not be aware of the need for prompt healthcare and advice at this stage.
- Susan's fear that she may have a sexually transmitted disease.
- The possibility that if the relationship was with an older man, it has involved a sexual offence and child protection will be a concern (see Resource File: Suspicion or Disclosure of Child Abuse, at the end of Chapter 49).
- The need for Susan to receive counselling as to the choice between an abortion or having the baby, in the event that she may be pregnant.

It would be desirable for Susan to have a pregnancy test. There are a number of tensions for the workers dealing with Susan's situation:

- *Susan's request for a confidential discussion and the need to intervene where a sexual offence has been committed against a young person under the age of consent, currently 16 years:* Professionals have a duty to report an offence and deal with a child protection matter according to agency child protection procedures. There is a need for the doctor to respect Susan's privacy but there is a duty to deal openly between professionals with the child protection issue. The child protection team would investigate.
- *Judging the man as having committed a sexual offence, while not judging Susan for a relationship she may regard as normal and consensual:* Under Section 5 of the Sexual Offences Act 2003, which repealed the Sexual Offences Act 1956, even if a child of 12 or under consents to sex, this is still treated by the law as rape.
- *Susan's wishes and the parent's responsibility:* The professionals may decide it is in Susan's best interest not to inform her mother, whose religious beliefs absolutely forbid sexual relationships before marriage (Article 2.2 of the UN Convention on the Rights of the Child).
- *The rights of Susan and the rights of the parents:* Under the Children Act 1989, parents and statutory agencies should work in partnership together. However, Susan can take advice from healthcare staff, including the doctor and nurse at

the medical centre, and continue to have a sexual relationship with the boy aged 15, which is not defined as a sexual offence, because there is no age difference between the two people concerned.

■ *The rights of Susan and her unborn baby:* There is a tension between Susan's rights and the right to life of her unborn baby.

Next Actions

The framework for assessment (DoH, 2000a) enables the worker to find out in more detail about Susan's circumstances. It provides a structure for gathering information about three aspects:

■ Susan's developmental needs
■ her mother's capacity to parent her
■ wider environmental issues, including potential religious and cultural issues, such as her mother's views about children and young people entering relationships, as well as potential support provided by the family.

The worker needs to explain about confidentiality, about which information needs to be shared and which can and cannot be shared with others.

The worker needs to decide what to do about the sexual relationship with the older man. Is it over or does it present a current risk to Susan's safety? If the worker does not believe the relationship is over, he or she has a statutory obligation to contact the police.

The worker needs to judge whether Susan has the capacity to make informed choices, for example about consenting to a medical examination and applying for an abortion. If Susan is assessed as able to do this, she will be judged as *Gillick competent.* In 1985, the Gillick case established that the capacity of a child under 16 years of age to be given advice about contraceptives without the consent of parents should depend on the child possessing the intelligence and understanding rather than being determined by an age limit laid down by law.

Supposing Susan is judged to be Gillick competent, the worker can refer her for a paediatric assessment. The purpose would be to find out whether she had been sexually active, whether there was any sexually transmitted disease and whether she was pregnant. Assuming Susan is Gillick competent, the aim should be to treat her as having rights, able to make decisions, ensuring that she is made aware of the consequences of her choices and decisions and is given information so that her actions are properly informed.

If there was positive evidence corroborating Susan's statement that she had been sexually active with the older man, the worker would need to pass this information on to the police.

The Data Protection Act 1998 protects confidentiality and the rights of the person. If Susan's mother asks, the worker can explain that under this Act she cannot share with her any information about Susan's relationship.

Throughout the process, the worker would need to be aware of his or her own beliefs and values, so that these did not affect the decisions made to the detriment of the best interests of Susan.

Summary of tensions:

- Health and social care workers may have to decide between supporting the paramountcy of Susan's welfare under the Children Act 1989, including supporting the right of Susan to receive confidential advice and, if she agrees, medical treatment for her condition, on the one hand, and respecting her mother's right to be informed of what is happening to her underage daughter on the other hand.
- The Human Rights Act 1998 gives Susan the right to freedom and security of person. The worker may state to her mother that Susan's relationship with the young man gives her that sense of security and freedom as a person. Susan has the right to have relationships with people, but she must be protected against child abuse.
- There is a tension between Susan's right to confidentiality regarding the identity of the older man with whom she had the sexual relationship, and her right and that of other children and young people to be safeguarded from harm.
- There is a tension between Susan's right to be empowered and the risk of a paternalistic approach by a worker. The worker should strive to achieve anti-discriminatory and anti-racist practice at the same time as carrying out his or her accountability to agency practice, including health, social services and police.
- There is a tension between Susan's immaturity in years and her own view that she is quite capable of making her own judgements and avoiding being drawn into a continuing, abusive relationship with the older man.
- Susan may decide not to pursue taking advice from the agencies, because she fears they will treat her as a child protection case and information may reach her mother.
- There is the uncertainty about whether Susan's interests would be better met by having the baby or having an abortion.

Practice study

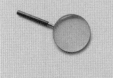

Susan (cont'd)

Susan has been persuaded to have a full examination. She does have a sexually transmitted disease (STD). The workers arrange treatment of Susan's sexually transmitted disease and this is successful. Meanwhile, Susan receives counselling from the nurse and other staff and decides to have the baby.

GPs and Midwives

Once the pregnancy is confirmed either by a home test or through the GP, Susan will be cared for by the antenatal service of her local hospital, supported by her GP and the midwife assigned to that GP's practice. Regular antenatal visits will commence and routine observations will be performed such as blood tests, urine tests and blood pressure checks. Regular monitoring of both Susan's and the baby's wellbeing will take place to ensure that any problems and complications are avoided. This type of healthcare is essential from an early stage in the pregnancy; it will also ensure that Susan receives the help and support she may need to help her to come to terms with the pregnancy and some of the emotions that she may be trying to deal with, such as how she tells her family, what will happen with her education and how she will deal with the baby once it is here.

Midwives play an important role in caring for pregnant women, their partners and subsequent families. Susan's GP will also play a key role in her maternity care. GPs are the first port of call for many patients. Approximately 20,000 GPs perform one million consultations per day. Children and young adults become familiar with their GP and this helps them to develop a trusting relationship with them. Visits by Susan to her GP will have commenced when she was a newborn baby and she may know her GP very well. GPs need to be aware of all the care options available to patients so that they use NHS resources appropriately and ensure that patients, regardless of their age, receive the correct care and treatment for their problem.

Many teenagers consider the doctors' surgery the place to go if you are ill or injured, which is obviously a good assumption. Rarely do they think of it as the place to go for advice on alcohol abuse, smoking and matters of a sexual nature. Recent research (Gleeson, 2003) has found that teenagers feel that the doctors' surgery is not an appropriate place to seek such advice because they fear a lack of confidentiality, worring that receptionists may reveal information to friends or relatives, or if they are accompanied by a parent that they may be able to view information of a confidential nature on the computer screen. Further concerns highlighted by the research are teenagers fearing that they are being judged by older people who may disapprove of sexual activity in young people, that the consultation is not long enough to receive the information they want and that they may not be able to attend appointments outside school hours.

Activity 52.2

1. Make brief notes of reasons why young people may not seek advice if they are having difficulties dealing with their health.
2. Take a few minutes to write down your thoughts about the people you may encounter within your local doctors' surgery.
3. Include some suggestions for why a teenager may not want to seek advice there.

School Nurses

GPs work closely with other healthcare professionals including school nurses and health visitors. Let us see how they work.

School nurses work closely with local education authorities, schools, teachers and parents to ensure that pupils are cared for appropriately and are offered health education and initiatives that promote and maintain their health and wellbeing. As part of a number of government strategies, school nurses became involved in many aspects of children's health within the school environment. You may remember what the school nurse did for you while you were at school – giving injections and checking for head lice and scabies. Although these preventive activities are important, the role of the school nurse has expanded to meet the legislative requirements of safeguarding and promoting the health of children and young people.

Activity 52.3

Adolescence (11–15-year-olds) is recognised as a time of risk-taking behaviour, but it is also a time for laying down the foundations of good health.

What do you think risk-taking behaviour is? How do you think the school nurse can help to reduce adolescent risk-taking behaviour?

Improving personal health and relationship education within primary schools and increasing young people's trust in the confidentiality of health advice are both important factors that the government hopes will halve the rate of teenage pregnancies. The government set up an Independent Advisory Group on Teenage Pregnancy in 2000 and responded to the first annual report of this group with these policy targets to reduce teenage pregnancies endorsed by many government departments (DoH, 2002e). Although some of this policy guidance may be a little late for Susan, she may develop a relationship with her school nurse that will help her to deal with the psychological and emotional problems she may be experiencing while coming to terms with being pregnant. School nurses play a key role providing this care requirement of developing trusting relationships with children and young adults. They work closely with teachers by assisting with the presentation of lessons on personal, social and health education within the school environment and they also remain available to offer advice to parents and teachers.

Further health promotion issues that school nurses are involved in include healthy eating advice, drug education, relationship advice and maintaining healthy lifestyles by tackling issues such as obesity, bullying, skin cancer awareness and the reduction of alcohol, drug and nicotine abuse. Working within schools and alongside the education service, school nurses can develop pupils' confidence in the NHS and offer advice on how to access other health services should the need arise, remembering at all times that the relationship they provide for individual pupils is of a confidential nature.

The contact that children and young people have with their school nurses will hopefully alleviate some of the difficulties identified earlier and help them to seek appropriate help as soon as possible. School nurses can help children and young people living in the local community to make healthy lifestyle choices, which will hopefully lead to the reduction of risk-taking behaviours such as drug, alcohol and nicotine abuse and teenage pregnancy.

Part VIII

Health Visitor

After the birth of Susan's baby and when the midwives have finished providing the care Susan needs, then the care of mother and baby will be provided by the health visitor. Of course, parents also have a huge span of parental responsibilities, including providing health and social care for their children from birth until they are 18.

Activity 52.4

What different health and social care support services do you think the health visitor will be able to provide for Susan and her new baby?

The role of the health visitor has changed significantly over the past few years. The majority of health visitors are attached to doctors' surgeries and provide health and social care to all family members, although the majority of their attention tradition-ally has been paid to children under five.

Health visitors have numerous partnerships with various organisations to assist families with their health and social care requirements. They are expected to work closely with social services in matters of child protection, housing and financial benefits for deprived families, and also with social services and local education authorities in the provision of Sure Start. It is essential that all these groups of people work closely together to ensure the health and social wellbeing of such a vulnerable group of people who cannot voice an opinion of their own due to their age.

The government has expressed numerous concerns about the health and social wellbeing of children, reflected in the major publication of *Every Child Matters* (HM Treasury, 2003). To try and tackle children's health and social problems, the govern-ment issued an NSF for children (DfES and DoH, 2004), which explored issues such as children's rights to appropriate healthcare delivered in the correct place by quali-fied people, appropriate services for children with mental health or learning disabili-ties and assisting parents who may require parenting support to bring up their children in a healthy and safe way. The government also decided to tackle poverty in an attempt to deal with the health and social wellbeing of children and young people.

Activity 52.5

Poverty creates a number of difficulties which affect a person's need for a range of health and social care services.

Write down what effects being poor would have on the health of a child.

The government thinks that children living in poverty are less likely to do well at school, they get into trouble with the police from a young age, are less likely to gain employment when they leave school and, as you have identified, suffer more health-related problems. In an attempt to reduce some of these things happening, the government introduced Sure Start, which was targeted at the under-four age group and aims to improve health, improve the children's ability to learn, improve social development and strengthen families. Poverty may be a key factor in why some people are unable to access the correct service to meet their needs. By introducing Sure Start, the government hopes that families will be able to gain access to all care providers to reduce poverty and maintain good health, have opportunities to develop their children's education and so lead to better prospects for them in later life.

Conclusion

Within this chapter, we have explored a number of issues that may arise from birth through to adolescence. You have briefly explored the roles of the people involved in working with children and young people, and you should have collected information from the activities that you will find useful in working through the next chapter.

REVIEW QUESTIONS

1   What are the three components of the framework for assessment of children and families?

2   What tensions are created for Susan and her mother by the Human Rights Act 1998?

3   Which health and social care professionals are likely to be working with Susan?

FURTHER READING

Bagnall, P. (1997) 'Children's Health: Taking it Seriously', *British Journal of Community Nursing*, 2(2): 68

DfES and DoH (2004) *The National Service Framework for Children, Young People and Maternity Services*, London, DoH

Logan, S. and Spencer, N. (2000) 'Inequality and Children's Health', *Child: Care, Health and Development*, **26**: 1–3

While, A. (2003) 'Child Health Services for the Future', *British Journal of Community Nursing*, 8(7): 336

WEBSITE: www.teenagepregnancyunit.gov.uk

Resource file

Dealing with a complaint

People who wish to make a complaint do not always state this openly from the start. They may be

- fearful of the reaction of people who know them
- worried about whether they can complain safely in confidence
- scared of being excluded from services

- nervous of a punitive response from somebody in authority.

There are commonly five levels or stages of seriousness of complaint:

- *Level 1: Informal resolution*
  At the first level, the person may talk to the pract-

itioners who deliver the service. They may be able to resolve the matter so that the person complaining no longer feels dissatisfied with the service.

■ *Level 2: Formal complaint*

If unhappy with the informal response, the person can ask for the complaint to be referred to the appropriate manager, who attempts to resolve it.

■ *Level 3: Second stage resolution*

If still dissatisfied, the person can ask for the complaint to be referred to the head of the Customer Service Centre, who should reply in writing, either to respond to the complaint or indicate why not and set a new deadline.

■ *Level 4: Independent adjudication*

If still dissatisfied, the person can have the complaint referred to an independent person with relevant knowledge and expertise outside the department, who will review how it has been handled.

■ *Level 5*

If still dissatisfied, the person can ask for the independent parliamentary commissioner for administration (the ombudsman) to investigate the complaint.

FURTHER READING

NHS Statutory Instrument 2006 No. 2084, The National Health Service (Complaints) Amendment Regulations 2006, www.opsi.gov.uk/si/si2006/20062084.htm

Social Care, England, Statutory Instrument 2006 No. 1681, The Local Authority Social Services Complaints (England) Regulations 2006, www.opsi.gov.uk/si/si2006/20061681.htm

Health and Social Care Work with Adults

JACQUIE HORNER and ALISON MULVIHILL

Learning outcomes

By the end of this chapter, you should be able to:

■ CONSIDER issues arising in health and social care work with adults

■ WORK through the stages of practice

■ TAKE INTO ACCOUNT tensions and dilemmas of practice

■ KNOW how to act in response to a complaint or need to protect a vulnerable adult.

This chapter examines how health and social care services are provided for service users over the age of 18 until they die. In order that you can explore such care, this chapter will present you with activities centred upon the care of three different people from different age groups.

Practice study

Hamid

Hamid is 22 years old and was seriously injured when he was knocked off his motorbike. He lives at home with his parents and was about to start a new job the day after his accident as a healthcare assistant at the local hospital where he is now a patient. He has been in hospital for a number of weeks with numerous serious fractures of his pelvis, legs and right arm; he also suffered a head injury that has left him a little short-tempered and forgetful. The ward staff have told his parents that Hamid will be ready for discharge soon, but he will need quite a few things doing for him when he first comes out of hospital until he is fully recovered. Hopefully he will be able to return to work once his rehabilitation is complete, but until then he is going to need help physically, emotionally and financially.

Numerous difficulties could arise as a result of this accident. Hamid has needed the services of doctors, nurses and other health and social care professionals while he has been in hospital and that care will need to continue, to ensure he makes a full recovery.

Activity 53.1

Refer back to the list you completed in Chapter 52 and respond to the following questions.

1. Write down who you think will have helped Hamid to date and who will be able to help him to fully recover.
2. What kind of physical, emotional and financial help do you think Hamid will need?
3. How do you think Hamid might feel having his parents looking after him at his age?

These three questions are important in understanding what it feels like to be cared for by somebody and what is involved in caring for another person. Care by parents reduces as a person reaches maturity and becomes increasingly independent, and at a certain age the person may even reject the care as too claustrophobic. You have now had the opportunity to explore some of these issues within this activity. Well-managed team care helps patients and their families to cope in situations like Hamid's on their way to full recovery and rehabilitation.

Practice study

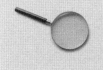

Leroy

Leroy is a 42-year-old lorry driver, married with four children aged between 19 and 8. Leroy smokes 20 cigarettes a day and he usually eats his meals while on the road in motorway cafes. He is overweight but he always seems to be hungry and tends to eat foods that fill him up. Leroy's partner has lost her job and he has been working overtime to make up for the loss of earnings. This is making him very tired and the only way he can unwind is to go to the pub with his friends for a few beers a couple of nights a week.

Leroy is having headaches, which a friend has told him is a sign of high blood pressure. Today, as Leroy returns from work feeling unwell with one of his headaches, he decides to go to the pub. On the way there he starts to feel sick, his right hand goes numb, he is finding it difficult to breath and has a pain in his chest as though somebody is tying a rope around him.

Activity 53.2

1. Why do you think Leroy is feeling unwell?
2. What kinds of daily problems may be making him feel unwell?

This incident is not uncommon; many people feel stressed by numerous things happening in their lives that will eventually affect their health. Leroy's situation may suggest that he is having a heart attack brought on by a number of key factors: having a stressful job; working long hours; a poor diet leading to obesity; and risk-taking behaviours that are life threatening such as smoking. These can all lead to changes in health and ultimately a heart attack. Heart disease is a significant killer in this country and the government has introduced numerous strategies to reduce the number of deaths associated with coronary heart disease within the NSF for coronary heart disease (DoH 2000c).

Leroy will require immediate medical assistance to deal with this life-threatening situation and needs emergency admission to hospital through the A&E department.

Activity 53.3

Revisit your list of practitioners from Chapter 52 and respond to the following questions.

1. Who will be the main practitioners as Leroy is admitted to hospital?
2. What are Leroy's major problems identified in the account?
3. What services should Leroy receive?

When Leroy is admitted to hospital, the health and social care professionals working with him will need to assess his situation immediately so that treatment can commence as soon as possible. Diagnosis of his problems will be carried out using various tests so that staff caring for him can stabilise him and prevent another attack from happening. This will be done by a careful assessment that takes into account all of Leroy's story of what has happened, when and where it happened and the events leading up to the suspected heart attack occurring. All this information will be documented accurately to ensure that Leroy receives appropriate treatment and care from practitioners.

Activity 53.4

1. What type of lifestyle advice do you think Leroy will need and why?
2. Write down what you think health promotion/health education is.
3. Who do you think will provide this information? Give reasons for your answer.

As a result of a good assessment at the outset, Leroy should recover quickly because the appropriate people have been involved in his care. Leroy will need lifestyle advice as a result of this attack, referred to as health promotion or health education.

Health promotion (see Chapter 38) is an important part of all our lives. It is provided by everybody who comes into contact with a patient, regardless of what their health problem may be, what kind of care they need and who gives them that care. As you have seen from the previous chapter, health promotion starts at a very young age, by helping children to adapt to healthy lifestyles to reduce risk-taking behaviour, and continues until a person dies. Health promotion and education are provided to service users regardless of where they need their care, be it home, hospital, school, nursing and residential homes, or wherever they seek the advice. However, not everybody accesses health promotion/health education. Ethnicity, fear of service providers, financial expectations, fear of illness and subsequent consequences are all key factors that influence people's ability to access appropriate health and social care. Lifestyle advice and help through health promotion may involve an occupational therapist or life coach. Life coaches help people build their capacity to develop and achieve their goals in life (Nelson-Jones, 2007).

Our third example from practice is more complex and includes responding to questions about the quality of practice.

Practice study

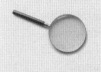

Mary and Rose

Mary is a widow aged 72 years who lives in her own home, which she owns outright. She also owns a shop and lives off the income from this. She invited her unemployed, penniless, only daughter Rose, aged 39, to live with her several years ago. Mary has had several strokes, which her daughter has coped with, but the latest was more serious, led to hospital admission and has left her with some loss of mobility on the right-hand side of her body. As a result of this she can only walk short distances but she has recovered to a certain extent. At the end of her hospital treatment, a meeting between medical and nursing staff, the hospital discharge coordinator, the care manager from adult services and Mary and Rose decides that Mary should be referred for intermediate care. Intermediate care is a short period of intensive care, treatment or rehabilitation at home or in another setting, so as to reduce, delay or prevent the need for a long-term stay in hospital.

There are two main issues which need tackling. First, before Mary can be discharged, the intermediate care assessment team will need to meet with her and her family to assess her needs and how best they can be met in her own environment. This case conference ensures that everybody involved in Mary's care knows what is to be provided for her, who will provide it and when it is likely to take place. It provides essential coordination of care to ensure that Mary's health and wellbeing are maintained in a safe and stable manner. Mary is admitted to Hopeland Court, a community-based short-term residential home, where she will have occupational therapy, speech therapy and physiotherapy services. This service is provided for her free for six weeks and her access to it is based on the Fair Access to Care eligibility framework (DoH, 2003a). The team at Hopeland Court work with Mary to help her to regain her strength and independence. They note that Mary is becoming confused, shows anger and increasingly criticises the services she receives.

Practice study

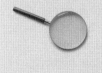

Mary and Rose (cont'd)

Mary is due to leave Hopeland Court and go home in a few days and keeps asking about the arrangements. At the last minute, Rose tells the worker she is unwilling to have her mother home, because she is selfish, bossy and tries to control her daughter's life and relationships. Rose says she has met a man whom her mother makes unwelcome in the house, but she wants this chance to have her own life. This complication raises several issues and tensions.

There is a tension between meeting Mary's needs and Rose's needs. Mary has needs as a patient and as a person likely to use social care services. Mary's needs are reviewed by the intermediate care team, the care manager and the domiciliary care team. Rose has needs as a carer. There is a need to ensure that Mary remains at Hopeland Court while her needs are reassessed. The plan for Mary to return home and live independently needs to take account of her apparently increasing confusion and her daughter Rose's attitude. This also involves assessing the extent of Mary's impairment following the latest stroke and, if she is to return home, finding a way to promote her independence as far as possible, while simultaneously safeguarding her against risks, such as accidents in the kitchen. Mary has a growing problem of incontinence, mainly at night, so this will need management too.

There is a need to meet Rose and discover her wishes, expectations and needs. In effect, this means carrying out a carer's assessment. It may be advantageous to ensure that one worker in the home support team works with Rose and another with Mary.

In one sense, Mary offered Rose a home and security, so perhaps her expectation was that Rose would care for her in return. Rose, however, has begun to see opportunities to have a life beyond caring for Mary.

There are other tensions, between:

- the role of the worker to work in partnership but also to enforce and carry out legislation – in other words between empowering the person and intervening
- working in a team of professionals at the same time as advocating on behalf of Mary
- acting so as to preserve Mary's independence, dignity and self-esteem, while protecting her from harm
- being accountable to the service user/carer and also to the agency, colleagues and professional values
- pressure to save time and find short cuts to completing arrangements and informing senior manager and hospital of difficulties following Rose's statement of views, and asking for more time to identify, agree with everybody and carry out alternative arrangements.

Practice study

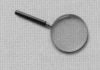

Mary and Rose (cont'd)

On the day Mary leaves Hopeland Court to go home, as she is about to get into the taxi, Mary thanks the care assistant and whispers to her about the incidents involving staff dealing with her at Hopeland Court. The care assistant sits with Mary in the back of the taxi and listens to her experiences. These incidents run against the view that Mary's rights should be preserved and her independence promoted, while protecting her from harm. The practitioner asks questions and becomes aware from Mary's response that she is confused and seems to be slipping back into events that occurred when her daughter was a child. The worker has a responsibility to challenge established ways of working that are oppressive, discriminatory or abusive. Mary goes on to criticise the latest prescription from the doctor, saying she hasn't felt right since she

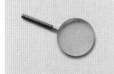

was on the new medication. The worker is aware of guidelines governing problems linked with questionable or poor clinical performance in the NHS (DoH, 2001e). The worker has a duty to inform the employer of adverse or unsatisfactory practice. The worker discusses this with Mary to see whether she wishes to make a complaint either about the incidents or her medication and outlines the procedure (see Resource File: Dealing with a Complaint, at the end of Chapter 52). After considering, Mary decides she does not want to pursue a complaint. The practitioner decides that in view of Mary's mood changes and confusion, she will discuss with other members of the team the possibility of referring Mary to the specialist who deals with Alzheimer's. The practitioner is aware of the need to balance Mary's perception of a grievance against her growing confusion and to ensure that her comments are not dismissed, just because her mental state is deteriorating. The practitioner considers that she may need continuing care in future. Continuing care is the routine use of healthcare resources where the nature, complexity and unpredictability of a person's needs require regular supervision by a member of the NHS team.

Practice Issues: Points Arising from the Three Cases

It is important to remember that service users need to be in control of their requirements and need to be asked what they want and how it can be achieved. They have rights to privacy, protection from harm, respect from others, freedom from inhuman and degrading treatment, dignity and independence under the Human Rights Act 1998. In Hamid and Leroy's cases, you may feel that the care they received was a key factor in helping them on the road to full recovery. However, the success of this care was dependent upon everybody involved doing what they had to correctly and taking the patients' needs into consideration at all times. In Leroy's case, it would not be a realistic idea to expect him to stop smoking if we were not going to give him help and support to do so. Hamid and Mary had similar requirements, they both needed personal things doing for them to assist in the recovery process, but they both needed to be involved in those decisions. Hopefully, because Hamid is younger and healing is possible, he will eventually recover fully. Unfortunately for Mary, her recuperation will be slow and she will never fully recover; as she ages things may become more difficult for her to achieve and her family may find it hard to support the changes as they happen. Any future intermediate or residential care Mary receives will need to safeguard her rights and should be an extension of the care Mary received at home. Again, the government has introduced strategies to assist service users, families and carers to deal with issues associated with ageing and deterioration in health and social care through the NSF for older people (DoH, 2001a). Clearly, we have only touched the surface of the case of Mary and Rose. There are complex issues for decision-making and coordinating health and social care practice.

Unfortunately not all care packages go to plan, difficulties may arise and a service user's requirements may increase as their health and social care needs change. Some families cannot cope with the demands that caring for a person can bring, regardless of the health and social care support they receive. In some cases, the service user may become vulnerable and subject to physical, psychological and emotional abuse. Finally, we need to add that the health and social care worker is responsible for the quality of the work and for improving his or her knowledge and skills.

Conclusion

This chapter has explored the care of three people over the age span and with different health and social care needs. Completion of the activities will also have helped you to think about the care that different people may need and how this will be achieved.

REVIEW QUESTIONS

1 What particular tensions arise in agreeing and implementing a care plan?

2 What kinds of shortcomings in service do you need to watch out for, in health and social care?

3 What action do you take where a person wishes to make a complaint?

FURTHER READING

Braye, S. and Preston-Shoot, M. (1999) *Empowering Practice in Social Care*, Buckingham, Open University Press

Brechin, A., Brown, H. and Eby, M.A. (eds) (2000) *Critical Practice in Health and Social Care*, London, Sage

DoH (2000) *Good Practice for Continence Services*, London, DoH

DoH (2000) *Care Homes for Older People: National Minimum Standards*, London, TSO

DoH (2001) *National Service Framework for Older People*, London, DoH

Hugman, R. (2005) *New Approaches in Ethics for the Caring Professions*, Basingstoke, Palgrave Macmillan

Nelson-Jones, R. (2007) *Life Coaching Skills: How to Develop Skilled Clients*, London, Sage

Roe, B. and Beech, R. (2005) *Intermediate and Continuing Care: Policy and Practice*, Oxford, Blackwell

Tetlow, R. (2006) *Continuing Care Retirement Communities: A Guide to Planning*, York, Joseph Rowntree Foundation

54 Residential and Daycare Practice

ROBERT ADAMS

In conjunction with this chapter, read Chapter 3 on the development of health and social care services, Chapter 37 on Goffman and the Resource File: Theories and Models of Residential Care at the end of this chapter.

Day and Residential Services: Neglected and Inadequate?

This chapter deals with an aspect of health and social care that is simultaneously personal and private – our domestic life – and the very public spaces of daycare services and residential care. Our discussion needs to be in the context of restrictions on services that limit people's choice and consequently their chances of continuing to live independently. The authoritative Wanless Report (2004) on the future of care services for older people provides detailed arguments and evidence. We focus here, however, on the quality of care itself. When we think of residential homes, what image do we conjure up? Is it an idealised picture of family life, transported to a room where the relatives sit around a dining table and chat in a beautiful mansion in a countrified setting? Or is it a rather busy, impersonal corridor between a stretch of dormitories and double rooms with their identical outer doors all open to allow access to the cleaners on one side, and on the other side a large lounge with forty chairs pushed back round its perimeter and the television blaring at one end, while forty residents sit like statues in their seats waiting for the bell to ring for the next tea break or meal?

To put the question another way, what kind of residential care would you want for yourself – a home where you had choices about where to sit and relax through the day and night, privacy to entertain in your own room decorated to your choice and crammed with your own ornaments, furniture, photographs and books, and the freedom to eat and brew a drink when you choose? Or would you be content to share a double room with a bed, locker and small pin board on the wall for a few postcards and a regime based around the needs of staff rather than the wishes of residents? These questions are loaded and the contrasting examples are extreme caricatures, but their ingredients are based on actual cases. We need to recognise that numerous research, inspections and inquiry reports over the past half century have drawn attention to glaring defects in residential care.

Daycare has tended to be neglected, by researchers, members of the public and, until latterly, agencies. It is still clear that access to daycare depends on where you live rather than on your needs and wishes (Tinker, 1999, p. 41). Day services for older people tend not to cater for people from ethnic minorities (Tester, 1996, p. 144). Day services tend to cater for people excluded from participation in wider society and do little or nothing to lessen that exclusion (Walker, 1997). An official review of the scope and future of daycare services in Scotland, for example, concludes that they need to become more flexible, in order to meet people's needs by becoming more inclusive, that is, by including people more in the community (Scottish Executive, 2000, p. 2).

Changing Context of Residential and Day Services

Fortunately, residential and day services are changing. Residential childcare (Levy and Kahan, 1991; Kirkwood, 1993; Waterhouse, 2000; Corby et al., 2001) has been shaken by successive inquiry reports into scandals and shortcomings. Training for staff has been recognised as crucial and moves are afoot for the sector skills body Skills for Care (skillsforcare.org.uk) to extend its existing registration of social workers to include all social care workers with adults and children. Under the Children Act 1989, a child should only be moved to a children's home as a last resort and, unfortunately, the history of residential establishments tends to live down to their image as institutions rather than living up to the ideal of providing, as their title suggests, a 'home'. Residential homes for older people have a rather negative image (Clough, 2000, p. 18) and are not places most people want to live in (Sinclair, 1988, p. 247). Nevertheless, residential and day services for older people are expected to meet minimum standards (DoH, 2001a). Peace et al. (1997, pp. 115–16) note that residential care services for older people are changing, for three reasons. Their points are applicable more generally to residential and day services. There is:

1. A growing tendency for carers and service users to exercise their opinions and assert their critical views about service.
2. A groundswell of policies and practices enabling people to empower themselves.

3. A growing awareness that conditions in residential care and daycare are not fixed and unable to be fundamentally reformed, but are part of the way in which the realities of people's lives and living conditions are socially constructed. As these social constructions change, so positive changes in residential and day services become more likely. For instance, in today's world of people living longer and developing new careers and activities after retirement, being older may be defined less in terms of being infirm, dependent and incapable and more in terms of being capable, energetic and independent.

Residential Care

Residential work relates to sociological theories about organisations and institutions and also to social psychological ideas about how individuals interact in small groups (see Chapters 7 and 32). The terms 'group care' and 'group living' are often used in connection with residential work. Sometimes attempts are made to build therapeutic experiences into the group care regime. There is a wide gulf between a traditional institution where some group activities take place and building an entire institution around therapeutic goals.

What are called 'group dynamics' – the processes of interaction between members contributing to the life of the group – are held by Tom Douglas (2000, p. 6), in his classic book about groupwork, to be similar in all groups. In residential work, it is true that different residential settings show a remarkably similar set of preoccupations. For instance, the so-called 'disruptive' consequences for the existing group of residents arriving and leaving, the conflicts between residents, and the tensions between meeting the needs of the individual and maintaining the orderly running of the establishment tend to be perpetual issues among successive generations of residents. It makes sense, therefore, to try to understand what is going on in the residential setting, not simply in terms of the complaint of Mrs X about staff member Y, but in terms of the application of group dynamics to the processes in the institution. The work of Douglas helps with this (Douglas, 2000).

What is Good Residential Care?

For many years, it has been recognised that the key to a good residential home is high-quality relationships and interaction between staff and adult or child residents. It is difficult to define this, since on one hand the treatment model of 'care' may go too far and treat the residents as unable to manage, while on the other hand the regime may require the residents to be independent to an extent that some people find uncomfortable and unsupportive.

The aim of care should be to enable people to live independently and to the full. Independence is not much use if a person's quality of life is less than when they were in residential care, for example. Some service users need a flexible home care package alongside their basic care package. The example of Zac below shows how this can work.

Practice study

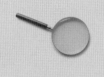

Zac

Zac lives in a relatively isolated situation and his physical mobility is restricted. His home care worker has been visiting Zac for some time and Zac has grown used to managing his small home, so he can use the remaining time flexibly when necessary. So sometimes Zac asks his home care worker to take him shopping, at other times to go for a walk down the lane with him or to take him to hospital for an appointment.

Activity 54.1

Thelma

Thelma's mother insisted that Thelma's learning disabilities required her to stay in a residential home. Thelma's key care worker in the home sensed that Thelma found this frustrating. Thelma's mother developed a terminal illness entailing an immediate stay of several months in hospital.

- Write brief notes on how the staff might have enabled Thelma to cope and move forward?

The care staff worked with Thelma to provide counselling and support. After Thelma's mother died, the staff ensured that a review meeting with Thelma discussed ways of her becoming more independent. Thelma opted for direct payments so that she could buy the services to enable her to live independently in her mother's house. She achieved this independence over a period of several months.

Activity 54.2

Mavis

Mavis wanted to visit several old people's homes before going further with the plan she had developed with Rose, her mother, to move her from her small second-floor flat to residential care.

- Make a list of what Mavis and Rose should look for when visiting each home.

We have grouped some of the questions they might consider under four headings.

Structure:
- Was the layout of the residents' rooms, lounges, toilets, bathrooms and eating areas fully accessible to all residents?
- Was there more than one place where residents could gather, for example, apart from a lounge with the television?
- Were residents mostly in their rooms, in day areas inside or outside the building (if in fine weather), or mostly in other communal areas where they could meet and interact?

Quality of staffing:

- Were any of the managing staff qualified either in caring or nursing?
- Were there signs of sufficient staff on duty, day and night, to cater for the residents' needs?

Quality of staff–residents' relationships:

- Were the staff moving (often, occasionally or never) in and out of the communal areas with residents, such as the lounge?
- Were staff sitting and standing among the residents or separated in an office or 'supervisory' area?
- Were staff eating or having their tea or coffee breaks with the residents or in a separate area?
- Were staff spending time chatting informally with residents or only speaking to them when they needed to, for example to ensure they moved to a dining area for a meal?

Regime (that is, daily programme for the life and work of the home):

- Were meals provided in a single, 'institutional' large eating area on large tables, or were there different eating areas and/or small, family-style tables for two, three or four residents?
- Was there a choice of menus for people of different faiths and diets?
- Were there regular activities brought into the home and were there regular activities taking residents out of the home?
- Were there facilities for residents to cook and make their own hot and cold drinks or was everything provided centrally at times determined by staff?

This last question is interesting because there could be a difference of view between those who advocate totally safe practice and those who advocate maximising the quality of life of the residents. There is a tension between maintaining health and safety regulations and giving residents choices, including the scope to do minor cooking and make their own drinks.

Activity 54.3

Spend a few minutes making a list of the values and principles Mavis and Rose may consider important in a residential home for Rose.

Here is our list of values and principles that we consider important:

- Respect for service users' rights
- Ensuring privacy
- Maintaining dignity
- Meeting residents' wishes
- Physical comfort
- Personal safety
- Different lounges (non-TV)
- Single or sharing room by choice
- Balancing risks against freedom of residents
- Empowering residents
- Caring for residents

- En suite toilet and wash basin
- Facilities to make hot drinks in room
- Freedom to entertain in own room
- A trusting, warm, caring atmosphere
- Flexible meal times
- Access to own room at any time.

Rights of People in Residential Care

The rights of people who use services often are considered *after* the services have been commissioned, contracted and delivered. Service users should be able to influence the quality of the residential care they receive.

Activity 54.4

Don't look at the list below. Now spend up to 30 minutes making a list of all the rights Mavis and Rose would consider to be important for Rose as a new resident in a residential home.

Here is a list drawn from official documents, staff papers and the views of residents and carers.

A resident in a residential home has the right to:

- not lose rights as I become older and more frail
- eat and drink what I want, when I choose
- have an advocate when I need one to speak up for me
- assessment and review of my needs on regular basis
- be cared for by trained staff
- have needs and wants met
- be treated with dignity and humanity
- not go into residential care except as an informed choice
- not be moved from my room or home without choice
- be formally consulted over the management of the home
- attend regular meetings of residents to discuss the home
- hold meetings without staff present
- care
- have a positive experience
- complain without being penalised
- lead as fulfilling life as possible
- have a better quality of life than I could expect elsewhere
- lose no more rights on admission than if staying in a hotel
- positive attitudes from staff towards my debilitating symptoms
- alleviation of my distressing conditions
- have my special diet
- have influence over rules and routines
- flexibility of the daily timetable
- choose when I get up and go to bed
- flexibility of meal times
- choose to sit in a TV or non-TV lounge

- make tea when I want
- entertain visitors in my room
- entertain day and evening visitors in a small private room and have relationships
- marry
- continue to manage my own money
- receive pension and pay bills, not being given 'pocket money'
- hang up pictures in wall space/room
- not lose my personal autonomy
- privacy (personal, room and property)
- remain part of local community
- follow my faith and worship in the community
- join local groups and societies
- attend the local day centre
- go to lunch clubs.

The Human Rights Act 1998 (Butler, 2006, pp. 26, 29) can also be used to enable people to:

- complain about shortcomings in services to which they are entitled
- expose neglect and abuse
- challenge vulnerability through exclusion
- resist multiple disadvantage
- claim redress.

The Equality Act 2006 dissolved the Equal Opportunities Commission, the Commission for Racial Equality and the Disability Rights Commission and in their place set up the Commission for Equality and Human Rights (CEHR). The aim of this was to promote equality through a single body tackling all aspects of discrimination – age, race, gender, disability, religion and belief and sexual orientation.

Frances Butler's (2006) important report for Age Concern examines major aspects of the application of human rights law to older people. She finds that despite the intention of the Human Rights Act 1998 to safeguard citizens' rights in the UK, across the board, vulnerable people's human rights were still being breached (Butler, p. 16). Butler proposes four fundamental human rights – the 'FRED' principles (pp. 20–2):

- *Fairness:* balancing people's rights equitably in a fair society
- *Respect:* for people's way of life, privacy, diversity and individuality
- *Equality:* protection against discrimination
- *Dignity:* preserving people's sense of self-worth, respect for privacy and family life.

The two important features of Butler's work lie in:

1. Developing principles that can be used as a benchmark against which to judge the quality of residential care

2. Firmly rooting these principles in European and worldwide (UN) statements about human rights.

Butler (2006, p. 31) extracts the following details from the European Convention on Human Rights (1950):

- article 2: right to life
- article 3: prohibition of inhuman and degrading treatment
- article 8: right to respect of family life and correspondence
- article 9: freedom of religion, conscience and thought
- protocol 1, article 1: right to enjoyment of possessions in peace.

Butler (p. 31) gives details of the five headings under which the UN principles for the advancement and protection of older persons' human rights are set out: independence, care, participation, self-fulfilment and dignity. She states:

> Human rights are intended to be transformative. They should empower people to stand up for their rights and help bring about long-term improvements in the provision of public services. (Butler, p. 28)

Despite these laudable aims, Butler (pp. 35–9) analyses the situation of vulnerable, including older, people and finds that neither international conventions nor the UK's Human Rights Act 1998 protect them from three major problems: ageism, discrimination and elder abuse.

In 2006, widespread concerns about shortcomings in the human rights of older people in healthcare led to the parliamentary Joint Committee on Human Rights beginning an inquiry into how human rights issues affect the ways in which older people are treated in hospital and residential care (www.parliament.uk/parliamentary_committees/joint_committee_on_human_rights).

Relatives and carers have rights, too. The Office of Fair Trading (Northern Ireland) (2005) investigated how people choose a care home and drew conclusions of relevance across the UK, namely that people often lack sufficient information and that the information about fees and contracts needs to be more transparent.

Day Services

Daycare services lie between full residential care and community support or care for people at home. Day services may fit alongside intermediate care and domiciliary care to contribute to a person's care package. In many parts of Britain, cuts in services, the tightening of eligibility criteria excluding people with so-called 'low level' learning disabilities and increased charges mean that many people no longer have access to daycare.

The term 'daycare' conjures up the picture of care available only during the daytime, presumably when 'normal' people would be at work, thus implying that users of daycare are unemployed. Daycare all too often has been seen as a neglected, low status service, a means of maintaining people with chronic problems for whom nothing more positive can be done. Traditionally, daycare means attendance at an institution, the day centre, with service users having to travel there in order to receive support. This suffers from the obvious disadvantage that the resources available are spread evenly across the population of users of the day centre, rather than allocated according to the various needs of the individual service users.

Imagine Mavis and Rose want some day services for the present and have identified four aspects they seek:

- More than day 'care'
- More than warehousing
- More than fitting people into a routine, to fitting the routine around the needs of people
- Flexibility of services.

Activity 54.5

Spend no more than 10 minutes writing down what Mavis and Rose may think of under the two headings of 'Strengths' and 'Weaknesses' of daycare services.

Our two lists are as follows:

Strengths:
- Somewhere to meet other people
- Warm in winter
- A friendly atmosphere
- A hot meal at lunchtime
- Not having to worry about transport
- Interesting things to do.

Weaknesses:
- Only available when the centre is open
- I have to travel a distance
- Crowded atmosphere
- No privacy
- Limited choice of activities.

Rethinking Day Services

Increasingly, there has been a move away from services revolving round the regime of the day centre, towards the notion of day services provided flexibly to meet the needs of people. Day services tackle a wide range of needs (Clark, 2001, p. 10):

- physical care and shelter
- companionship
- rehabilitation
- new achievements
- promoting independence.

Activity 54.6

Spend a few minutes devising a poster advertising day services, making it sound as attractive as possible to Mavis and Rose.

Here are some thoughts about the content of the poster. Day services could be made totally flexible, geared to the needs of individual people, run under the banner of a general aim with a coherent philosophy of high-quality service to the users and their carers, aiming to prepare users for having a life in work or leisure rather than just passing the time. Thus, rather than being cut off from other services, day services could be the means of including formerly socially excluded people.

Research evidence shows that the key to improving people's vocational success is not individual factors related to their ability and motivation so much as the approach of the day services (Grove and Membrey, 2001, p. 222). This puts the onus squarely on the staff in daycare to improve their working practices.

Practice study

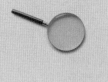

Ron

Ron has cerebral palsy, with profound and multiple impairments and restricted mobility. He spends most of his days and nights confined to his parents' ground floor flat. He is unable to move independently, except by using his motorised wheelchair. His parents both looked after him, alternating between home care and their part-time jobs until his forty-fourth birthday last year, when his father died. His mother, Jean, who retired two years ago, has struggled since then to cope with caring full time for Ron.

The worker took care to discuss respite care with both Jean and Ron together. She said it could be helpful for Jean and provide a new environment for Ron. She organised a visit for them both, with a lunch, to a nearby day centre providing specialist therapeutic services for people with impairments. Staff at the centre were encouraged by the manager to take part in staff development that promoted creative and imaginative therapeutic work with profoundly disabled people. Over a period of months, regular, weekly respite care proved beneficial for both Jean and Ron. Ron found many of the activities stimulating and became happier and more communicative. Jean found time to resume a small part-time job, one day a week.

In summary, the criteria for judging quality in day services (Clark, 2001, pp. 13–14) include the extent of:

- flexibility in time of day available
- flexibility in place offered
- responsiveness to people's requirements
- matching to varying, complex needs
- cultural and ethnic sensitivity
- inclusiveness
- support for social integration into the wider community.

Part VIII

Conclusion

This chapter has referred to some of the strengths and weaknesses of residential and day provision. It has pointed to some aspects where improvements in regimes can be be made and illustrated how these services can contribute to meeting people's needs.

REVIEW
QUESTIONS

1   What are the main strengths and weaknesses of residential services?

2   What are the main strengths and weaknesses of day services?

3   What major factors would you take into account if asked to evaluate a day or residential service?

FURTHER
READING

Atkinson, D. (1998) 'Living in Residential Care', in A. Brechin, J. Walmsley, J. Katz and S. Peace (eds) *Care Matters: Concepts, Practice and Research in Health and Social Care*, London, Sage, pp. 131–26

Booth, T. (1985) *Home Truths: Old People's Homes and the Outcome of Care*, Aldershot, Gower

Butler, F. (2006) *Rights for Real: Older People, Human Rights and the CEHR*, London, Age Concern, www.ageconcern.org.uk

Clarke, C. (ed.) (2001) *Adult Day Services and Social Inclusion*, London, Jessica Kingsley

Clough, R. (1998) *Living in Someone Else's Home*, London, Counsel and Care

Clough, R. (2000) *The Practice of Residential Work*, Basingstoke, Palgrave – now Palgrave Macmillan

Council of Europe (1950) European Convention on Human Rights, Strasbourg, Council of Europe

Johnson, J. (1993) 'Does Group Living Work?', in J. Johnson and R. Slater (eds) *Ageing and Later Life*, London, Sage, pp. 120–7

Oldman, C. (2000) *Blurring the Boundaries: A Fresh Look at Housing and Care Provision for Older People*, Brighton, Pavilion
This imaginative report explores whether enhanced sheltered housing can effectively replace some residential care for older people.

Sinclair, I. (ed.) (1988) *Residential Care: The Research Reviewed* (Wagner Report) London, HMSO
Provides very useful, wide-ranging reviews.

UN (1991) *Principles for Older Persons*, Geneva, UN

UN (1948) *Universal Declaration of Human Rights*, Geneva, UN

Wagner, G. (1988) *Residential Care: A Positive Choice. Report of the Independent Review of Residential Care* (Wagner Report) NISW, London, HMSO

Theories and models of residential care

According to Roger Clough (2000, pp. 74–81), four types of theories apply to residential care.

Theories about the worlds of residents

These attempt to describe, interpret and explain how and why residents act as they do. Clough suggests that there are three groups of these theories:

- *Biological and maturational:* these rely on linking changes in the body and mind with behaviour, for instance as a person ages. They tend to ignore social and environmental factors.
- *Psychological development:* these relate to how people feel, think and perceive themselves to how they act. They tend to neglect sociological factors.
- *Sociological perspectives:* these link the societal factors that influence people's lives, such as their age, ethnicity, disability, social class, family and work status, with how they act. They tend to emphasise 'top-down' factors from society to the individual, rather than the reverse.

Theories about intervention

These focus on the different effects that techniques such as counselling (see Chapter 45) or cognitive-behavioural programmes (see Chapter 42) might have.

Theories about the functions and tasks of residential establishments

These functionalist explanations focus on the links between policies and debates about the most appropriate ways to treat residents and what residential establishments do. Functionalist perspectives and approaches in sociology focus on the way in which societies and the institutions within them, such as the family, the factory, the residential home for older people, function. The emphasis is on how things are, the status quo, rather than on ques-

tioning, critically, how they might change dramatically, perhaps for the better. Miller and Gwynne (1972) have carried out a classic study of the tasks of residential institutions dealing with people with physical disabilities and identify three main models (a model is a way of understanding and categorising what they actually do):

- *Warehousing model:* The warehouse operates like a factory. The emphasis is on hygiene and efficiency. People may enter dirty and needing clothing. They leave clean and tidy. The warehouse does not empower people or encourage independence. In the warehouse, they tend to be stored during the period between their social death and their physical death.
- *Horticultural model:* The priority is to identify people's potential and encourage them to develop new skills. Despite its seeming attractions, the model is less appropriate where residents either cannot or do not want to take courses, experience personal development or acquire new skills (Clough, 2000, pp. 79, 141).
- *Organisational model:* This refers to settings where both independent people and dependent people are catered for. It can be said that this approach puts the needs of the residential establishment as a kind of factory before the needs of residents.

Theories that view residential establishments as systems

While we may initially be drawn to the horticultural model, we may find it oppressive and disempowering for some residents. It may be preferable on their behalf to adopt the organisational model, regarding the residential home from a systems perspective both as a product of the home and as a resource to be drawn on in ensuring staff and residents carry out the tasks of the establishment (Clough, 2000, p. 148). This is not necessarily better, as each group of ideas has its drawbacks. A systems approach has the strength of emphasising what staff and residents share and believe in common, but the defect of glossing over fundamental differences of interest between them, in the same way that managers and workers in a factory may agree to work together, but recognise that in some ways their interests differ.

FURTHER READING

Miller, E. and Gwynne, C. (1972) *A Life Apart*, London, Tavistock

Clough, R. (2000) *The Practice of Residential Work*, Basingstoke, Palgrave – now Palgrave Macmillan

Futures for Practice

Continuing Professional Development

55

DIANE HOWARD and RUTH HAMILTON

Learning outcomes

By the end of this final chapter in the book, you should be able to:

■ REVIEW and evaluate your learning to date

■ RECORD your personal and professional development

■ ASSESS what work and study you may consider next.

The end of your programme of study is an important milestone in your personal and professional development. It is a time of change and opportunity. It is useful to ask yourself some key questions :

■ Where am I now?

■ Where do I want to go from here?

■ How can I get to where I want to go?

This chapter is designed to help you to find your own answers to these questions and to know the resources available to support you.

Where You Have Been

As a student on a vocational course of study, you will have developed your competence as a student and a practitioner. In considering the key questions, it is useful to remind yourself of the scope of the learning you have already achieved. The learning outcomes of your particular course of study are likely to match with the aims and objectives listed below.

An ability to critically examine and develop your practice, for example:

- have knowledge and understanding of the theories that underpin health and/or social care practice
- possess an evidence base you can use to explain and justify your practice
- use a wide range of methods and skills
- have a clear professional identity
- have the habit of critical reflection and self-evaluation
- are committed to the implementation of professional values and recognise the need for ethical decision-making.

An ability to identify and use transferable personal skills, for example:

- increased confidence in expressing your views
- a wide range of intellectual and study skills (gathering and analysing information, discussion, assignment writing, working with others on projects, report writing)
- communication and interpersonal skills
- self-management
- time and task management, including problem-solving
- flexibility and the ability to manage change
- ICT skills.

In order to fully recognise your individual achievements, it is important to finish the course in a planned and positive way and to review and record your own personal learning.

Where Am I Now?

When your course of study is ending, opportunities are available to consolidate and further develop the learning you have gained by becoming and being a student.

By doing and recording the following activities, you will have an up-to-date port-folio demonstrating your achievements and evidence of your ability to reflect and self-evaluate.

At the end of your course, your tutors should provide you with:

- Opportunities for individual and group review and evaluation, which usually involves formal and informal activities that enable you and your learning group to clearly identify:
  - the strengths and weaknesses of the learning provision (teaching, support services, assessment)
  - to what extent students have achieved the personal and professional goals common to the student group
  - how well you have met your individual personal and professional goals.
- An individual 'exit' tutorial in which you are given personal feedback, guidance and advice for future planning; you should record this and put it in your port-folio (dated and signed).

■ An opportunity for the students and staff to formally recognise the end of the course. This is often an event to mark the final time that you and the other course participants will get together as a learning group. This is an important symbolic occasion. It allows you to 'complete' the course and bid farewell to your roles and responsibilities as a student. Even if you are busy and tired, you may well find it beneficial to attend.

At the end of your course, you should reflect on your achievements and review and evaluate your learning. When you became a student, you successfully moved out of an established comfort zone of familiar people, places, activities, demands and rewards. You have gained experience and coping skills in this new role and in managing your student, worker and family/community responsibilities. Now you need to make another adjustment. Attitudes towards change differ from person to person and so at the end of your course, you may experience one or more of a range of feelings from relief and regret to hope and threat. Self-awareness will enable your planning and management of the loss of this now familiar identity as a learner and course member.

Good interpersonal and communication skills will enable you to successfully navigate the process of 'ending the course'. For instance, you will:

■ Decide who you want to keep in touch with and plan and organise when and where you will meet.
■ Be realistic about relationships that are likely to end, while being aware that you may become colleagues in the future.
■ Use your interpersonal skills to acknowledge and validate the benefits of the relationships you have had with each individual and to wish people well. This redefines your relationship and provides clear boundaries.
■ Gain feedback from others about how you have contributed to their learning experience (you may wish to include testimonials in your portfolio).

Activity 55.1

Take time to reflect on your feelings about ending this course of study.

Example: Kath

This was completed by Kath at the end of a two-year part-time higher education course.

■ *I'll gain:* extra time for family, friends and leisure; five days to do my work instead of four; space on my dining room table
■ *I'll lose:* worry about failing; that awful feeling when I'm not sure how to do an assignment; always feeling that I have something to do
■ *I'll miss:* the other students; the tutors; finding out new things; the feeling when I've succeeded and got good feedback; knowing about other workplaces; getting up later on a Thursday.

Recording your Personal and Professional Development

To consolidate your personal and professional development and know where you are now, it is important at this stage to identify and record your learning achievement. If you have recorded personal tutorials and kept professional logs showing how you have developed your practice, it is worth rereading these in order to clearly know what you have achieved.

You should also carefully review how well you have achieved the stated aims and objectives of the course. Keep a record of them in your personal and professional development portfolio with your evidence of how they have been met and the standards you achieved. You will need to consult course and module information to do this properly. You will also need to take copies of all assessment and assignment feedback.

Activity 55.2

Review your learning and record where you are now by redoing the SWOT analysis completed at the start of the course. At this stage, concentrate on your strengths and weaknesses as a learner and as a practitioner.

Example: Kath

Strengths:

- Confidence
- Knowing the importance of my own values
- Being able to articulate what I do at work and why I do it.

Weaknesses:

- I still need to be able to evaluate the validity and reliability of research papers
- I struggle with some sociology and its relevance, for example globalisation
- I'm still a bit intimidated by 'academic' writing
- I need to be more assertive when I can't meet service users' needs because of lack of resources.

Kath's review identified new strengths, which she expected. She realised that she could also identify new weaknesses because while on the course she had become more aware of what else she could learn. This ability to maintain a cycle of review and development goals indicates that Kath is a reflective and continually developing practitioner.

Paulo Freire (2002) described education as an unending process, because people are constantly changing. 'The unfinished character of human beings and the transformational character of reality necessitate that education be an ongoing activity' (p. 84). Through the emancipating experience of education, as 'critical co-investigators'

(p. 81) with our tutors, we gain a thirst for knowledge so that we increasingly gain understanding of ourselves and our world (Freire, 2002, pp. 85–6).

Kath may have begun the course 'unconsciously competent' in many areas. She now believes that she will continue to build on her strengths and address her weaknesses because she believes in being 'consciously competent' and using times of uncertainty as opportunities for learning. She is intent on staying informed about the political context of care, saying, 'who would have thought that I'd be reading (a quality broadsheet) and listening to Radio 4!'

Where Do I Want to Go from Here?

You may know the answer to this question before your present course of study ends or you may be unable to think clearly about this immediately and need more time for your new learning to become embedded. The changes you want to make may be motivated by employment or career development or by personal development and lifestyle change. When you are ready to consider your next steps, you should begin by gaining background information and advice about the options available. You may decide on one or more of the following:

1. To progress to a degree course/professional qualification.
2. To progress your career by applying for other posts.
3. To remain in your current post and further develop your professional expertise by job enrichment activities, such as joining agency working parties, shadowing colleagues, taking on new responsibilities, mentoring others, or attending short courses/in-house training.
4. To investigate opportunities in other vocational areas.

When you have chosen your new direction, you will need to clarify your goal(s), again using the SMART methods explored in Chapter 1. To do this it is useful to:

- Find out about any finance/fee implications and the help available.
- Review your responses to the activities suggested in this chapter. They may help you to decide which general direction is right for you at this time.
- Recognise that you will be making decisions in a rapidly changing professional environment. It is difficult to predict what lies ahead for health and social care professionals. Gain as much information as possible about policy changes and the likely future directions of service provision.
- Identify a mentor. This is someone who is more experienced in the workplace than yourself. She or he will know you and your work and also have current understanding of the educational, training and careers opportunities available. If mentoring is not common in your workplace, consult the person responsible for staff training and development.
- Be aware that the achievement of your award has given you new options.

Part IX

Activity 55.3

Clearly identify your next goal. Complete a new SWOT analysis with reference to your readiness to work towards this goal.

Example: Kath

Kath decided to use the advanced standing progression route from her recent qualification at level 4 to a professional qualification course at a university. This entailed one year of portfolio building while also working full time plus one year full time at university (including a practice placement). Below is Kath's SWOT analysis.

Strengths	Weaknesses
Did well in my level 4 assessments My personal tutor thinks I can achieve at degree level I've got good study skills and habits I'm very experienced in practice I'm well organised I like learning	I still worry too much about failing
Threats	Opportunities
Will I have enough time/energy for my studies and to be a good mother? My earnings will be reduced in the second year. Can we manage? Do I want the responsibility of being a qualified worker (but I've got a qualified worker's caseload now!)? Will my husband be supportive of two more years of college work and not resent my new friends and ideas? Will my husband find it difficult when my job prospects are better than his?	My employer is willing to support me (some time in year 1, a trainee salary in year 2) My line manager and team are all for it and will be supportive I want to do it now

How Can I Get to Where I Want to Go?

Having a goal is the most effective way that you can help yourself to get to where you want to be. It is also useful to test out whether you have the resources to achieve your goal. A useful methodology is that of the force field analysis.

Activity 55.4

Do a force field analysis to map out what will help and hinder you in achieving your goal.

The steps are simple:

1. What is your goal?

2. What 'forces' could prevent you from achieving this?
3. What 'forces' could help you to combat the hindering forces?
4. What other resources do you have that would contribute to you achieving your goal?
5. Look at the force field map and decide whether you can achieve your goal.

Example: Kath

Kath's goal is to progress to a professional qualification training at a university. Below is Kath's force field analysis.

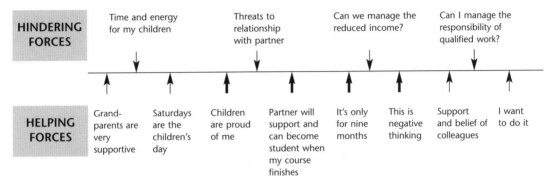

GOAL   To gain my professional qualification (completed in two years' time)

The thin arrows indicate Kath's first thoughts. At this stage it looked as if she would not have enough 'force' to achieve her goal. She discussed the force field analysis with her partner and children and they added the thicker arrows. Kath thought that 'I want to do it' was a powerful force and combined with the family's support, she decided to continue with her studies.

It is also useful to consider who are the people who will offer you support.

| Activity 55.5 |

Write down all the people who could support you at work, at home and elsewhere. Contact them and tell them what you want to achieve and ask if/how they are willing to help you.

What Now?

Many people feel a sense of anticlimax on completion of a course of study and it is important to have a positive view of the next steps so that we can overcome this feeling. If you do ask and answer the questions posed in this chapter, you will fully use your current course and feel in control of your future. You are now more aware of yourself, more aware of how you learn, more aware of how to improve your performance at work and you know how to cope with transition. In your portfolio, you have a new CV, new information of your competences as a student and a worker, new contacts, new life and/or work aims and a clear idea of where you are and where you want to move to. Your achievements, and the credit you give yourself for them, will support you in moving on. The education bug is catching and, like Kath (and possibly her partner and children), you may well find yourself itching to learn more and to become a 'lifelong learner'.

Conclusion

It is proper that this is a conclusion without an end, because in a real sense your continuing personal and professional development should have no ending. It should be a moment of transition and choices should open up for you to which you didn't previously have access. The Resource File below offers some leads that may help you decide what to do next.

FURTHER READING

Brown, R.A. (1995) *Portfolio Development and Profiling for Nurses*, Salisbury, Dinton Books

Cottrell, S. (2003) *Skills for Success: The Personal Development Planning Handbook*, Basingstoke, Palgrave Macmillan

Cottrell, S. (2003) *The Study Skills Handbook* (2nd edn) Basingstoke, Palgrave Macmillan

Northedge, A. (2005) *The Good Study Guide*, Buckingham, Open University Press

Quinn, F.M. (1998) *Continuing Professional Development in Nursing: A Guide for Practitioners and Educators*, Cheltenham, Stanley Thornes

Wallace, M. (1990) *Lifelong Learning: PREP in Action*, Edinburgh, Churchill Livingstone

RESOURCE FILE: Continuing Education and Training, below

Resource file

Continuing education and training

Information that should be made available during your studies should include clear briefings about costs and financial help, including options for what you can do next. This is often not well established, as David Simms (1997) points out. The information should also include progression pathways to a range of other programmes of learning. Employers may be invited to present information about in-house training and other employer-supported training opportunities. If there is an articulated progression route to qualification training and/or an honours degree, someone from the university may well contribute to your preparation for leaving and progressing. Visits to the university will have been organised to acquaint you with people, places and procedures. The options for you include:

- topping up to an honours degree
- progression to a professional vocational award such as the degree in social work or nursing
- progression to another level 4 or above qualific-

ation in a relevant subject such as management, training, practice assessment or counselling

■ progression or change in your career by applying for a different post

■ consolidation of your learning in your current post with development through new activities and responsibilities such as mentoring others or contributing to service or practice development.

You will find information and advice on education and training opportunities in your learning support centre or library at your college, university or in your nearest local authority library at home. Some sources are listed below.

Careers advice

You can find careers advice in several places: the learning resources centre of your college or university, the staff development and training departments of your agency or employer. You can also contact the relevant professional body in health and social care, by email, post or telephone.

Employer support and key people

Many employers are committed to providing staff with opportunities for development, through further training at work or linked with colleges and universities. It is important that you ask questions at work of colleagues, your line manager and any other staff with responsibilities for staff development and training. Opportunities for staff development often arise and you need to make sure that you are aware of them. You need to assert yourself and make your enthusiasm and commitment known to others. This will improve your chances of receiving information and being put forward as a person who may benefit from short courses, conferences and study days. These may lead to longer courses of study linked to further qualifications.

Professional bodies

Professional bodies in health, social care and social work are important sources of relevant information and will suggest ways of progressing your career, your training and your promotion prospects through continuing professional development. The two main bodies related to health and social care work are Skills for Health and Skills for Care.

Skills for Health (SfH) is a trust, part of the NHS, but working independently with its own board and management to cover the four UK health departments, in England, Wales, Scotland and Northern Ireland. It does not provide training directly but is responsible for improving the skills of the workforce and developing education and training by employers, colleges and universities. Skills for Health is working to ensure the modernisation of academic and vocational qualifications in the health sector, including developing national occupational standards, vocational qualifications and foundation degrees.

Skills for Health, www.office@skillsforhealth.org.uk 2nd Floor, Goldsmiths House, Broad Plain, Bristol, BS2 0JP, Tel. 0117 922 1155

Skills for Care (SfC) is responsible for the skills development of the adult care workforce in England, children's services being the responsibility of the new Children's Workforce Development Council (CWDC). Adult social care in the rest of the UK is covered by the Scottish Social Services Council, Care Council for Wales and Northern Ireland Social Care Council. Skills for Care works through nine regions and has regional and national arrangements to involve carers and service users (whom it calls 'people who use services') in all its work.

Skills for Care, www.info@skillsforcare.org.uk 5 Albion Court, Leeds, LS1 6JL, Tel. 0113 245 1716

Qualifying, continuing professional development (CPD) and post-qualifying

1. Nursing, midwifery and social work
The level of education and professional training immediately beyond the foundation degree is the professional undergraduate (honours degree) programme

linked either with a professional nursing/midwifery qualification or a professional social work qualification. Further information is available from the following.

The Nursing and Midwifery Council (NMC) is the statutory regulatory body for nursing, midwifery and health visiting in the UK.

NMC, www.nursingnetuk.com
23 Portland Place, London, W1N 4JT, Tel. 0207 333 6600

The General Social Care Council (GSCC) is the regulator and guardian of standards for the social care workforce in England; the rest of the UK being covered by the Scottish Social Services Council, the Care Council for Wales and the Northern Ireland Social Care Council.

General Social Care Council, www.secretariat@gscc.org.uk
Goldings House, 2 Hay's Lane, London, SE1 2HB, Tel. 0207 397 5100

Scottish Social Services Council, www.enquiries@sssc.uk.com
Compass House, 11 Riverside Drive, Dundee, DD1 4NY, Tel. 01382 207101

Care Council for Wales, www.info@ccwales.org.uk
6th Floor, West Wing, South Gate House, Wood Street, Cardiff, CF10 1EW, Tel. 02920 226257

Northern Ireland Social Care Council, www.info@niscc.n-nhs.uk
7th Floor, Mill House, 19–25 Great Victoria Street, Belfast, BT2 7AQ, Tel. 02890 417600

2. Professions allied to medicine

The Chartered Society of Physiotherapy, www.csp.org.uk/director/about.cfm

The Society of Chiropodists and Podiatrists, www.feetforlife.org

The British Association/College of Occupational Therapists, www.cot.org.uk

The Society of Radiographers, www.sor.org

The British Psychoanalytic Council, www.mail@psychoanalytic-council.org. This is the umbrella organisation for the following four groups of practitioners: psychoanalytic psychotherapy, psychoanalyis, analytical psychology, psychoanalytic psychotherapy and child psychotherapy.

3. Complementary health professions

For information see Appendix 3.

FURTHER READING

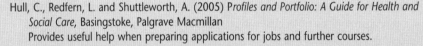

Hull, C., Redfern, L. and Shuttleworth, A. (2005) *Profiles and Portfolio: A Guide for Health and Social Care*, Basingstoke, Palgrave Macmillan
Provides useful help when preparing applications for jobs and further courses.

Simms, D. (1997) *Reflections on Guidance and Learning: A Study of Adults' Experience*, Slough, National Foundation for Educational Research (NFER)

Appendices

Legislation

1948 National Assistance Act
1959 Mental Health Act
1968 Health Services and Public Health Act
1968 Social Work (Scotland) Act
1968 Medicines Act
1970 Chronically Sick and Disabled Persons Act
1970 Equal Pay Act
1971 Misuse of Drugs Act
1972 Poisons Act
1974 Health and Safety at Work etc. Act
1975 Sex Discrimination Act
1976 Race Relations Act
1977 National Health Service Act
1977 Housing Act
1983 Mental Health Act
1983 Health and Social Services and Social Security Adjudications Act
1984 Police and Criminal Evidence Act
1986 Disabled Persons (Services, Consultation and Representation) Act
1989 Children Act
1990 National Health Service (NHS) and Community Care Act
1995 Disability Discrimination Act
1995 Mental Health (Patients in the Community) Act
1995 Carers (Recognition and Services) Act
1996 Community Care (Direct Payments) Act
1996 Family Law Act

1998 Human Rights Act
1998 Crime and Disorder Act
1998 Social Security Act
1998 Data Protection Act
1999 Health Act
2000 Carers and Disabled Children Act
2000 Care Standards Act
2000 Children (Leaving Care) Act
2000 Freedom of Information Act
2000 Local Government Act
2000 Race Relations (Amendment) Act
2000 Road Traffic Act
2000 Youth Justice and Criminal Evidence Act
2001 Criminal Justice and Police Act
2001 Health and Social Care Act
2001 Health Service Act (Care Homes)
2002 Homelessness Act
2002 NHS Reform and Health Care Professions Act
2002 Adoption and Children Act
2003 Sexual Offences Act
2004 Children Act
2004 Domestic Violence, Crime and Victims Act
2004 Carers (Equal Opportunities) Act
2005 Mental Capacity Act
2006 Equality Act
2006 Childcare Act
2006 Health Act
2007 Mental Health Act

Regulations

Control of Substances Hazardous to Health Regulations (COSHH) 1999
Employers' Liability (Compulsory Insurance) Regulations 1969
Employment Equality (Religion or Belief) Regulations 2003
Employment Equality (Sexual Orientation) Regulations 2003
Health and Safety (First Aid) Regulations 1981
Health and Safety Information for Employees Regulations 1989
Management of Health and Safety at Work Regulations 1999
Manual Handling Operations Regulations 1992
Personal Protective Equipment (PPE) Regulations 1992
Provision and Use of Work Equipment Regulations (PUWER) 1999
Reporting of Injuries, Diseases and Dangerous Occurrences Regulations
    (RIDDOR)1985
Workplace (Health, Safety and Welfare) Regulations 1992

Useful Contacts

Advocacy
www.advocacy.org.uk

Barnardo's
www.barnardos.org.uk

British Council of Disabled People
www.bcodp.org.uk

British Library Catalogue (records of books/journals
available on loan through your college or university
library)
www.bl.uk

Carers UK
www.carersuk.org

Centre for Policy on Ageing
www.cpa.org.uk

Children's Commissioner
www.childrenscommissioner.org

Children's Legal Centre
www.childrenslegalcentre.com

Children's Rights Alliance for England
www.crae.org.uk

Children's Rights Officers and Advocates (CROA)
www.croa.org.uk

Children's Society
www.childrenssociety.org.uk

Commission for Social Care Inspection
www.csci.org.uk

Crisis (homelessness charity)
www.crisis.org.uk/single

Department of Health
www.dh.gov.uk/en/Policyandguidance/
Healthandsocialcaretopics

DoH NSF for older people
www.dh.gov.uk/en/Policyandguidance/Healthand
socialcaretopics/Olderpeoplesservices/
DH_4073597

Headway (the Brain Injury Association)
www.headway.org.uk

Healthcare Commission
www.healthcarecommission.org.uk

HMSO publications
www.legislation.hmso.gov.uk

HMSO publications
www.scotland-legislation.hmso.gov.uk

Joseph Rowntree Foundation (for research
publications)
www.jrf.org.uk

Mind (mental health charity)
www.mind.org.uk

National Audit Office
www.nao.org.uk, 020 7798 7999 (to make a disclosure), 020 7798 7000 (enquiries)

National Children's Homes
www.nch.org.uk

National Institute for Clinical Excellence
www.nice.org.uk

National Youth Advocacy Service
www.nyas.net

NHS Direct (24-hour information about health
problems) 0845 4647
www.nhsdirect.nhs.uk

NSPCC
www.nspcc.org.uk

Office of Children's Rights Director
www.rights4me.org.uk

Office of Public Sector Information
www.opsi.gov.uk

Ofsted
www.ofsted.gov.uk

Parenting Plus
www.parentlineplus.org.uk

Sane (mental illness charity)
www.sane.org.uk

Save the Children
www.savethechildren.org.uk

Scope (cerebral palsy organisation)
www.scope.org.uk, helpline 0808 8003333

Sense (deaf blind charity)
www.sense.org.uk

Social Care Institute for Excellence
www.scie.org.uk

Speakability (national charity for people with aphasia)
www.speakability.org.uk

Terrence Higgins Trust
www.tht.org.uk

The King's Fund Information and Library Service, 11–13 Cavendish Square, London, W1M OAN
www.kingsfund.org.uk/elibrary/html/index.html
A useful source of reports, research and audits of health and social services.

The Stroke Association
www.stroke.org.uk, 0845 3033100

Complementary Health Information

The following is a selected list from many complementary health approaches and sources that may be used in conjunction with, or as an alternative to, conventional healthcare, where practitioners, people using services and carers regard it as appropriate.

Acupuncture
A holistic form of traditional Chinese medicine using needles inserted into the skin at potentially over 300 'acu' points, so as to balance the energy ('chi') of the body, thereby improving health (for example reducing pain) and preventing health problems.

British Acupuncture Council www.acupuncture.org.uk

Alexander technique
Not a therapy but a self-empowering method for learning how to stand, move and be more self-aware and coordinated in order to avoid discomfort, reduce wear and tear on the body and perform better.

Society of Teachers of the Alexander Technique www.stat.org.uk

Aromatherapy
Uses essential oils (aromatic substances distilled or squeezed from specific plants) holistically, through bathing, massage and inhaling (the latter not for asthmatic people) to improve a person's emotional and physical well-being.

Aromatherapy Council info@aromatherapycouncil.co.uk

Chiropractic
A profession diagnosing and treating through manipulation (or manual adjustment) of joints, enabling the body, particularly through the nervous system, to self-heal problems such as neck and back pain resulting from dysfunctions of joints.

The General Chiropractic Council enquiries@gcc-uk.org

Chiropractic and Osteopathy (online journal) info@biomedcentral.com

Homeopathy
As the word suggests, treats like with like. It uses natural substances to treat people for particular medical conditions, diluting to an extreme

degree and administering to the person the same toxin that is considered to create the condition.

www.trusthomeopathy.org/contact.html

Light therapy (Phototherapy)	A non-invasive therapy used to alleviate pain and skin conditions, for cosmetic reasons or in psychiatry to combat weather-related depression. It involves exposing people to specific wavelengths of light, using diodes emitting light, lasers, bright lights or fluorescent lamps.
Macrobiotics	Macrobiotics, from Greek 'great life', is a diet based on principles of polarity (opposites) between yin and yang, each food contributing to one of these, balanced to meet the person's yin–yang needs. It is used to treat depression, skin disorders and arthritis.
Massage	A traditional, Eastern and Western way of manipulating muscles and soft tissue to improve health and wellbeing, tackling injuries, circulation difficulties, problems of stiffness and the relief of stress. Head massage is used to release stress in the muscles and nerves of the head, neck and shoulders, as a way of rebalancing the three linked but distinct aspects of mind, body and spirit. Thai massage, Thai foot massage and hand, foot and leg massage originated more than 5,000 years ago in China and are holistic treatments. They aim to achieve balance and prevent stress and health problems.
Meditation	An approach to relaxation of the body by focusing on something in order to achieve inner peace and harmony.
Osteopathy	Identifies and treats damaged joints, muscles, nerves and ligaments, tackling, for example, injuries, repetitive strains and problems of posture. General Osteopathic Council info@osteopathy.org.uk
Pranic healing	An ancient treatment for physical illness based on the healer directing 'prana' (vital energy) towards the endocrine system of the person, to revitalise it.
Reflexology	A holistic therapy derived from similar origins to Chinese acupuncture. Each reflex point in the hand and foot is linked with each specific area and organ in the body and it is held that massaging each point in the hand or foot can stimulate that body part to self-heal. Association of Reflexologists info@aor.org.uk International Institute of Reflexology (UK) www.reflexology-uk.co.uk
Reiki	Reiki, Japanese word for the life energy surrounding us, is non-invasive and non-manipulative. The practitioner acts as channel for the life energy rather than as a healer, the aim being to restore the emotional and physical balance and enable the body to heal itself. The Reiki Association www.reikiassociation.org.uk
Sahaj marg	A healing practice rooted in spiritual traditions of meditation.
Shiatsu	A form of Eastern massage, rooted in the principles of acupuncture, which aims to restore balance to the body and is used to treat stress, indigestion and poor posture.

Infinite t'ai chi	Refers to forms of graceful movements based on the rhythm of life and including breathing exercises, aiming to promote self-awareness, personal and spiritual development, balanced health and inner strength.
Yoga	A collective term for ancient practices from India, associated with Hindu philosophy, intended to bring about relaxation and bring harmony to the person's body, mind and spirit. It is used for managing stress and may be claimed as a by-product to improve muscular flexibility, tone and strength.
	British Wheel of Yoga www.bwy.org.uk

FURTHER READING

March-Smith, Rosie (2005) *Counselling Skills for Complementary Therapists*, Buckingham, Open University Press

WEBSITES: www.bcma.co.uk (British Complementary Medicine Association)
www.internethealthlibrary.com (Internet Health Library)
http://bmj.com/cgi/collection/complementary_medicine (British Medical Journal articles since January 1998 on complementary medicine)

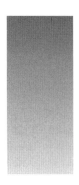

Bibliography

Abraham, A. (2005) *NHS Funding for Long-term Care: Follow up Report*, HC 348, Session 2005–6, London, TSO

Abraham, S. and Llewellyn-Jones, D. (2001) *Eating Disorders: The Facts (5th edn)* Oxford, Oxford University Press

Abrams, P., Braivas, J.G. and Stanton. S.L. (1988) 'Standardisation of Terminology of Lower Urinary Tract', *Neurological Urodynamics*, **7**: 403–27

Acheson Report (1998) *Independent Inquiry into Inequalities in Health*, London, TSO

Achterberg, J. (1990) *Woman as Healer*, Boston, MA, Shambhala Publications

ACMD (Advisory Council on the Misuse of Drugs) (2005) *Further Consideration of the Classification of Cannabis under the Misuse of Drugs Act 1971*, London, ACMD

Adams, R. (2002) 'Social Work Processes', in R. Adams, L. Dominelli and M. Payne (eds) *Social Work: Themes, Issues and Critical Debates*, Basingstoke, Palgrave Macmillan

Adams, R. (2003) *Social Work and Empowerment* (3rd edn) Basingstoke, Palgrave Macmillan

Adams, R. (2007) *Social Work and Empowerrment* (4th edn) Basingstoke, Palgrave Macmillan

ADSS (Association of Directors of Social Services) (2005) *Safeguarding Adults: A National Framework of Standards for Good Practice and Outcomes in Adult Protection Work*, London, ADSS

Aggleton, P. and Chalmers, H. (2000) *Nursing Models and the Nursing Process* (2nd edn) Basingstoke, Palgrave – now Palgrave Macmillan

Ainsworth, M. (1967) *Infancy in Uganda: Infant Care and the Growth of Love*, Baltimore, John Hopkins University Press

Albrecht, H., Shearen, C., Degalau, J. and Guay, D.R.P. (2002) 'Team Approach to Infection Prevention and Control in the Nursing Home Setting', *American Journal of Infection Control*, February

ALG (Association of London Government et al.) (2003) *All London Child Protection Procedures*, London, London Child Protection Committee

Andrews, M.M. and Hanson, P.A. (2003) 'Religion, Culture and Nursing', in M.M. Andrews and J.S. Boyle (eds) *Transcultural Concepts in Nursing Care* (4th edn) Philadelphia, Lippincott, Williams & Wilkins

AOTA (American Occupational Therapy Association) (1994) 'Uniform Terminology for Occupational Therapy' (3rd edn) *American Journal of Occupational Therapy*, **48**(11): 1047–59

Argyle, M. (1969) *Social Interaction*, London, Methuen

Argyle, M. (1972) *The Social Psychology of Work*, London, Allen Lane/Penguin

Argyle, M. (1988) *Bodily Communication* (2nd edn) London, Methuen

Armstrong, E. (1995) *Mental Health Issues in Primary Health Care: A Practical Guide*, Basingstoke, Macmillan – now Palgrave Macmillan

Arnstein, S. (1969) 'A Ladder of Citizen Participation', *Journal of the American Institute of Planners*, **35**(4): 216–22

Atherton, H. (2003) 'A History of Learning Disabilities', in B. Gates (ed.) *Learning Disability: Towards Inclusion*, London, Churchill Livingstone, Chapter 4

Ayliffe, G.A.J., Babb, J.R. and Quoraishi, A.H. (1978) 'A Test for Hygienic Hand Disinfection', *Journal of Clinical Pathology*, 31: 923

Bailey, R. and Brake, M. (eds) (1975) *Radical Social Work*, London, Arnold

Baker, K. (2005) 'Assessment in Youth Justice: Professional Discretion and the Use of ASSET', *Youth Justice*, **5**(2): 106–22

Baker, S. and Read, J. (1996) *Not Just Sticks and Stones: A Survey of the Stigma, Taboos and Discrimination Experienced by People with Mental Health Problems*, London, MIND

Baldwin, S. (1990) 'Helping Problem Drinkers – Some New Developments', in S. Collins (ed.) *Alcohol, Social Work and Helping*, London, Tavistock/Routledge, pp. 67–95

Bandura, A. (1977) *Social Learning Theory*, New York, General Learning Press

Bandura, A. (1986) *Social Foundations of Thought and Action: A Social Cognitive Theory*, Englewood Cliffs, NJ, Prentice-Hall

Banks, L., Haynes, P., Balloch, S. and Hill, M. (2006) *Changes in Communal Provision for Adult Social Care 1991–2001*, York, Joseph Rowntree Foundation

Barnes, C., Mercer, G. and Din, I. (2003) *Research Review on User Involvement in Promoting Change and Enhancing the Quality of Social Care Services for Disabled People*, Final Report for SCIE, Leeds, Centre for Disability Studies, University of Leeds, disability-studies@leeds.ac.uk

Bartlett, H.M. (1970) *The Common Base of Social Work Practice*, New York, National Association of Social Workers

Bartlett, S. (2005) 'The Healing Starts Here', *Community Care*, 1561: 41

Barton, R. (1976) *Institutional Neurosis* (3rd edn) Bristol, Wright

Batty, D. (2003) Catalogue of Cruelty, http://Society.guardian.co.uk/print/0,3858,4271108-108861,00.html

Beckett, C. (2002) *Human Growth and Development*, London, Sage

Beckett, C. and Maynard, A. (2005) *Values and Ethics in Social Work: An Introduction*, London, Sage

Berger, K.S. (2004) *The Developing Person Across the Lifespan* (6th edn) New York, Worth

Berridge, D. (1998) *Foster Care: A Research Review*, London, TSO

Berridge, D. and Brodie, I. (1988) *Children's Homes Revisited*, London, Jessica Kingsley

Biddle, D. and Gardiner, D. (1986) 'Working with Chronic Solvent Misusers', in R. Ives (ed.) *Solvent Abuse in Context*, London, National Children's Bureau, pp. 43–51

Biehal, N., Mitchell, F. and Wade, J. (2003) *Lost from View: Missing Persons in the UK*, Bristol, Policy Press

Biestek, F. (1961) *The Casework Relationship*, London, Allen & Unwin

Bion, W.R. (1968) *Experiences in Groups and Other Papers*, London, Tavistock

Birchenall, M., Baldwin, S. and Morris, J. (1997) *Learning Disability and the Social Context of Care*, Edinburgh, Open Learning Foundation/Churchill Livingstone

Black Report (1980) *Inequalities in Health*, London, DHSS

Blackburn, I., Twaddle, V. and Associates (1996) *Cognitive Therapy in Action: A Practitioner's Casebook*, London, Souvenir Press

Blom-Cooper, L. (1985) *A Child in Trust: the Report of the Panel of Inquiry into the Circumstances Surrounding the Death of Jasmine Beckford*, London, London Borough of Brent

Bloom, L. and Tinker, E. (2001) The Intentionality Model and Language Acquisition: Engagement, Effort and the Essential Tension in Development, *Monographs of the Society for Research in Child Development*, **66**(4) Serial No. 267

Blunt, J. (2001) 'Wound Cleansing: Ritualistic or Research-based Practice', *Nursing Standard*, **16**(1): 33–6

BMA (1999) *Growing up in Britain: Ensuring a Healthy Future for our Children*, London, British Medical Association

BMA (2003) *Adolescent Health*, London, British Medical Association

BMA (2005) *Preventing Childhood Obesity*, London, British Medical Association

Bornat, J. and Walmsley, J. (2004) 'Biography as Empowering Practice: Lessons from Research', in P. Chamberlayne, J. Bornat and U. Apitzsch (eds) *Biographical Methods and Professional Practice: An International Perspective*, Bristol, Policy Press, pp. 221–36

Bowlby, J. (1969) *Attachment and Loss*, vol. I, *Attachment*, Harmondsworth, Penguin

Bowlby, J. (1973) *Attachment and Loss*, vol. II, *Separation: Anxiety and Anger*, Harmondsworth, Penguin

Bowlby, J. ([1980]1991) *Attachment and Loss,* vol. III, *Loss: Sadness and Depression,* Harmondsworth, Penguin

Bowlby, J. and Parkes, C.M. (1970) 'Separation and Loss within the Family', in E.J. Anthony and C. Koupernick (eds) *The Child in His Family: International Yearbook of Child Psychiatry and Allied Professions,* New York, Wiley, pp. 197–216

Bradshaw, J. (1972) 'A Taxonomy of Social Need', *New Society* (March): 640–3

Brearley, C.P. (1982) *Risk and Social Work,* London, Routledge & Kegan Paul

Broad, B. (1998) *Young People Leaving Care: Life after the Children Act 1989,* London, Jessica Kingsley

Bronfenbrenner, U. (1979) *The Ecology of Human Development,* Cambridge, MA, Harvard University Press

Brown, G.W. (1996) 'Life Events, Loss and Depressive Disorders', in T. Heller, J. Reynolds, R. Gomm, R. Muston and S. Pattison (eds) *Mental Health Matters: A Reader,* Basingstoke, Macmillan – now Palgrave Macmillan, pp. 36–45

Brown, G.W. and Harris, T.O. (eds) (1978) *Social Origins of Depression: A Study of Psychiatric Disorder in Women,* London, Tavistock

Brown, H. (1999) 'Abuse of People with Learning Disabilities', in N. Stanley, J. Manthorpe and B. Penhale (eds) *Institutional Abuse: Perspectives Across the Life Course,* London, Routledge, pp. 81–109

Brown, H. Cosis (2005) 'Counselling', in R. Adams, L. Dominelli and M. Payne (eds) *Social Work: Themes, Issues and Critical Debates,* Basingstoke, Palgrave Macmillan, pp. 139–48

Browner, B.D., Pottack, A.N. and Gupton, C. (eds) (2002) *Emergency Care and Transportation of the Sick and Injured,* Sudbury, MA, Jones & Bartlett

Buck, T. and Smith, R.S. (2003) (eds) *Poor Relief or Poor Deal? The Social Fund, Safety Nets and Social Security,* Aldershot, Ashgate

Buckinghamshire County Council (1998) *Independent Longcare Inquiry,* Buckinghamshire, County Council

Burnard, P. (2005) *Counselling Skills for Health Professionals* (4th edn) Cheltenham, Nelson Thornes

Burns, T. and Sinfield, S. (2003) *Essential Study Skills: The Complete Guide to Success at University,* London, Sage

Burns, T. and Stalker, G.M. (1961) *The Management of Innovation,* London, Tavistock

Butler, F. (2006) *Rights for Real: Older People, Human Rights and the CEHR,* London, Age Concern, www.ageconcern.org.uk

Butler Sloss, E. (1988) *Report of the Inquiry into Child Abuse in Cleveland,* Cm 412, London, HMSO

Cambridgeshire County Council (2006) *Protection of Vulnerable Adults from Abuse. Annual Report April 2005–March 2006,* Cambridgeshire County Council, www.cambridgeshire.gov.uk

Camden and Islington NHS Trust (1999) *Beech House Inquiry – Report of the Internal Inquiry Relating to the Mistreatment of Patients Residing at Beech House, St Pancras Hospital during the period March 1993–April 1996,* London, Camden and Islington NHS Trust

Campbell, D., Draper, R. and Huffington, C. (1991) *A Systemic Approach to Consultation,* London, Karnac

Campbell, P. (1996) 'The History of the User Movement in the United Kingdom', in T. Heller, J. Reynolds, R. Gomm, R. Muston and S. Pattison, (eds) *Mental Health Matters: A Reader,* Basingstoke, Macmillan – now Palgrave Macmillan

Caplan, G. (1961) *A Community Approach to Mental Health,* London, Tavistock

Caplan, G. (1964) *Principles of Preventive Psychiatry,* New York, Basic Books

Carey, L. (ed.) (2006) *Expressive and Creative Arts Methods for Trauma Survivors,* London, Jessica Kingsley

Carnwell, R. and Buchanan, J. (eds) (2004) *Effective Practice in Health and Social Care: A Partnership Approach,* Maidenhead, Open University Press

Caroline, N.L. (1995) *Emergency Care in the Streets* (5th edn) Boston, MA, Little, Brown

Carr, E. and Mann, E. (2000) *Pain: Creative Approaches to Effective Management*, Basingstoke, Palgrave – now Palgrave Macmillan

Carr, S. (2004) *Has Service User Participation Made a Difference to Social Care Services?* Position Paper 3, London, Social Care Institute for Excellence (SCIE)

Challis, D., Chessum, R., Chesterman, J., Luckett, R. and Woods, R. (1988) 'Community Care for the Frail Elderly: An Urban Experiment', *British Journal of Social Work*, 18 (Supplement): 13–42

Chambers, H. (2005) *Healthy Care Programme Handbook*, London, National Children's Bureau

Chambers, H. with Howell, S., Madge, N., Olle, H. (2002) *Healthy Care: Building an Evidence Base for Promoting the Health and Wellbeing of Looked After Children and Young People*, London, NCB

Chesner, A. (1995) *Dramatherapy for People with Learning Disabilities: A World of Difference*, London, Jessica Kingsley

Children's Society (2004) *Thrown Away: The Experiences of Children Forced to Leave Home*, London, The Children's Society

Chomsky, N. (1968) *Language and Mind*, New York, Harcourt Brace Jovanovich

Christensen, P.J. and Kenney, J.W. (eds) (1995) *Nursing Process: Applications of Conceptual Methods*, St Louis, MO, Mosby

Clark, C. (2001) 'The Transformation of Day Care', in C. Clark (ed.) *Adult Day Services and Social Inclusion: Better Days*, Research Highlights in Social Work 39, London, Jessica Kingsley, pp. 9–18

Clarke, M. and Ogg, J. (1994) 'Recognition and Prevention of Elder Abuse', *Journal of Community Nursing*, May, pp. 4–6

Clough, R. (2000) *The Practice of Residential Work*, Basingstoke, Palgrave – now Palgrave Macmillan

Clyde, J.J. (1992) *Report of the Removal of Children from Orkney in February 1991*, Edinburgh, HMSO

Cole, E. (2003) 'Wound Management in A&E Departments', *Nursing Standard*, **17**(46): 45–52

Collins, S. (ed.) (1990) *Alcohol, Social Work and Helping*, London, Tavistock/Routledge

Commission for Health Improvement (2003) *Investigation into Matters Arising from Care on Rowan Ward, Manchester Health and Social Care Trust*, London, Commission for Health Improvement

Corby, B. (2005) *Child Abuse: Towards a Knowledge Base*, Buckingham, Open University Press

Corby, B., Doig, A. and Roberts, V. (2001) *Public Inquiries into Abuse of Children in Residential Care*, London, Jessica Kingsley

Corr, C. (1992) 'A Task-based Approach to Coping with Dying', *Omega*, **24**(2): 81–94

Coulan, E. (1997) *Advocacy: A Code of Practice*, London, DoH

Crawford, D. and Jeffery, R.W. (eds) (2005) *Obesity Prevention and Public Health*, Oxford, Oxford University Press

Crawford, M., Rutter, D. and Thelwall, S. (2003) *User Involvement in Change Management: A Review of the Literature*, Report to NHS Service Delivery Organisation, London, Department of Psychological Medicine

Creek, J. (2003) *Occupational Therapy Defined as a Complex Intervention*, London, College of Occupational Therapists

CSCI (Commission for Social Care Inspection) (2004) *Inspecting for Better Lives: Modernising the Regulation of Social Care*, London, CSCI

CSCI (Commission for Social Care Inspection) (2005a) *Direct Payments. What are the Barriers?*, London, CSCI

CSCI (Commission for Social Care Inspection) (2005b) *Making Every Child Matter: Messages from Inspections of Children's Social Services*, London, CSCI

CSCI (Commission for Social Care Inspection) (2005c) *Performance Ratings for Social Services in England*, London, CSCI

CSCI (Commission for Social Care Inspection) (2006a) *An Overview of Home Care Services for Older People in England*, London, CSCI

CSCI (Commission for Social Care Inspection) (2006b) *Performance Ratings for Adults' Social Services in England*, London, CSCI

CSCI (Commission for Social Care Inspection) (2006c) *Handled with Care? Managing Medication for Residents of Care Homes and Children's Homes – A Follow-up Study*, London, CSCI

Danso, C., Greaves, H., Howell, S., Ryan, M., Sinclair, R. and Tunnard, J. (2003) *The Involvement of Children and Young People in Promoting Change and Enhancing the Quality of Services*, Research Report for SCIE, London, NCB

Darves-Bornoz, J., Lepine, J., Choquet, M., Berger, C., Degiovanni, A., and Galliard, P. (1998) 'Predictive Factors of Chronic Stress Disorder in Rape Victims', *European Psychiatry*, **13**(6): 281–7

Davey, B. (ed.) (2001) *Birth to Old Age: Health in Transition*, Buckingham, Open University Press

Davis, N. (1990) *Once Upon a Time: Therapeutic Stories to Heal Abused Children*, Psychological Associates

Dearden, C. and Becker, S. (2000) 'Listening to Children: Meeting the Needs of Young Carers', in H. Kemshall and R. Littlechild (eds) *User Involvement and Participation in Social Care: Research Informing Practice*, London, Jessica Kingsley

Dent, A. and Stewart, A. (2004) *Sudden Death in Childhood: Support for the Bereaved Family*, Edinburgh, Elsevier Science

Department for Communities and Local Government (2006) *Strong and Prosperous Communities: The Local Government White Paper*, Vol. II, Cm 6939-II, London, TSO, www.communities.gov.uk

DfES (1998) *Meeting the Childcare Challenge: A Framework and Consultation Document*, Green Paper, Cm 3959, London, TSO

DfES (2004a) *Every Child Matters: The Next Steps*, London, DfES

DfES (2004b) *Every Child Matters: Change for Children in Social Care*, London, DfES

DfES (2004c) *Common Core of Skills and Knowledge for the Children's Workforce*, London, DfES

DfES (2005) *Youth Matters*, Green Paper, Cm 6629, London, HMSO

DfES (2006a) *Working Together to Safeguard Children: A Guide for Inter-agency Working to Safeguard and Promote the Welfare of Children*, London, TSO

DfES (2006b) *The Common Assessment Framework for Children and Young People: Practitioners' Guide*, London, DfES

DfES and DoH (2004) *The National Service Framework for Children, Young People and Maternity Services*, London, DoH

DfES and DoH (2006) *Options for Excellence Final Report: Building the Social Care Workforce of the Future*, London, DoH

DHSS (1969) *Report of the Committee of Inquiry into Allegations of Ill-treatment of Patients and Other Irregularities at the Ely Hospital*, Cardiff, Cmnd 3975, London, HMSO

DHSS (1971) *Better Services for the Mentally Handicapped*, Cmn 4683, HMSO, London

DHSS (1982) *Child Abuse: A Study of Inquiry Reports*, London, HMSO

Doel, M. and Marsh, P. (1992) *Task-Centred Social Work*, Aldershot, Ashgate

DoH (1989) *Caring for People: Community Care in the Next Decade and Beyond*, London, HMSO

DoH (1991a) *Child Abuse: A Study of Inquiry Reports: 1980–1989*, London, HMSO

DoH (1991b) *Care Management and Assessment: Practitioner's Guide*, London, HMSO

DoH (1991c) *The Children Act Guidance and Regulations*, vol. 2, *Family Support, Day Care and Educational Provision for Young Children*, London, HMSO

DoH (1991d) *The Children Act Guidance and Regulations*, vol. 3, *Family Placements*, London, HMSO

DoH (1993) *Standards for the Residential Care of Elderly People with Mental Disorders*, Inspecting for Quality Series, London, HMSO

DoH (1995a) *Building Bridges: A Guide to Arrangements for Inter-Agency Working for the Care and Protection of Severely Mentally Ill People*, London, DoH

DoH (1995b) *Child Protection: Messages from Research*, London, HMSO

DoH (1998a) *Working Together: Securing a Quality Workforce for the NHS*, London, DoH

DoH (1998b) *Modernising Social Services: Promoting Independence, Improving Protection, Raising Standards*, Cm 4169, London, TSO

DoH (1998c) *People Like Us: The Review of Safeguards for Children Living Away from Home*, London, TSO

DoH (1999a) *National Service Framework for Mental Health: Modern Standards and Service Models*, London, DoH

DoH (1999b) *Effective Care Co-ordination in Mental Health Services: Modernising the Care Programme Approach*, London, DoH

DoH (1999c) *Working Together to Safeguard Children: A Guide to Inter-agency Working to Safeguard and Promote the Welfare of Children*, London, TSO

DoH (2000a) *Framework for the Assessment of Children in Need and their Families*, London, TSO

DoH (2000b) *Care Homes for Older People: National Minimum Standards*, London, TSO

DoH (2000c) *National Service Framework for Coronary Heart Disease*, London, DoH

DoH (2000d) *The Management and Control of Hospital Infection*, Health Service Circular, London, HMSO

DoH (2000e) *The NHS Plan: A Plan for Investment, A Plan for Reform*, London, TSO

DoH (2000f) *Good Practice for Continence Services*, London, DoH

DoH (2001a) *National Service Framework for Older People*, London, DoH

DoH (2001b) *Valuing People: A New Strategy for Learning Disabilities in the 21st Century*, White Paper, Cm 5068, London, HMSO

DoH (2001c) *Social Care for Deafblind Adults and Children*, London, DoH

DoH (2001d) *The Expert Patient: A New Approach to Disease Management for the 21st Century*, London, DoH

DoH (2001e) *Assuring the Quality of Medical Practice: Implementing 'Supporting Doctors Protecting Patients'*, London, DoH

DoH (2001f) *The Carers and Disabled Children Act 2000: A Practitioners' Guide to Carers' Assessments*, London, DoH

DoH (2001g) *The Protection of Vulnerable Adults: Inter-agency Policy, Procedures and Practice Guidance*, London, DoH

DoH (2001h) *Better Prevention, Better Services, Better Sexual Health: The National Strategy for Sexual Health and HIV*, London, DoH

DoH (2002a) *Care Homes for Older People: National Minimum Standards* (2nd edn) London, TSO

DoH (2002b) *The Single Assessment Process Guidance for Local Implementation*, London, DoH

DoH (2002c) *Health Action Plans and Health Facilitation*, London, DoH

DoH (2002d) *Sign of the Times: Modernising Mental Health Services for People Who are Deaf*, London, DoH

DoH (2002e) *Government Response to the First Annual Report of the Independent Advisory Group on Teenage Pregnancy*, London, DoH

DoH (2003a) *Fair Access to Care Services: Guidance on Eligibility Criteria for Adult Social Care*, London, DoH

DoH (2003b) *Fairer Charging Policies for Home Care and other Non-residential Social Services*, London, DoH

DoH (2003c) *Homes for Older People: National Minimum Standards: Care Homes Regulations 2001* (3rd rev. edn) London, TSO

DoH (2003d) *Our Inheritance, Our Future: Realising the Potential of Genetics in the NHS*, White Paper, Cm 5791-II, London, TSO

DoH (2003e) *Winning Ways: Working Together to Reduce Healthcare Associated Infection in England*. Report from the Chief Medical Officer, London, DoH

DoH (2003f) *Direct Payments Guidance: Community Care, Services for Carers and Children's Services (Direct Payments) Guidance England 2003*, London, DoH

DoH (2004a) *Standards for Better Healthcare*, London, DoH

DoH (2004b) *A Guide to Receiving Direct Payments from your Local Council: A Route to Independent Living*, London, DoH

DoH (2004c) *Choosing Health: Making Healthy Choices Easier*, White Paper, Cm 6374, London, TSO

DoH (2004d) *The NHS Improvement Plan: Putting People at the Heart of Public Services*, London, DoH

DoH (2004e) *Towards Cleaner Hospitals and Lower Rates of Infection: A Summary of Action*, London, DoH

DoH (2004f) *The Community Care Assessment Directions*, LAC 24, London, TSO

DoH (2004g) *National Standards, Local Action: Health and Social Care Standards and Planning Framework 2005/06–2007/08*, London, DoH

DoH (2005) *Independence, Well-being and Choice: Our Vision for the Future of Social Care for Adults in England*, Green Paper, London, DoH

DoH (2006a) *Our Health, Our Care, Our Say: A New Direction for Community Services*, Cm 6737, London, TSO

DoH (2006b) *The Health Act 2006: Code of Practice for the Prevention and Control of Healthcare Associated Infections*, London, DoH

DoH Adoption and Permance Taskforce (2001) *Adoption: Adoption and Permanence Taskforce Annual Report*, London, DoH

DoH and Home Office (2000) *No Secrets: Guidance on Developing and Implementing Multi-Agency Policies and Procedures to Protect Vulnerable Adults from Abuse*, London, DoH

DoH, Scottish Office, Welsh Office (1996) *Choice and Opportunity: Primary Care: The Future*, London, TSO

Dossey, B.M. (2000) *Florence Nightingale: Mystic, Visionary, Healer*, Springhouse, PA, Springhouse

Douglas, T. (2000) *Basic Groupwork* (2nd edn) London, Routledge

Dryden, W. and Feltham, C. (1992) *Brief Counselling: A Practical Guide for Beginning Practitioners*, Buckingham, Open University Press

Dustin, D. and Davies, L. (2007) 'Female Genital Cutting (FGC) and Children's Rights: Implications for Social Work Practice', *Journal of Child Care Practice*, **13**(1): 3–16

East, P. (1995) *Counselling in Medical Settings*, Buckingham, Open University Press

Efraimsson, E., Sandman, P., Hydén, L.-C. and Rasmussen, B.H. (2004) 'Discharge Planning: "Fooling Ourselves?" – Patient Participation in Conferences', *Journal of Clinical Nursing*, **13**: 562–70

Egan, G. (1998) *The Skilled Helper: A Problem Management Approach to Helping* (6th edn) Boston, MA, Brooks Cole

EOC (Equal Opportunities Commission) (2005) *Carers and Work–Life Balance*, London, EOC, www.eoc.co.org

Esson, K. and Leeder, S.R. (2004) *The Millenium Development Goals and Tobacco Control: An Opportunity for Global Partnership*, Geneva, WHO

Etkin, P. (1999) 'The Use of Creative Improvisation and Psychodynamic Insights in Music Therapy with an Abused Child', in T. Wigram and J. de Backer (eds) *Clincial Applications of Music Therapies in Developmental Disability, Paediatrics and Neurology*, London, Jessica Kingsley

Ettore, E. (1992) *Women and Substance Abuse*, Basingstoke, Macmillan – now Palgrave Macmillan

Exworthy, M., Stuart, M., Blane, D. and Marmot, M. (2003) *Tackling Health Inequalities since the Acheson Inquiry*, Bristol, Policy Press

Eysenck, H. (1963) *Uses and Abuses of Psychology*, Harmondsworth, Penguin

Falkov, A. (1996) *A Study of Working Together: Part 8 Reports: Fatal Child Abuse and Parental Psychiatric Disorder*, London, DoH

Fanti, G. (1990) 'Helping the Family', in S. Collins (ed.) *Alcohol, Social Work and Helping*, London, Tavistock/Routledge, pp. 125–52

Fennell, G., Phillipson, C. and Evers, H. (1988) *The Sociology of Old Age*, Milton Keynes, Open University Press

Ferall, B.R., McCaffery, M. and Rhiner, M. (1992) 'Pain and Addiction: An Urgent Need for Change in Nurse Education', *Journal of Pain and Symptom Management*, 7: 141–8

Foucault, M. (1982) *Discipline and Punish: The Birth of the Prison*, London, Allen Lane

Frampton, P. (2003) *Golly in the Cupboard*, London, Tamic (available from Blackwells Bookshop, Ladbroke House, Highbury Grove, London N5)

Freire, P. (2002) *Pedagogy of the Oppressed*, New York, Continuum

Freud, S. (1933) 'Anxiety and Instinctual Life' Lecture 32, *New Introductory Lectures on Psycho-Analysis*, London, Hogarth Press, pp. 107–43

Gilbert, P. (2000) *Overcoming Depression: A Self-help Guide using Cognitive Behavioural Techniques*, London, Robinson Press

Gilbert, P. (2006) 'Breathing Space', *Community Care*, 1606: 36–7

Gill, O. (1983) *Adoption and Race: Black, Asian and Mixed Race Children in White Families*, London, Batsford Academic

Gitterman, A. (2004) 'Interactive Andragogy: Principles, Methods, and Skills', *Journal of Teaching in Social Work*, **24**(3/4): 95–112

Glasby, J. and Littlechild, R. (2004) *The Health and Social Care Divide: The Experiences of Older People* (2nd edn) Bristol, Policy Press

Gleeson, C. (2003) 'Improving Teenagers' Access to Health Services', *Practice Nursing*, **14**(6): 263–6

Glendenning, F. (1999) 'The Abuse of Older People in Institutional Settings', in N. Stanley, J. Manthorpe and B. Penhale (eds) *Institutional Abuse: Perspectives across the Life Course*, London, Routledge, pp. 173–90

Goffman, E. (1961) *Asylums: Essays on the Social Situation of Mental Patients and Inmates*, Harmondsworth, Penguin

Golan, N. (1978) *Treatment in Crisis Situations*, New York, Free Press

Goldson, B. and Coles, D. (2005) *In the Care of the State? Child Deaths in Penal Custody in England and Wales*, London, Inquest

Gould, D. (2000) 'Infection Control: Principles for Safe Practice of Older Adults', *Elderly Care*, **12**(5): 18–23

Grant, A., Mills, G., Mulhern, R. and Short, N. (2004) *Cognitive Behavioural Therapy in Mental Health Care*, London, Sage

Gray, B. and Jackson, R. (2002) *Advocacy and Learning Disability*, London, Jessica Kingsley

Green, S. and Jackson, P. (2006) 'Nutrition', in M.R. Alexander, J.N. Fawcett and P.J. Runciman (eds) *Nursing Practice: Hospital and Home* (3rd edn) Edinburgh, Churchill Livingstone

Greig, R. (2005) *Valuing People: The Story So Far … A New Strategy for Learning Disability in the 21st Century*, London, DoH

Grove, B. and Membrey, H. (2001) 'Effective Mental Health Day Services and Employment: Evidence and Innovations', in C. Clark (ed.) *Adult Day Services and Social Inclusion*, London, Jessica Kingsley

Grubin, D. and Gunn, J. (1990) *The Imprisoned Rapist and Rape*, London, Institute of Psychiatry

GSCC (General Social Care Council) (2002) *Code of Practice for Social Care Workers and Code of Practice for Employers of Social Care Workers*, London, GSCC

Habenstein, R.W. and Christ, E.A. (1963) *Professionaliser, Traditionaliser and Utiliser* (2nd edn) Columbia, MO, University of Missouri

Hammersley, R. (1999) 'Substance Use, Abuse and Dependence', in D. Messer and F. Jones (eds) *Psychology and Social Care*, London, Jessica Kingsley

Harkreader, H. and Hogan, M.A. (2004) *Fundamentals of Nursing: Caring and Clinical Judgement* (2nd edn) Philadelphia, Saunders

Hart, R. (1992) *Children's Participation: From Tokenism to Citizenship*, UNICEF Innocenti Essays, No. 4, Florence, International Child Development Centre

Harway, M. and O'Neill, J.M. (1999) 'What Causes Men to Be Violent Against Women? The Unanswered and Controversial Question', in M. Harway and J.M. O'Neil (eds) *What Causes Men's Violence Against Women?*, London, Sage

Hastings, G., Stead, M., McDermott, L., MacKintosh, A., Rayner, M., Godfrey, C., and Caraher, M. (2003) *Review of Research on the Effects of Food Promotion to Children (2002–2003)*, Glasgow, Institute for Social Marketing

Hawton, K., Salkovskis, P.M., Kirk, J. and Clark D.M. (eds) (1991) *Cognitive-Behaviour Therapy for Psychiatric Problems: A Practical Guide*, Oxford, Oxford University Press

Healthcare Commission (HC) and Commission for Social Care Inspection (CSC) (2006) *Joint Investigation into the Provision of Services for People with Learning Disabilities at Cornwall Partnership NHS Trust*, London, Commission for Healthcare Audit and Inspection

Help the Aged (undated) Preventing Falls: Don't Mention the F-Word, Help the Aged, www.helptheaged.org.uk

HM Government (2006) *Working Together to Safeguard Children: A Guide to Inter–agency Working to Safeguard and Promote the Welfare of Children*, London, TSO

HM Treasury (2003) *Every Child Matters*, Green Paper, Cm 5860, London, TSO

HM Treasury, DfES, DTI, DWP (2004) *Choice for Parents, the Best Start for Children: a 10-year Strategy for Childcare*, London, TSO

Home Office Drug Strategy Directorate (2004) *Tackling Drugs, Changing Lives: Keeping Communities Safe from Drugs*, Drug Strategy Progress Report, London, Home Office

Honey, P. and Mumford, A. (1992) *The Manual of Learning Styles* (3rd edn) Maidenhead, P. Honey Publications

Horton, R. and Parker, L. (2002) *Informed Infection Control Practice* (2nd edn) Edinburgh, Churchill Livingstone

Horwath, J. (ed.) (1991) *The Child's World: Assessing Children in Need*, London, Jessica Kingsley

House of Commons Health Committee (2004) *Elder Abuse*, 2nd Report of Session 2003–4, London, TSO

Hucker, K. (2001) *Research Methods in Health, Care and Early Years*, Oxford, Heinemann

Hunter, M. (2005) 'Hoping for Rethink', *Community Care*, 1567: 53–6

ICNA (Infection Control Nurses Association) (2002) *Hand Hygiene Guidelines*, http://www.icna.co.uk

Institute of Alcohol Studies (2002) *What is Problem Drinking*, IAS Factsheet, St Ives, IAS

International Association for the Study of Pain (1986) 'Classification of Chronic Pain: Descriptions of Chronic Pain Syndromes and Definitions of Pain Terms', *Pain*, S1–S226

Ives, R. (ed.) (1986) *Solvent Abuse in Context*, London, National Children's Bureau

Jackson, E. and Jackson, N. (1999) *Learning Disability in Focus: The Use of Photography in the Care of People with a Learning Disability*, London, Jessica Kingsley

James, A. (2005) 'A Sense of Sound', *Openmind*, 133: 24

Janzon, K. and Law, S. (2003) *Older People Influencing Social Care: Aspirations and Realities*, Brighton, Care Equation, Kjanzon@care-equation.org.uk

Jenkins, G., Asif, Z. and Bennett, G. (2000) *Listening is not Enough*, London, Action on Elder Abuse

Jones, K. (1993) *Asylums and After: A Revised History of the Mental Health Services: From the Early 18th Century to the 1990s*, London, Athlone

Jones, K. (2000) *The Making of Social Policy in Britain: From the Poor Law to New Labour*, London, Athlone

Jones, K. and Fowles, A.J. (1984) *Ideas on Institutions: Analysing the Literature on Long-term Care and Custody*, London, Routledge & Kegan Paul

Jones, M. (1968) *Beyond the Therapeutic Community*, New Haven, CT, Yale University Press

Kadushin, A. and Kadushin, G. (1997) *The Social Work Interview: A Guide for Human Service Professionals* (4th edn) New York, Columbia University Press

Kavaler, F. and Spiegel, A.D. (1997) *Risk Management in Health Care Institutions: A Strategic Approach*, Sudbury, MA, Jones & Bartlett

Kelly, G.A. (1955) *The Psychology of Personal Constructs*, New York, Norton

Kelly, G.A. (1970a) 'A Brief Introduction to Personal Construct Theory,' in D. Bannister (ed.) *Perspectives in Personal Construct Theory*, London, Academic Press, pp. 1–29

Kelly, G.A. (1970b) 'Behaviour is an Experiment', in D. Bannister (ed.) *Perspectives in Personal Construct Theory*, London, Academic Press, pp. 255–69

Kelly, M. (1996) *A Code of Ethics for Health Promotion*, London, Social Affairs Unit

Kemm, J. and Close, A. (1995) *Health Promotion: Theory and Practice*, Basingstoke, Macmillan – now Palgrave Macmillan

Kennard, D. (1998) *Introduction to Therapeutic Communities*, London, Jessica Kingsley

Kennedy, I. (2001) *Learning from Bristol: The Inquiry into the Management of Care of Children Receiving Complex Heart Surgery at the Bristol Royal Infirmary*, Cm 5207, London, TSO

Kent, R. (1990) 'Focusing on Women', in S. Collins (ed.) *Alcohol, Social Work and Helping*, London, Tavistock/Routledge, pp. 96–124

Kidd, A. (1999) *State, Society and the Poor in Nineteenth-Century England*, Basingstoke, Macmillan – now Palgrave Macmillan

Kilbrandon Report (1964) *Children and Young Persons Scotland*, Edinburgh, HMSO

King, I.M. (1981) *A Theory for Nursing: Systems, Concepts, Process* (2nd edn) New York, John Wiley & Sons

King's Fund Centre (1992) *A Positive Approach to Nutrition as Treatment*, London, Multiplex Medway

Kirkwood, A. (1993) *The Leicestershire Inquiry 1992*, Leicester, Leicestershire County Council

Klein, M. (1997) *The Psycho-analysis of Children*, London, Vintage

Klosko, J.S. and Sanderson, W.S. (1999) *Cognitive-Behavioural Treatment of Depression*, Northvale, NJ, Jason Aronson

Kubler-Ross, E. (1970) *On Death and Dying*, London, Tavistock

LAC (2002) 17 *Children Missing from Care and From Home: a Guide to Good Practice*, London, DoH

Laming, H. (2003) *The Victoria Climbié Inquiry: Report of an Inquiry by Lord Laming*, London, TSO

Larson, E. (1988) 'A Causal Link between Hand Washing and Risk of Infection? Examination of the Evidence', *Infection Control and Hospital Epidemiology*, 9: 28–36

Larson, E. (1997) 'Social and Economic Impact of Infectious Diseases – United States', *Clinical Performance and the Quality of Health Care,* 5: 31–7

Lawrence, J. and May, D. (2003) *Infection Control in the Community*, Edinburgh, Churchill Livingstone

Leason, K. (2006) 'Keep Off the Grass', *Community Care,* 1611: 28–9

Leece, J. and Bornat J. (eds) (2006) *Developments in Direct Payments*, Bristol, Policy Press

Levy, A. and Kahan, B. (1991) *The Pindown Experience and the Protection of Children: The Report of the Staffordshire Child Care Inquiry 1990*, Stafford, Staffordshire County Council

Lewis, P. (2007) 'Missing 48 trafficked children taken into care', *Guardian*, 15 January

LGO (Local Government Ombudsman) (2006) *Delivering Public Value: Annual Report of Local Government Ombudsman*, London, LGO

Liebmann, M. (ed.) (1994) *Art Therapy with Offenders*, London, Jessica Kingsley

Lishman, J. (1994) *Communication in Social Work*, Basingstoke, BASW/Macmillan

Lister, R. (1997) *Citizenship: Feminist Perspectives*, Basingstoke, Macmillan – now Palgrave Macmillan

Littlewood, J. (1992) *Aspects of Grief: Bereavement in Adult Life*, London, Routledge

Lloyd, L. (2003) 'Caring Relationships: Looking beyond Welfare Categories of "Carers" and "Service Users"', in K. Stalker (ed.) *Reconceptualising Work with 'Carers': New Directions for Policy and Practice*, London, Jessica Kingsley, pp. 37–55

London Borough of Greenwich and Greenwich Health Authority (1987) *A Child in Mind: Protection of Children in a Responsible Society. The Report of the Commission of Inquiry into the Circumstances Surrounding the Death of Kimberley Carlisle*, London, London Borough of Greenwich

London Borough of Lambeth (1987) *Whose Child? The Report of the Panel Appointed to Inquire into the Death of Tyra Henry*, London, London Borough of Lambeth

Lorenz, W. (1994) *Social Work in a Changing Europe*, London, Routledge

Lustbader, W. (1991) *Counting on Kindness: The Dilemmas of Dependency*, New York, Free Press

McCaffery, M. and Beebe, A. (1994) *Pain: A Clinical Manual of Nursing Practice*, London, Mosby

McDonald, A. (2006) *Understanding Community Care: A Guide for Social Workers* (2nd edn) Basingstoke, Palgrave Macmillan

MacDonald, Z., Tinsley, L., Collingwood, J., Jamieson, P. and Pudney, S. (2005) *Measuring the Harm from Illegal Drugs Using the Drug Harm Index*, Home Office Online Report 24/5 London, Home Office, http://www.homeoffice.gov.uk/rds/pdfsos/rdsolr2405.pdf

McLeod, E. and Bywaters, P. (2000) *Social Work, Health and Equality*, London, Routledge

Macpherson Report (1999) *The Stephen Lawrence Inquiry*, Cm 4262-1, London, TSO

McWhirter, J.P. and Pennington, C.K. (1994) 'Incidence and Recognition of Malnutrition in Hospital', *British Medical Journal*, 308: 945–8

Madden, P. (2005) 'Open Forum', *Community Care,* 6–12 October, p. 22

Manthorpe, J. and Iliffe, S. (2005) *Depression in Later Life*, London, Jessica Kingsley

Marieb, E.N. (2004) *Human Anatomy and Physiology* (6th edn) San Francisco, Pearson

Marlatt, G.A. and Gordon, J.R. (1985) *Relapse Prevention*, New York, Guildford Press

Marsh, P. and Doel, M. (2005) *The Task-Centred Book*, London, Routledge/Community Care

Marshall, F. (1993) *Losing a Parent*, London, SPCK

Marshall, S. and Turnbull, J. (eds) (1996) *Cognitive Behaviour Therapy: An Introduction to Theory and Practice*, London, Ballière Tindall

Maslow, A. (1943) 'A Theory of Human Motivation', *Psychological Review*, 50: 370–96

Maslow, A. (1970) *Motivation and Personality*, London, Harper & Row

Maslow, A. (1987) *Towards a Psychology of Being*, London, HarperCollins

Medicines Resource Centre (1999) 'The Management of Constipation', *Medicines Resource Centre Bulletin*, **10**(9): 33–6

Metropolitan Police (2003) *Operation Paladin Child: A Partnership Study of Child Migration into the UK via London Heathrow,* London, Metropolitan Police

Miller, E. and Gwynne, C. (1972) *A Life Apart*, London, Tavistock

Ministry of Health (MoH) (1962) *A Hospital Plan for England and Wales*, Cmd 1604, London, HMSO

Monckton, W. (1945) *Report of Sir Walter (later Viscount) Monckton on the Circumstances which Led to the Boarding out of Dennis and Terence O'Neill at Bank Farm, Misterley, and the Steps Taken to Supervise their Welfare*, Cmnd 6636, London, HMSO

Morgan, R. (2006) *Young People's Views on Leaving Care: What Young People in, and formerly in, Residential and Foster Care Think about Leaving Care*, London, CSCI

Morris, J. (1991) *Pride Against Prejudice: Transforming Attitudes to Disability*, London, The Women's Press

Morris, J. (1993) *Independent Lives: Community Care and Disabled People*, Basingstoke, Macmillan – now Palgrave Macmillan

Morris, M. (2004) *Dangerous and Severe: Process, Programme and Person: Grendon's Work*, London, Jessica Kingsley

Moss, B. (2005) *Religion and Spirituality*, Lyme Regis, Russell House

Mullender, A. and Ward, D. (1991) *Self-directed Groupwork: Users take Action for Empowerment*, London, Whiting & Birch

Munafò, M., Drury, M., Wakley, G. and Chambers, R. (2003) *Smoking Cessation Matters in Primary Care*, Abingdon, Radcliffe Medical Press

Munro, E. (2002) *Effective Child Protection*, London, Sage

NAO (National Audit Office) (2000) *The Management and Control of Hospital Acquired Infection in Acute NHS Trusts in England*, London, TSO

National Assembly for Wales and Home Office (2000) *In Safe Hands: Implementing Adult Protection Procedures in Wales*, Cardiff, National Assembly for Wales

NCB (National Children's Bureau) (2005) *Healthy Care Training Manual: A Health Promotion Training Programme for Foster Carers and Residential Social Workers*, London, NCB

Nelson-Jones, R. (2007) *Life Coaching Skills: How to Develop Skilled Clients*, London, Sage

NHS (2004) *A Matron's Charter: An Action Plan for Cleaner Hospitals*, London, NHS

NHS Executive (1999) *Primary Care Trusts: Establishing Better Services*, London, NHS Executive

NICE (National Institute for Health and Clinical Excellence) (2005) *The Management of Pressure Ulcers in Primary and Secondary Care*, Clinical Practice Guideline, London, TSO

Nicholas J. (1992) 'The Inside Story: Seeing Clients Inside their Own Homes', in E. Noonan and L. Spurling (eds) (1992) *The Making of a Counsellor,* London, Routledge

NIMHE (2005) *NIMHE Guiding Statement on Recovery*, London, DoH

NMC (Nursing and Midwifery Council) (2004) *The NMC Code of Professional Conduct: Standards for Conduct, Performance and Ethics*, London, NMC, www.nmc-uk.org

NSPCC (1997) *Turning Points: A Resource Pack for Communicating with Children*, London, NSPCC

Nutbeam, D. (1998) *Health Promotion Glossary*, Geneva, WHO

O'Hagan, K. (1986) *Crisis Intervention in Social Services*, Basingstoke, Macmillan/BASW

Office of Fair Trading (Northern Ireland) (2005) *Care Homes for Older People in the UK: A Market Study,* Belfast, Department of Health, Social Services and Public Safety

Ofsted (2003) *Annual Report of Her Majesty's Chief Inspector of Schools: Standards and Quality in Education 2001/02*, London, TSO

Ofsted (2005) *Framework for the Regulation of Childminding and Day Care*, London, Ofsted

Oliver, M. (1983) *Social Work with Disabled People*, Basingstoke, Macmillan – now Palgrave Macmillan

Oliver, M. (1990a) 'The Individual and Social Models of Disability', paper presented at Joint Workshop of the Living Options Group and the Research Unit of the Royal College of Physicians, http://www.leeds.ac.uk/disability-studies/archiveuk/Oliver/in%20soc%20dis.pdf

Oliver, M. (1990b) *The Politics of Disablement*, Basingstoke, Macmillan – now Palgrave Macmillan

Oliver, M. and Sapey, B. (2006) *Social Work with Disabled People* (3rd edn) Basingstoke, Palgrave Macmillan

Oliviere, D. Hargreaves, R. and Monroe, B. (1998) *Good Practices in Palliative Care: A Psychosocial Perspective*, Aldershot, Ashgate

ONS (2005) News Release: Projected Increase of 7.2m in UK Population by 2031, Office for National Statistics/Government Actuary's Department

Orme, J. (2001) *Gender and Community Care: Social Work and Social Care Perspectives*, Basingstoke, Palgrave – now Palgrave Macmillan

Ousey, K. (2005) *Pressure Area Care*, Oxford, Blackwell

Parton, N. (1985) *The Politics of Child Abuse*, Basingstoke, Macmillan – now Palgrave Macmillan

Parton, N., Thorpe, D. and Wattam, C. (1997) *Child Protection: Risk and the Moral Order*, Basingstoke, Macmillan – now Palgrave Macmillan

Patel, N., Naik, N. and Humphries, B. (1998) *Visions of Reality: Religion abd Ethnicity in Social Work*, London, CCETSW

Patient and Public Involvement Team (2006) *A Stronger Local Voice: A Framework for Creating a Stronger Local Voice in the Development of Health and Social Care Services*, London, DoH

Pavlov ([1897] 1982) *The Work of the Digestive Glands*, Delran, New Jersey, Gryphon

Payne, M. (1995) *Social Work and Community Care*, Basingstoke, Macmillan – now Palgrave Macmillan

Payne, M. (2000) *Teamwork in Multiprofessional Care*, Basingstoke, Palgrave – now Palgrave Macmillan

Payne, M. (2005a) *The Origins of Social Work: Continuity and Change*, Basingstoke, Palgrave Macmillan

Payne, M. (2005b) *Modern Social Work Theory* (3rd edn) Basingstoke, Palgrave Macmillan

Payne, M. (2006) *What is Professional Social Work?* (2nd edn) Bristol, Policy Press

Peace, S., Kellaher, L. and Willcocks, D. (1997) *Re-evaluating Residential Care*, Buckingham, Open University Press

Peake, A. and Rouf, K. (1989) *My Body My Book*, London, The Children's Society

Pearson, A., Vaughan, B. and Fitzgerald, M. (1996) *Nursing Models for Practice* (2nd edn) Oxford, Butterworth Heinemann

Perlman, H.H. (1957) *Social Casework: A Problem Solving Process*, Chicago, University of Chicago Press

Piaget, J. (1963) *The Origins of Intelligence in Children*, New York, W.W. Norton

Piaget, J. and Inhelder, B. (1969) *The Psychology of the Child*, London, Routledge

Pike, S. and Forster, D. (1995) *Health Promotion for All*, Edinburgh, Churchill Livingstone

Pillemer, K. (1986) 'Risk Factors in Elder Abuse: Results from a Care Control Study', in K. Pillemer and R. Wolf (eds) *Elder Abuse: Conflict in the Family*, Dover, MA, Auburn House, pp. 239–63

Pincus, A. and Minahan, A. (1973) *Social Work Practice: Model and Method*, Itasca, IL, Peacock

Plowman, R., Graves, N. and Griffin, M. et al. (2001) 'The Rate and Cost of Hospital Acquired Infections Occurring in Patients Admitted to District General Hospitals', *Journal of Hospital Infection*, **4**(3): 198–209

Potter, J. Norton, C. and Cottenden, A. (eds) (2002) *Bowel Care in Older People: Research and Practice*, London, Royal College of Physicians

Pratt, R.J., Pellowe, C., Loveday, H.P., Robinson, N., Smith, G.W. and the Epic Guideline Development Team (2001) The Epic Project: Developing National Evidence-based Guidelines for Preventing Healthcare Associated Infections, phase 1: Guidelines for Preventing Hospital-acquired Infections, *Journal of Hospital Infection*, 47 (suppl): S1–82

Preston-Shoot, M. (1987) *Effective Groupwork*, Basingstoke, BASW/Macmillan

Prime Minister's Strategy Unit (2004) *National Alcohol Harm Reduction Strategy*, London, Cabinet Office

Prince, K. (1996) *Boring Records? Communication, Speech and Writing in Social Work*, London, Jessica Kingsley

Princess Royal Trust (2004) *Directory of Carers Support Groups in the Leeds Area*, Leeds, Carers Leeds

Pringle, K. (1995) *Men, Masculinities and Social Welfare*, London, UCL Press

Prochaska, J.O. and DiClimente, C.C. (1984) *The Transtheoretical Approach: Crossing Traditional Boundaries of Therapy*, Homewood, IL, Dow Jones/Irwin

Progoff, I. (1953) *Jung's Psychology and its Social Meaning*, London, Routledge & Kegan Paul

Raynes, N.V. (2001) *Quality at Home for Older People: Involving Service Users in Defining Home Care Specifications*, Bristol, Policy Press

Read, J. and Reynolds, J. (eds) (1996) *Speaking our Minds: An Anthology of Personal Experiences of Mental Distress and its Consequences*, Basingstoke, Macmillan – now Palgrave Macmillan

Reder, P., Duncan, S. and Gray, M. (1993) *Beyond Blame: Child Abuse Tragedies Revisited*, London, Routledge

Reid, W.J. (1963) *An Experimental Study of Methods Used in Casework Treatment*, Columbia University School of Social Work

Reid, W.J. (1978) *The Task-Centred System*, New York, Columbia University Press

Reid, W.J. and Shyne, A.W. (1969) *Brief and Extended Casework*, New York, Columbia University Press

Reid, W.J. and Epstein, L. (1972) *Task-Centred Casework*, New York, Columbia University Press

Reith, M. (1998) *Community Care Tragedies: A Practice Guide to Mental Health Inquiries*, Birmingham, Venture

Residential Forum (1996) *Create a Home from Home: A Guide to Standards*, London, NISW

Richards, M., Payne, C. and Shepard, A. (1990) *Staff Supervision in Child Protection Work*, London, NISW

Robertson, J. and Bowlby, J. (1952) 'Responses of Young Children to Separation from their Mothers', *Courier of the International Children's Centre*, Paris, 2: 131–40

Robinson, C. (2000) *Adoption and Loss: The Hidden Grief*, Christie's Beach, South Australia, Clova Publications

Robinson, J. (2005) *Mary Seacole: The Charismatic Black Nurse who became a Heroine of the Crimea*, London, Constable

Roer-Strier, D. (2005) 'Human Development Education for Social Workers in Multicultural Societies', *Social Work Education*, **24**(3): 311–26

Rogers, C. (1942) *Counselling and Psychotherapy*, Boston, Houghton Mifflin

Rogers, C. (1951) *Client-Centred Therapy*, London, Constable

Rogers, C. (1961) *On Becoming a Person: A Therapist's View of Psychotherapy*, London, Constable

Rogers, C. (1980) *A Way of Being*, Boston, Houghton Mifflin

Rosdahl, C.B. and Kowalski, M.T. (2003) *Textbook of Basic Nursing* (8th edn) Philadelphia, Lippincott, Williams & Wilkins

Rose, D., Fleischmann, P., Tonkiss, F., Campbell, P. and Wykes, T. (2003) *Review of the Literature: User and Carer Involvement of Change Management in a Mental Health Context*, Report to NHS Service Delivery Organisation, Service User Research Enterprise, London, Institute of Psychiatry

Rowe, D. (1996) *Depression: The Way Out of your Prison*, London, Routledge

Rutter, M. (2006) *Genes and Behaviour: Nature–Nurture Interplay Explained*, Oxford, Blackwell

Salaman, G., Adams, R. and O'Sullivan, T. (1994) *Managing Personal and Team Effectiveness*, Milton Keynes, Open University Press

Saleeby, D. (2002) *The Strengths Perspective in Social Work Practice* (3rd edn) New York, Allyn & Bacon

Sanderson, L., Long, T. and Hale, C. (2004) 'Evaluation of Educational Programmes for Paediatric Cancer Nursing in England', *European Journal of Oncology Nursing*, **8**(2): 138–47

Sanderson, M. (2003) 'Person Centred Planning', in B. Gates (ed.) *Learning Disability: Towards Inclusion*, London, Churchill Livingstone, Chapter 19

Saunders, P. (2000) *Mosby's Paramedic Text Book* (2nd edn) St Louis, Mosby

Scott, M. (1989) *A Cognitive-Behavioural Approach to Clients' Problems*, London, Tavistock/Routledge

Scottish Executive (2000) *The Same as You? A Review of Services for People with Learning Disabilities*, Edinburgh, Scottish Executive

Scottish Executive (2001) *Guidance on Single Shared Assessment of Community Care Needs*, Circular No. CCD8/2001, Edinburgh, Scottish Executive

Scrutton, S. (1989) *Counselling Older People*, London, Edward Arnold

Seager, P. and Kebbell, M. (1999) 'Pitfalls in Interviewing: A Psychological Perspective', in D. Messer and F. Jones (eds) *Psychology and Social Care*, London, Jessica Kingsley

Secretary of State for Social Services (1974) *Report of the Committee of Inquiry into the Care and Supervision Provided in Relation to Maria Colwell*, London, HMSO

Seddon, D. and Robinson C.A. (2001) 'Carers of Older People with Dementia: Assessment and the Carers Act', *Health and Social Care in the Community*, **9**(3): 151–8

Seebohm Report (1968) *Report of the Committee on Local Authority and Allied Personal Social Services*, Cmnd 3703, London, HMSO

Seed, P. (1990) *Introducing Network Analysis in Social Work*, London, Jessica Kingsley

Shannon, C.E. (1949) *The Mathematical Theory of Communication*, Urbana, University of Illinois

Sheldon, B. (1995) *Cognitive Behavioural Therapy: Research, Practice and Philosophy*, London, Routledge

Sheldon, F. (1997) *Psychosocial Palliative Care*, Cheltenham, Nelson Thornes

Simmons, K. (2000) *A Place At The Table*, Kidderminster, British Institute of Learning Disabilities

Simms, D. (1997) *Reflections on Guidance and Learning: A Study of Adults' Experience*, Slough, National Foundation for Educational Research (NFER)

Sinclair, I. (1988) 'The Elderly', in I. Sinclair (ed.) *Residential Care: The Research Reviewed*, London, HMSO

Skinner, B.F. (1953) *Science and Human Behaviour*, New York, Macmillan

Skinner, B.F. (1974) *About Behaviourism*, New York, Random House

Smale, G. and Tuson, G. with Biehal, N. and Marsh, P. (1993) *Empowerment, Assessment, Care Management and the Skilled Worker*, London, HMSO

Stainton, T. (2002) 'Taking Rights Structurally: Disability Rights and Social Work Responses to Direct Payments', *British Journal of Social Work*, 32: 751–63

Steel, R. (2004) *Involving the Public in NHS, Public Health and Social Care Research*, Eastleigh, Involve

Stein, M. (2004) *What Works in Leaving Care*, Ilford, Barnardo's

Stein, M. (2005) *Resilience and Young People Leaving Care*, York, Joseph Rowntree Foundation

Stein, M. and Carey, K. (1986) *Leaving Care*, Oxford, Blackwell

Stein, M. and Dixon, J. (2006) 'Young People Leaving Care in Scotland', *European Journal of Social Work*, **19**(4): 407–23

Stevenson, O. (1996) *Elder Protection in the Community: What can we Learn from Child Protection?*, London, Age Concern Institute of Gerontology

Stott, F.E. and Bowman, B. (1996) 'Human Development Knowledge: A Slippery Base for Practice', *Early Childhood Research Quarterly*, 11: 169–83

Striker, S. (2004) *Anti-Colouring Book*, London, Scholastic

Sugarman, L. (2004) *Counselling and the Life-Course*, London, Sage

Sure Start (2006) *Sure Start Children's Centres, Practice Guidance*, London, DfES

Teasdale, K. (1998) *Advocacy in Healthcare*, Oxford, Blackwell

Tester, S. (1996) *Community Care for Older People: A Comparative Perspective*, Basingstoke, Macmillan – now Palgrave Macmillan

Thane, P. (1996) *Foundations of the Welfare State* (2nd edn) London, Longman

Thomas, N. (2002) *Children, Family and the State*, Bristol, Policy Press

Thompson, J. (1999) *Drama Workshops for Anger Management and Offending Behaviour*, London, Jessica Kingsley

Thompson, N. (2002) *People Skills* (2nd edn) Basingstoke, Palgrave Macmillan

Thompson, N. (2005) *Understanding Social Work: Preparing for Practice* (2nd edn) Basingstoke, Palgrave Macmillan

Thompson, N. (2006) *Anti-Discriminatory Practice* (4th edn) Basingstoke, Palgrave Macmillan

Thompson, S. (2005) *Age Discrimination*, Lyme Regis, Russell House

Thorndike, E.L. (1898) 'Animal Intelligence: An Experimental Study of the Associative Processes', Psychological Review Monograph Supplements 2 (4, whole edition) No. 8

Tinker, A., Wright, F., McCreadie, C., Askham, J., Handock, R. and Holmans, A. (1999) *Alternative Models of Care for Older People: Research*, vol. 2 of the Report by the Commission on Long Term Care, London, TSO

Tones, K. and Tilford, S. (2001) *Health Promotion: Effectiveness, Efficiency and Equity* (3rd edn) Cheltenham, Nelson Thornes

Tyrer, P. and Steinberg, D. (2005) *Models for Mental Disorder: Conceptual Models in Psychiatry* (4th edn) Chichester, Wiley

UNICEF (1990) *Convention on the Rights of the Child*, http://www.unicef.org/ccrc/fulltext.htm

Velleman, R. (1992) *Counselling for Alcohol Problems*, London, Sage

Vigotsky, L.S. (1978) *The Development of Higher Psychological Processes*, Cambridge, MA, Harvard University Press

Vroom, V.H. and Yetton, P.H. (1973) *Leadership and Decision-making*, Pittsburgh, PA, University of Pittsburgh Press

Walker, A. (1997) 'Introduction: The Strategy of Inequality', in A. Walker and C. Walker (eds) *Britain Divided: The Growth of Social Exclusion in the 1980s and 1990s*, London, Child Poverty Action Group

Wanless Report (2004) *Securing Good Health for the Whole Population: Final Report*, London, HMSO

Wanless, D. (2006) *Securing Good Care for Older People: Taking a Long-term View*, London, King's Fund

Ward, D. (2005) 'Groupwork', in R. Adams, L. Dominelli and M. Payne (eds) *Social Work: Themes, Issues and Critical Debates*, Basingstoke, Palgrave Macmillan, pp. 149–58

Ward, J., Henderson, Z. and Pearson, G. (2003) *One Problem Among Many: Drug Use among Care Leavers in Transition to Independent Living*, Home Office Research Study No. 260, London, Home Office

Waterhouse, Sir, R. (2000) *Lost in Care: Report of the Tribunal of Inquiry into the Abuse of Children in Care in the Former County Council Areas of Gwynedd and Clwyd since 1974*, HC 201, London, TSO

Watson, M., Lucas, C. and Hoy, A. (eds) *Oxford Handbook of Palliative Care*, Oxford, Oxford University Press

Whitaker, D.S. (1985) *Using Groups to Help People*, London, Routledge & Kegan Paul

White, C.A. (2001) *Cognitive Behaviour Therapy for Chronic Medical Problems: A Guide to Assessment and Treatment in Practice*, Chichester, John Wiley & Son

Whitehead, M. (1992) *Inequalities in Health: The Black Report and The Health Divide*, Harmondsworth, Penguin

WHO (World Health Organization) (1948) *Constitution*, Geneva, WHO

WHO (World Health Organization) (1986) *Ottawa Charter for Health Promotion*, Geneva, WHO

WHO (World Health Organization) (1997) *Jakarta Declaration on Leading Health Promotion into the 21st Century*, Geneva, WHO

Wilcox, D. (1994) *A Guide to Effective Participation*, York, Joseph Rowntree Foundation

Williams, J. and Keating, F. (1999) 'The Abuse of Adults in Mental Health Settings', in N. Stanley, J. Manthorpe and B. Penhale (eds) *Institutional Abuse: Perspectives across the Life Course*, London, Routledge, pp. 130–51

Williams, V. (2003) *Has Anything Changed? User Involvement in Promoting Change and Enhancing the Quality of Services for People with Learning Difficulties*, Final Report for SCIE, Bristol, Norah Fry Research Centre, University of Bristol

Willis, M. (2005) 'Defining Vision', *Community Care*, 1580: 32–3

Willow, C. and Hyder, T. (1998) *It Hurts You Inside*, London, Save the Children/NCB

Wilson, J. (2006) *Infection Control in Clinical Practice* (3rd edn) London, Ballière Tindall

Winnicott, D.W. (1991) *The Child, the Family and the Outside World* (new edn) Harmondsworth, Penguin

Winter, G. ([1962] 2003) 'Healing of Skin Wounds and the Influence of Dressings on the Repair Process', in J.P. Timmons, 'Local Factors and their Impact on the Wound Healing Process', *Primary Health Care*, **13**(9): 43–9

Wistow, G. (2006) 'A New Alliance Blooms,' *Community Care*, 1613: 34–5

Wolfensberger, W. (2003) 'What is Normalisation?', in D. Thomas and H. Woods (eds) *Working With People With Learning Disabilities. Theory and Practice*, London, Jessica Kingsley, Chapter 4

Wolverson, M. (2003) 'Challenging Behaviour', in B. Gates (ed.) *Learning Disability, Towards Inclusion*, London, Churchill Livingstone, Chapter 10

Woodbridge, K. and Fulford, K. (2004) *Whose Values? A Workbook for Values-based Practice Health Care*, London, Sainsbury Centre for Mental Health

Yelloly, M. and Henkel. M. (1995) *Learning and Teaching in Social Work: Towards Reflective Practice*, London, Jessica Kingsley

Young, A.F. and Ashton, E.T. (1956) *British Social Work in the Nineteenth Century*, London, Routledge & Kegan Paul

Youth Justice Board (2004) *National Standards for Youth Justice Services*, London, YJB

Yura, H. and Walsh, M.B. (1988) *The Nursing Process: Assessment, Planning, Implementing, Evaluating*, Norwalk, CT, Appleton & Lange

Name Index

Subject Index